A textbook of
Paediatric Orthopaedics

A textbook of
Paediatric Orthopaedics

From the

Royal Children's Hospital, Melbourne

Edited by

Nigel S Broughton FRCSEd, FRCS, FRACS

Consultant Orthopaedic Surgeon
Royal Children's Hospital
Melbourne, Australia

WB Saunders Company Limited
London   Philadelphia   Toronto   Sydney   Tokyo

WB Saunders Company Ltd   24–28 Oval Road
London NW1 7DX, UK

The Curtis Center
Independence Square West
Philadelphia, PA 19106–3399, USA

Harcourt Brace & Company
55 Horner Avenue
Toronto, Ontario M8Z 4X6, Canada

Harcourt Brace & Company, Australia
30–52 Smidmore Street
Marrickville, NSW 2204, Australia

Harcourt Brace & Company, Japan
Ichibancho Central Building, 22–1 Ichibancho
Chiyoda-ku, Tokyo 102, Japan

A catalogue record for this book is available from the British Library

ISBN 0-7020-1962-3

Typeset by Paston Press Limited, Loddon, Norfolk
Printed and bound at The Bath Press, Avon, UK

Contents

Contributors

Nigel S Broughton FRCSEd, FRCS, FRACS
Consultant Orthopaedic Surgeon, Royal Children's Hospital, Melbourne

D Robert V Dickens FRACS
Director of Orthopaedics, Royal Children's Hospital, Melbourne

Donnchadha G Gallagher M Eng Sc
Biomedical Engineer, Gait Analysis Laboratory, Royal Children's Hospital, Melbourne

H Kerr Graham MD, FRCSEd, FRACS
Professor of Orthopaedic Surgery, Royal Children's Hospital, Melbourne

Andrew J Herbert FRACS
Locum Orthopaedic Surgeon, Royal Children's Hospital, Melbourne

Malcolm B Menelaus MD, FRCS, FRACS
Senior Orthopaedic Surgeon, Royal Children's Hospital, Melbourne

Gary R Nattrass FRCS(C), FRACS
Consultant Orthopaedic Surgeon, Royal Children's Hospital, Melbourne

Mark D O'Sullivan FRACS
Consultant Orthopaedic Surgeon, Royal Children's Hospital, Melbourne

Susan M Randle FRACP
Consultant Rheumatologist, Royal Children's Hospital, Melbourne

Virginia J Saxton FRCR
Consultant Radiologist, Royal Childrens's Hospital, Melbourne

Ian P Torode FRACS, FRCS(C)
Consultant Orthopaedic Surgeon, Royal Children's Hospital, Melbourne

Foreword

Paediatric Orthopaedics represents an admirable team effort by the entire orthopaedic staff and some of their associates from the world renowned Royal Children's Hospital of Melbourne, Australia. It has been effectively edited by Nigel Broughton who has either authored, or co-authored, 4 of the 24 chapters.

Sir Isaac Newton wrote: 'We see so far because we stand on the shoulders of giants.' The orthopaedic giant upon whose shoulders the authors of *Paediatric Orthopaedics* have stood is Peter Williams who, in the 1950s, through his pioneering academic accomplishments created in the Royal Children's Hospital of Melbourne the leading paediatric orthopaedic unit in Australia. (The First Edition of his book *Orthopaedic Management in Childhood* in 1982 and the Second Edition co-authored by another outstanding academic orthopaedic surgeon, William Cole in 1991, are both excellent.)

With some notable exceptions it is only since the 1940s that all of orthopaedic surgery came to be practised by well-trained orthopaedic surgeons as opposed to very capable general surgeons who had 'an interest' in orthopaedics. This was especially true of children's orthopaedics – even within children's hospitals. During the past six decades, however, paediatric orthopaedic surgery has grown and developed tremendously from childhood through adolescence to adulthood. Indeed, even within this specialty there have emerged an increasing number of subspecialties to the extent that it is no longer possible for one paediatric orthopaedic surgeon to be an authoritative expert in all aspects of children's orthopaedics.

In general, undergraduate medical students prefer a single-author textbook with its inherent consistency concerning content, style, and underlying philosophy as an 'introduction' to a given specialty such as the broad field of orthopaedics for patients of all ages. Having been 'introduced' to the specialty however, most postgraduate students – registrars, residents, fellows – as well as practising orthopaedic surgeons are attracted to a multi-author book with the various aspects, including operative orthopaedics, being presented in separate chapters by highly specialized and respected academic orthopaedic surgeons who have special expertise in their own area of interest.

By preparing the multi-author book *Paediatric Orthopaedics* the eleven contributors from within a single institution have combined the advantages of a multi-author book with those of a single-author book. Having had the privilege of reading the 324 page proofs of this book, I can state that the content of each of the 24 chapters is clearly written, appropriately brief and includes reference to the most significant recent advances in children's orthopaedics. This book manages to present the combined policy and practice of all the orthopaedic surgical staff and their associates of one of the world's most outstanding departments of paediatric orthopaedics. In essence, the authors are stating: 'This is what we teach and what we practise.'

The postgraduate student who assimilates the clinical information provided by this excellent book will be able not only to pass any reasonable qualifying examination in the paediatric aspects of orthopaedic surgery (such as the Fellowship examinations of the Commonwealth countries and the American Board of Examinations) but also to begin a career that includes the sensitive, safe, sound practice of paediatric orthopaedic surgery.

It is a pleasure to be able to recommend highly and enthusiastically this splendid book to postgraduate students world-wide as well as to their teachers and also to those who practise paediatric orthopaedics.

Robert B Salter OC, OOnt, MD, MS, FRCSC, FACS
Professor of Orthopaedics,
The Hospital for Sick Children, Toronto, Canada

Preface

Paediatric orthopaedics is a wide-ranging subject covering many different areas. This textbook covers the whole spectrum of conditions presented by a single department.

The Orthopaedic Department at the Royal Children's Hospital, Melbourne, has developed, over the years, a unified philosophy of approach. The strengths of the Department have included strong leadership from Mr Peter Williams and Mr Malcolm Menelaus and the encouragement of expertise in the many varied fields of paediatric orthopaedics by the different contributors to this textbook.

The book is designed to provide a text for orthopaedic surgeons in training to a depth required for Fellowship or Board examinations. Many of the contributors have been examiners at this level and give a valuable insight into the knowledge required.

In using only contributors from one department we can provide the expertise in all areas and also combine in a consistency of philosophy and overall management. Appropriate editing has also produced a consistency of style and presentation so the facts can be easily understood and learned. The many illustrations of conditions collected over the years by our department have been used profusely to ensure ease of assimilation.

The book should appeal not only to trainees about to take examinations but also to general orthopaedic surgeons requiring an up-to-date overview of paediatric orthopaedics. Hopefully it will inspire some young surgeons to pursue a career in an area in which all the contributors feel privileged to be involved.

Acknowledgements

Many people have helped in different ways so this book could be produced. All the contributors have devoted many hours to the preparation of the material both written and illustrative.

The following colleagues have read and suggested improvements to the text; Dinah Reddihough, Harley Powell, David Sillence, Bert Thorbecke, Anne McCoy, Peter Renton and Lloyd Shield. I would particularly like to thank Peter Williams for the selfless task of reading many of the chapters and helping in matters of fact, grammar and style of expression.

All the contributors appreciate that this work is only possible as we work in a first class children's hospital with the help and support of many devoted and conscientious colleagues. We would like to acknowledge the support we receive from our nursing colleagues in theatre, on the wards and in out-patients, from physiotherapists, orthotists and medical records staff. Our experience is only possible with the collaboration of our medical colleagues in other units, particularly in the Department of Radiology.

As the editor of this book I am most appreciative of the people around me who have allowed me to devote so much time to this project; Peter McCombe, John Rehfisch, Reinhart Wuttke, Peter Hamilton, Margaret Manning, Nicola Evans, Wendy Wood and my paediatric colleagues at Frankston Hospital. My secretaries Anne Dalby and Nola Rayson have been unstinting and my wife Sheena, and children William, Andrew and Lucy are always supportive.

This book is dedicated to the many children who have put their trust in our judgement and surgery, in the hope that in the future we can better treat them.

Chapter I
Orthopaedic Assessment

D Robert V Dickens and Nigel S Broughton

The orthopaedic surgeon involved in paediatric orthopaedics is predominantly an orthopaedic physician. The majority of patients who come for consultation do not require surgery and the management consists of a simple explanation or reassurance for the parents.

When conducting a paediatric orthopaedic practice, one must consider the facilities available in the consulting area. There should be appropriate toys for children to play with, a friendly environment, an area where children can play unimpeded that will allow an interview with the parents while the child remains in view. Gaining the confidence of the child varies. Experience suggests that a direct approach is often successful for older children but for younger children from 2–4 years of age it is often wise to interview the parents first and allow the child to observe you in this situation. During this time the doctor can gauge how the child is going to cope with the situation.

Many of the children seen by a paediatric orthopaedic surgeon do not require treatment and are normal. Frequently the role of the orthopaedic surgeon is to exclude significant pathology and explain a variation of normal rather than make a definitive diagnosis. It is important to consider where the problem lies. In many circumstances the problem is a parental one, the child having no concern whatsoever about the condition that is causing anxiety in the family. It is also interesting and helpful to spend some time taking a history from the child. Not infrequently the history obtained from the parent conflicts with that of the child.

Since many of the conditions seen in orthopaedic practice are variations of normal the parents require a significant consultation time to provide an explanation of the condition and its natural history, and then reassurance that the expected outcome is likely to occur. For example, it is well recognized that flat feet in four-year-olds is a common variation of normal. Similarly knock knees in a four-year-old are to be expected, as are bow legs in a two-year-old.

The success of a paediatric orthopaedic consultation relies heavily on the surgeon's ability to communicate.

HISTORY TAKING

To achieve a successful outcome to the consultation it is important that the problem concerning the parents is explored. If both parents are present it is useful to ask each of them to describe the problem as they see it to appreciate it from their point of view. It is common for each parent to express their concern in different ways with varying emphasis on what they feel are the important issues.

When taking a history it often becomes apparent that the parents are attributing a delay in the normal developmental progress of their child, particularly an inability to walk, to a condition that is most unlikely to be significant. For example, intoeing is often blamed for a delay in walking. This must be noted in the history so that when discussing the child's condition, it can be stressed that this is not a significant factor.

Presenting Complaint

The history should start with the onset of the problem that has been noted by the parents, its duration, its severity, and whether it is worsening or improving. A description of the type of any pain and its exact position should be sought. Children as young as four years of age can sometimes usefully describe symptoms, and if the child is over seven years of age it is worth taking some time to elicit such information. The younger the child the less idea they will have of the timing of events, but the parents can help out with this. Any previous treatment and the response to it should be noted.

History of the Pregnancy

The history of the pregnancy including the duration of the pregnancy, the position (breech or vertex), the type of delivery and the immediate postnatal progress may be of significance in determining the diagnosis. Prematurity, a long spell in a special care nursery, and severe jaundice should be noted, particularly if developmental delay is suspected.

Developmental Milestones

The developmental milestones should be asked about, noting when the child started smiling, rolling, sitting, crawling, walking and talking, to assess any likely developmental delay (*Table 1.1*). The stage at which the child has reached in schooling and progress within the schooling system should be noted.

Growth

The child's growth is assessed and height is charted. Parents' knowledge about whether their child is the smallest or tallest in the class will give some general idea of growth and development. The height of the parents and any other siblings is noted. The onset of menarche is important as a guide to skeletal maturity, which is expected about two years after the onset of menarche.

Past History

The parents should be questioned about any significant disorders in the child in the past and how they relate to the present disorder.

Table 1.1 Developmental milestones

Milestone	Age
Rolling back to front	6 months
Sitting alone unsupported	9 months
Pulling up on furniture to stand	12 months
Walking alone	15 months
Running well	2 years
Hopping on individual legs	5 years

Family History

Other illnesses in the family should be documented, particularly if the presenting condition is congenital or a genetic disorder is suspected. Any illnesses running in the family and their mode of inheritance should be noted. The possibility of any consanguineous marriages should be asked about if an autosomal recessive condition is suspected. Problems running in the family that may be overlooked at this stage are reactions to anaesthesia and bleeding disorders. The history should always include a discussion about siblings: their ages, sex and general health, including illnesses.

Social History

The social background of the family can be highly significant in the management of chronic conditions, particularly if there is any suspicion of a non-organic component to the child's disorder.

The Vaccination History

The vaccination history should also be noted, particularly vaccination against polio and Haemophilus influenza B.

EXAMINATION

Examination should start as soon as the child enters the consulting room, firstly observing the child with the parents, and then at play with toys that have been provided.

Examination of a child requires adequate exposure of the patient, which can become a sensitive issue in younger boys and adolescent girls. These sensitivities must be recognized and appropriately managed to avoid confrontation or difficulty.

When observing the child it is helpful to observe the relatives at the same time: whether they have conditions that may have some genetic significance such as scoliosis, neurofibromatosis and flat feet.

It is important to recognize that children have marked degrees of ligamentous laxity and that it is often possible for them to perform party trick manoeuvres such as subluxing or even dislocating various joints or producing loud clunks or clicks. Subluxation of the shoulder is common. The ability to produce a loud clunking sensation around the trochanteric area of the hip, loud clunking and jerking movements within the knee joint, and loud clicking

Table 1.2   MRC grading of muscle strength

Power	Description	
0	Zero	No movement
1	Trace	Contraction can be felt, but no movement of joint
2	Poor	Movement with gravity eliminated
3	Fair	Movement takes place against gravity
4	Good	Movement against gravity and some added resistance
5	Normal	Normal strength

sensations in the cervical spine are not infrequent findings in normal children. In general these abnormalities are innocuous, and little management is required apart from discouraging the child from repeating them.

General Examination

The orthopaedic assessment should include a general examination, including a search for lymphadenopathy and an assessment of the circulation and peripheral pulses. An abdominal examination is also indicated to detect any tumours or tenderness.

In assessing the general appearance of the child any skin blemishes should be noted, particularly café au lait spots, haemangiomas and other cutaneous findings that might suggest a diagnosis.

The overall posture of the child is observed and any asymmetry or disproportion is noted, for example in hand span compared to height.

Neurological Assessment

Neurological assessment is an integral part of any orthopaedic examination and it is essential to test for power, sensation, vibration, position sense, the plantar response, and the tendon and superficial reflexes. In children the plantar response is a difficult assessment as a withdrawal response is frequently elicited by this manoeuvre. The plantar response may be upgoing in children up to 18 months of age, but after that an upgoing plantar response is abnormal. An assessment of the plantar responses and muscle tone is most important in those children suspected of having cerebral palsy.

In those for whom a neurological explanation is suspected the child is asked to lie on the floor and get up (Gowers test). A positive Gowers sign is produced when the child has to rely on using his hands to push down on his knees and then has to work his hands up his thighs to help him get up into the standing position. It is caused by proximal muscle weakness

and is most frequently seen in muscular dystrophy at the age of about four years.

If the child has a fixed deformity it is important to measure the strength of the muscle groups to assess whether it is due to muscle imbalance. The strength of the muscle groups is described according to the Medical Research Council (MRC) descriptions of muscle strength (*Table 1.2*). The aetiology of the muscle imbalance can then be deduced from further neurological testing.

Gait

The child is encouraged to walk as the first stage of the examination. Abnormal upper limb movements may suggest cerebral palsy, but any athetoid or spastic movements are noted. The degree of intoeing or outtoeing can be assessed as can the severity of any toe-walking. The way in which the foot strikes the ground is important in deciding on any surgical treatment for foot deformity.

Limp

Any asymmetry of the movement of the lower limbs is described as a limp and the correct interpretation of the limp is an important aspect of the assessment of the child. Limps may be due to pain, shortening or instability. Types of gait include the following:

- The **antalgic gait** or painful gait demonstrates a hurried stance phase of the affected limb and a quick swing phase of the other limb.
- A **short limb gait** shows a dip of the shoulder on the affected side.
- The **Trendelenburg gait** is due to instability of the hip. The abductors of the hip are unable to perform adequately, so instead of the abductors holding the pelvis level in the stance phase, the contralateral side of the pelvis dips. To compensate for this the ipsilateral shoulder sways over the

hip in the stance phase. This produces a characteristic waddling or swaying gait, which is particularly marked when bilateral, for example in the adult female with bilateral congenital dislocation of the hips.

It may be difficult to assess the type of limp as there is often a combination of these factors.

The stiff knee produces a limp. If the quadriceps is weak, patients often compensate for this by 'back-kneeing.' As the stance phase starts the child pushes the knee into recurvatum at the heel strike by hip extension and can thus prevent the knee from collapsing. A degree of fixed equinus helps to achieve this. Sometimes the child may use his hand to push back on the front of the thigh at the heel strike to achieve this 'back-kneeing.'

The child may walk in equinus. This may be a fixed equinus with no dorsiflexion when the ankle is examined, or a dynamic equinus with dorsiflexion of the ankle at rest, but the child walks on his toes. It may be that the child's foot falls into plantar flexion in the swing phase because of the lack of active dorsiflexors of the ankle. This causes a characteristic high stepping gait to clear the ground with the trailing toes known as a foot drop gait.

It is often helpful to ask the child to walk on the heels and then the toes to assess coordination and to determine whether there is any weakness or muscle imbalance that may become more apparent using this manoeuvre. Asking the child to hop on one leg can be helpful after the age of about four years to estimate agility and this manoeuvre may exaggerate any tendency to spasticity or increased tone.

Spine

Start by looking at the spine. Any variation of the normal contours of the spine are important. Looking from the side, the cervical spine has a natural lordosis, the thoracic spine, a kyphosis, and the lumbar spine, a lordosis (*Figure 1.1*). Looking from the back the spine should be straight; any lateral curvature is called a scoliosis. The inside of the curve is its concavity and the outside of the curve, its convexity. In deciding on how to manage a scoliosis it is important to assess whether the upper body lists to one side. This can be assessed by dropping a plumb line from the vertebral prominence at the lower end of the cervical spine and seeing where it falls in relation to the natal cleft. Any cutaneous lesions should be looked for. Café au lait spots can be seen in neurofibromatosis, and areas of pigmentation or excessive hair, particularly in the midline, in spinal dysraphism.

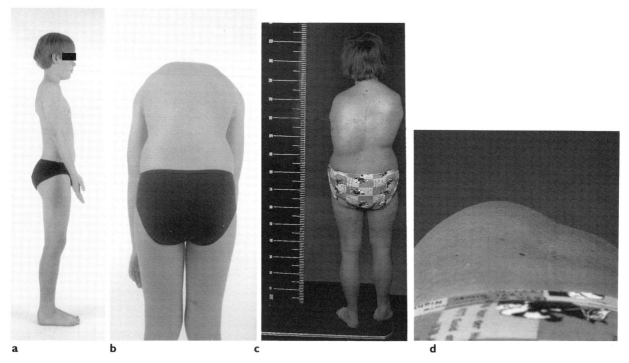

a   b   c   d

Figure 1.1   a From the side the normal cervical lordosis, thoracic kyphosis and lumbar lordosis is seen.   **b** In a normal spine on forward flexion there is no asymmetry.   **c** This patient has a structural scoliosis despite previous surgery.   **d** On forward flexion this patient has an asymmetrical rib hump due to the rotational deformity indicating a structural scoliosis.

Next feel the spine when the patient is standing normally, then when forward flexed, and then when prone on the couch. Any areas of tenderness on the spinous processes or in the adjacent muscle groups should be elicited. The forward slip of the vertebrae in spondylolisthesis may be felt.

Then move the spine. A structural scoliosis will demonstrate a rotational abnormality on forward flexion, with the development of an asymmetrical rib or lumbar hump (*Figure 1.1d*). A postural scoliosis does not show this. Postural scoliosis may be due to pain from nerve root entrapment or leg length inequality. Scoliosis due to leg length inequality can be corrected by blocks under the short leg to equalize leg length or by sitting. Fixed pelvic obliquity cannot be corrected by blocks or sitting and is due to a structural abnormality at the junction of the spine and pelvis.

Measure the range of movement in forward flexion, extension, lateral flexion and rotation. Forward flexion may appear to be normal, but watch the lumbar spine carefully to check that the movement is taking place in the spine and not at the hips. Any nerve root entrapment may result in a restriction of straight leg raising ability by performing a straight leg raising test.

Lower Limb

Trendelenburg Test

The child is observed from the back and asked to stand on one leg with the other leg flexed at the knee, but not at the hip. Normally the pelvis on the side of the non-weight-bearing leg rises (Trendelenburg negative). If there is instability and the hip abductors on the side of the weight-bearing leg are unable to perform normally the pelvis dips on the side of the non-weight-bearing leg (Trendelenburg positive). If the test is negative, the child is asked to stand like this for 30 seconds and if the pelvis dips during this time the test is a delayed positive. When standing on one leg, the body automatically brings its centre of gravity over the weight-bearing leg. Because the pelvis dips away from the weight-bearing leg in the Trendelenburg-positive child, the upper body has to sway in an exaggerated manner to achieve a position with the centre of gravity of the body over the weight-bearing limb. This produces the characteristic sway of the upper body in the Trendelenburg gait.

A positive Trendelenburg sign indicates that the abductors are unable to contract effectively. This may be due to instability of the hip, pain at the hip, weakness of the abductors, or shortening of the femoral neck.

Leg Length Inequality

A significant inequality causes a short leg gait.

The block test
Leg length inequality is best measured by blocks. The child stands with both knees fully extended and the feet together. The examiner stands behind the child with a thumb on each posterior superior iliac spine (PSIS) and assesses whether they are level. If not, blocks are placed under the short leg until the PSISs are level (*Figure 1.2*). The test cannot be carried out if there has been previous surgery or an abnormality of the PSIS, or if there is significant knee deformity.

True shortening
In true shortening the length of one leg is shorter than the other. This can be measured by the block test, but this is not valid if there is a fixed deformity at the hip or knee. If there is a fixed deformity the child is asked to lie on the couch and the distance between the anterior superior iliac spine and the tip of the medial malleolus is measured. The normal leg is then placed in the same degree of deformity and the measurement repeated to give an indication of the difference between the two legs.

Apparent shortening
In apparent shortening one leg appears shorter than the other due to a fixed deformity at the hip. When the child lies on the couch the apparent difference in lengths of the legs is noted by the relative positions of the heels or medial malleoli. Alternatively a tape measure can be used to measure the distance between the umbilicus and medial malleolus. If there is a fixed adduction deformity of the hip one leg will appear to be shorter, and if there is a fixed abduction deformity of the hip the leg will appear to be longer than the other (see *Figure 1.3*).

Galeazzi test
If there is true shortening, the Galeazzi test can be performed to determine whether the shortening is above or below the knee, or both. The child lies supine on the couch, the knees are flexed to a right angle, and the heels rest on the couch together. By looking from the side at the relative positions of the knees, it can be seen where the shortening lies.

Shortening in the hip region
If the shortening lies above the knee, ask the child to lie supine on the couch with the legs extended.

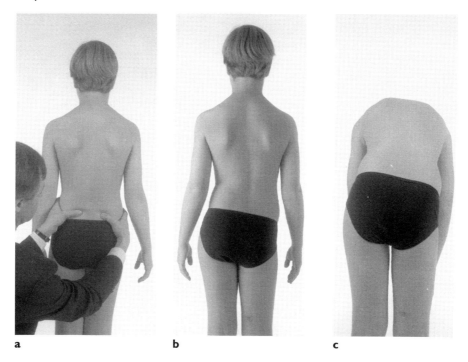

a   b   c

Figure 1.2 **a** The posterior superior iliac spines are palpated with the thumbs to determine whether the pelvis is level and the legs equal in length. **b** If there is leg length inequality there is pelvic obliquity and a postural scoliosis. **c** Because the scoliosis is not structural there is no rotational deformity and therefore no asymmetry to cause a rib hump on forward flexion.

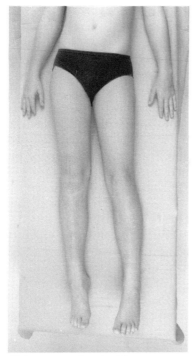

Figure 1.3 If there is a fixed adduction contracture, as in the right hip, the legs will be apparently unequal in length.

Palpation of the relative positions of the anterior superior iliac spines and the greater trochanters comparing both hips will demonstrate whether the shortening is above or below the trochanter (*Figure 1.4*).

Rotational Profile

The rotational profile of the leg is first assessed by watching the child walk to make an assessment of the foot progression angle (FPA). The FPA merely describes the direction in which the foot points during gait and can be altered by an abnormality at any level in the leg.

The child is then asked to lie supine on the couch, and the absence or presence of metatarsus adductus is noted.

By then asking the patient to lie prone the foot thigh angle (FTA) can be assessed to determine if there is any significant tibial torsion, either internal or external. By flexing the knee to a right angle and then looking down from above (short clinicians may require the use of a stool!), the angle made by an imaginary straight line along the axis of the femur and an imaginary line along the axis of the foot at

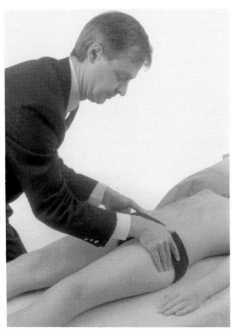

Figure 1.4 The relative positions of the greater trochanter and anterior superior iliac spine can be palpated directly and compared for asymmetry.

rest (*Figure 1.5a*) can be estimated. Normally the FTA demonstrates an external tibial rotation of approximately 10–15°. Alternatively tibial torsion can be assessed with the child sitting and the knee flexed to a right angle. Palpation of the malleoli will allow an assessment of the transmalleolar axis. Normally the lateral malleolus lies behind the medial malleolus by 20° and variations from this give a figure for tibial torsion; in other words if the transmalleolar axis is zero there is 20° of internal tibial torsion (*Figure 1.5b*).

Then ask the child to return to the prone position and elicit both internal and external rotation of the hips to determine whether there is any persistent femoral anteversion. The knee is kept at a right angle, the femur stabilized and the leg rolled out (internal rotation) and then in (external rotation). The assessment of the angle is helped by using the long straight line of the tibia as a goniometer (*Figure 1.5c & d*).

This method of observing the rotational profile is most important in determining the cause of any intoe gait and assessing whether the abnormality lies in the femur, tibia or feet.

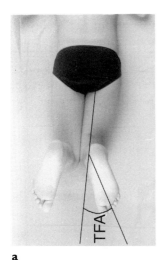

a

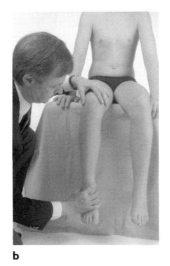

b

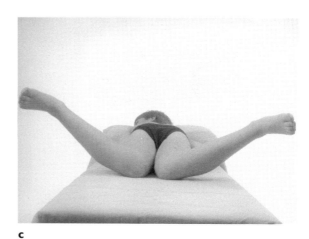

c

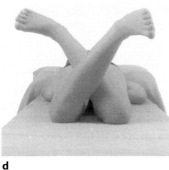

d

Figure 1.5 a The thigh foot angle is measured to determine tibial torsion. **b** The transmalleolar axis is determined by palpation of the medial and lateral malleoli. **c** The range of internal rotation of the femur. **d** The range of external rotation of the femur.

Hip

First look at the hip. There may be asymmetrical skin creases in developmental dysplasia of the hip (DDH). Note any scar from previous surgery or old sinuses indicating previous infection.

Feeling the hip may reveal areas of tenderness, particularly over the superficial greater trochanter. However, the hip is a difficult joint to feel because it is so deeply placed. The femoral head may be palpable in the groin if there is significant anteversion of the hip in partially-treated DDH. This is confirmed if the femoral head becomes more easily palpable on external rotation of the leg.

After observing the gait, the first movement of the hip when the child is lying on the couch should be to determine if there is any fixed flexion deformity of the hip by the Thomas test. The other hip is flexed to its limit and it is useful if the child can hold onto the flexed leg. A check is then made that this manoeuvre has flattened the lumbar spine against the couch. If the thigh cannot be placed onto the couch there is a fixed flexion deformity of the hip. The amount of fixed flexion deformity is the angle between the thigh and the couch. In order to ensure the lumbar spine is flat against the couch it may be necessary to flex the hip that is being tested and then to lower it to its limit to read off the fixed flexion deformity (*Figure 1.6a*).

The range of flexion, abduction and adduction can also be measured as the child lies supine, but the pelvis should be stabilized to give a true reading otherwise movement between the pelvis and lumbar spine may be interpreted as hip movement. For abduction, stabilization of the pelvis is best achieved by maximum abduction of the contralateral hip (*Figure 1.6b*). Internal rotation and external rotation of the hip can also be assessed in the supine position by looking at the direction in which the patellae point rather than the feet, but it is probably more accurate to do this when the patient lies prone, as described in the rotational profile section. Internal and external rotation of the hip can also be examined in 90° of hip flexion, but it is better to make the assessment in the functional position with the hips extended.

The hip can be stressed to elicit irritability if there is synovitis, as seen in arthritic conditions. The first movement to decrease in these circumstances is the ability to adduct in 90° of hip flexion; normally there should be at least 20° of adduction in this position and any decrease in this movement is indicative of significant irritability or contracture (*Figure 1.6c*).

In the very young child, stressing the hip by Ortolani and Barlow test to determine instability is important in assessing DDH and is discussed further in Chapter 16 on DDH. In the older age group, gross telescoping may be evident in DDH or dislocation due to an old septic arthritis.

Knee

First look at the knee for any swelling. This may be either generalized, as in synovitis due to an inflam-

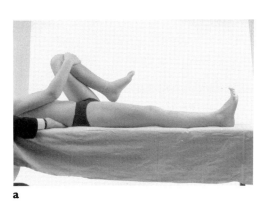
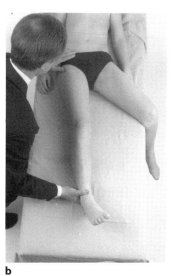
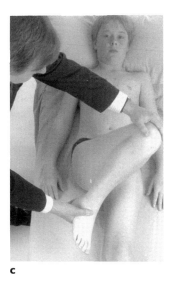

a   b   c

Figure 1.6 a The Thomas test of the right hip is performed with the left hip fully flexed and a hand to check that the lumbar spine is flat on the couch. There is no fixed flexion deformity. **b** The pelvis has been stabilized by maximally abducting the left hip. A hand is placed on the pelvis to check for any movement and the right leg can then be moved into abduction and adduction to obtain a true measurement of the maximum range of motion. **c** A useful test for hip irritability is the range of adduction in 90° flexion.

matory arthritis, or localized, as in the enlarged tibial tuberosity of Osgood–Schlatter disease. A large effusion is readily identified by swelling in the suprapatellar pouch, and a smaller effusion by filling in of the medial and lateral parapatellar gutters. Any colour change with redness and signs of inflammation should be noted. Deformities of valgus, varus or fixed flexion deformity can be observed while the child is walking. A normal two-year-old has a tendency to genu varum and a four-year-old has a tendency to assume a valgus position. In the adult there is a valgus angle of 5–10°.

The knee should be palpated to detect any lumps such as an exostosis over the medial side of the distal femoral metaphysis. A patellar tap may be elicited in moderate effusions or the fluid may have to be squeezed out of the suprapatellar pouch to elicit this sign. In the older child it is important to flex the knee to a right angle and palpate each joint line to elicit signs of tenderness over the menisci. In chondromalacia patellae there may be tenderness of the undersurface of the patella on palpation.

When moving the knee it is important to determine the active and passive range of movement. Careful inspection of the patellofemoral joint will reveal any patellar tilt or habitual dislocation in either extension or flexion. The patella may be high (patella alta) or low in position (patella baja). An apprehension test for patellar instability is performed by pressing the patellar laterally when the knee is in an extended position and then slowly flexing the knee (*Figure 1.7a*). A positive test is obtained when the child resists the movement rather than just finds it uncomfortable. Patellofemoral crepitus may be felt on flexion and extension of the knee in chondromalacia patellae. Compression of the patella against the femoral trochlea with the leg extended is also used to confirm crepitus.

At 30° of flexion both collateral ligaments are tested by a varus then a valgus strain. At 20° of flexion, the distal femur and proximal tibia should be held and stress applied (Lachman test) (*Figure 1.7b*). Any abnormal movement in an anteroposterior direction is noted. This may be present after a tear of the anterior cruciate in the older child, but is also seen in children with a congenital short femur associated with a deficiency of the anterior cruciate mechanism. There may also be a positive pivot shift test, but because this test is painful, it is often fiercely resisted by children so is less reliable. Defects or tears in the posterior cruciate ligament are best assessed by a posterior sag of the knee when the knees are flexed to a right angle in the supine position on the couch.

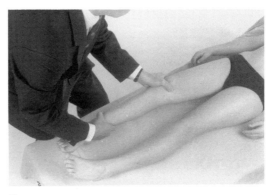

a

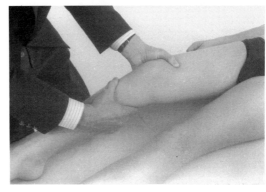

b

Figure 1.7 a The patella apprehension test is performed with a thumb on the medial side of the patella pushing laterally and the limb being pushed into knee flexion. **b** A Lachman test is performed at 20° flexion with one hand grasping the lower end of the femur and the other the upper end of the tibia. Any anteroposterior instability can be detected.

Ankle and Foot

Deformity of the foot can be described in ten ways. The ankle may be in calcaneus or equinus. The subtalar joint may be in varus or valgus. The medial arch may be flat (planus) or high (cavus). The forefoot may be deviated into adductus or abductus and may be twisted inwards into pronatus or outwards into supinatus. A combination of these deformities can therefore give a useful description of all the abnormalities in one foot. For example a common foot deformity in cerebral palsy is the calcaneovalgo-abductus foot and the typical foot of peroneal muscular atrophy is a cavo-varus foot.

First look at the foot both at rest and while walking. There is a normal tendency for the heel to be in a valgus posture in children. The ankle is not in any degree of valgus or varus, but the valgus position

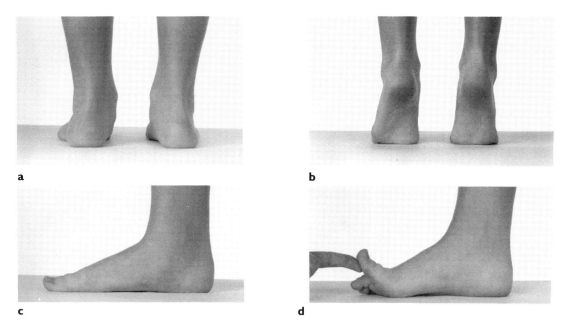

Figure 1.8 a Both heels are in valgus. **b** When the child goes on to tiptoes the position of the heel corrects. **c** Looking from the side on weight-bearing the arch is relatively flat. **d** On dorsiflexion of the big toe the arch is formed.

on standing is due to subtalar mobility (*Figure 1.8a & b*). The arch of the foot may appear either flat, normal or high in position. The weight-bearing surface of the foot should be observed as this is a good indication of any deformity as the foot strikes the ground. There may be thickened skin in an area taking the majority of the load, or if over a smaller area, there may be a callus. If there is a sensory neuropathy such as spina bifida these areas may develop neuropathic ulcers. When examining feet it is also important to observe the shoe wear pattern and any evidence of distortion of the shoe. Clawing of the toes and any forefoot deformity in the form of a metatarsus adductus or metatarsus varus may be noted.

The foot is palpated to elicit any areas of tenderness, such as over the calcaneal apophysis in Sever disease or over the second metatarsal head in Freiberg disease.

When moving the foot assess the mobility of the ankle and subtalar joint and note any deformity. It is important to note whether the deformity is fixed or correctable. Rigidity of the subtalar joint may suggest tarsal coalition or subtalar irritability due to some other cause such as juvenile chronic arthritis. Any deformity of the forefoot is assessed to see if it can be corrected.

Flat feet are best examined from behind, where the flat arch and valgus heel are seen. If the child then stands on tiptoe, the heel comes into neutral or varus and the arch is reconstituted in physiological flat feet. Flat feet can also be assessed by passive dorsiflexion of the great toe in the standing position. If the deformity is correctable this creates a medial arch with external rotation of the tibia and is a reassuring test for anxious parents of children with flat feet (*Figure 1.8c & d*).

Fixed pronation deformity, as seen in peroneal muscular atrophy, can produce a varus posture of the heel in weight-bearing that is fully correctable when not weight-bearing. This can be examined by the Coleman block test (see Chapter 20 on feet) in which a block is placed obliquely to support the heel and lateral border of the foot, but allowing the first metatarsal head to drop (*Figure 1.9*). If the heel varus is due to fixed pronation of the foot, the heel should be corrected to normal or valgus by this manoeuvre. Alternatively the child can stand on a step and then advance until he has offloaded the whole of the forefoot and is only weight-bearing through the heels.

The posture of the toes is important and it is possible to distinguish four characteristic toe deformities; the hammer toe, the mallet toe, the claw toe and the curly toe.

In foot deformity it is always important to examine the muscles of the foot to determine whether the foot deformity is due to muscle imbalance. The peroneal muscles are often weak in neuro-

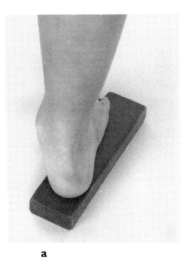
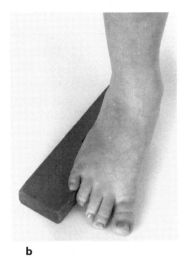
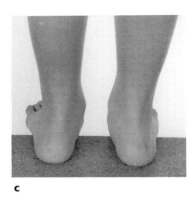

a   b   c

Figure 1.9 a,b The Coleman block test is performed by placing a block obliquely under the foot to support the heel and fifth metatarsal head and the heel is examined from behind. **c** The Melbourne modification of the Coleman test is to ask the child to stand on the edge of a step with the whole forefoot unsupported and to observe the position of the heels.

pathic foot deformity. The aetiology of foot deformity may be structural (e.g. old club foot) or muscular (e.g. Duchenne muscular dystrophy), or due to disorders of the peripheral nerves (e.g. peroneal muscular atrophy), nerve roots (e.g. spinal dysraphism) or brain (e.g. cerebral palsy).

Upper Limb

Shoulder

Observe the contour of the shoulder. Children with diaphyseal aclasia often have exostoses around the shoulder on the lateral aspect of the upper humeral metaphyses. A Sprengel shoulder or undescended scapula will be obvious, even when looking from the front.

Webbing of the neck and a low hair line should be noted.

Feel the shoulder for any tenderness or lumps. It may be useful to palpate the two shoulders at the same time to easily compare the two. There may be a defect of both clavicles in cleidocranial dysostosis, or a lump and abnormal movement over a pseudarthrosis of the clavicle.

Next move the shoulder to assess the movements at both the glenohumeral joint and then the scapulothoracic joint. The glenohumeral movement is evaluated by first stabilizing the scapula and then moving the arm. The arm is then moved without restricting the scapula to see if there is normal scapulothoracic movement. The range of movement

should be carried out using both active and passive ranges of movements.

Stability of the shoulder is assessed by stressing the shoulder forwards and backwards. An apprehension test – putting the arm up into abduction and external rotation – is helpful in detecting anterior shoulder instability. A positive test is obtained if the child resists being placed into that position. If the child complains of clunks or instability of the shoulder it is worth asking for a demonstration of the sign.

Elbow

Looking at the elbow is very informative because it is a relatively superficial joint and swelling and deformity are easily seen. In full extension the carrying angle can be assessed and compared to the other side. The normal carrying angle is 10–15° (more in females and less in males, *Figure 1.10*). An alteration in the carrying angle, which is best detected by a comparison with the normal side, may be seen in malunion after a supracondylar fracture. If the valgus carrying angle is lost and becomes varus it looks quite ugly and produces the so-called gun-stock deformity.

Feeling the elbow for areas of tenderness is important. Palpation of the triangle of medial and lateral epicondyles and the olecranon is useful for assessing a malunion when compared to the normal side. Palpation of the radial head can reveal abnormalities in its relationship with the capitellum, as in congenital dislocation of the radial head or an old missed Monteggia fracture.

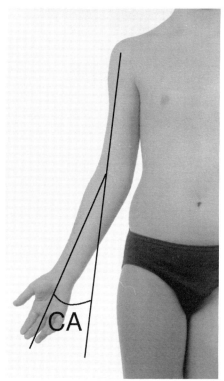

Figure 1.10   The carrying angle of the elbow.

as Madelung deformity with prominence of the ulna head) or generalized (as occurs in rheumatoid arthritis). Because of its accessibility one can palpate for swelling, synovial thickening and any increase in temperature. Movements of the wrist can be assessed and often the wrist is used as a measure of ligamentous laxity with hypermobility.

Hand

The overall appearance of the hand can be helpful in making a diagnosis (e.g. arachnodactyly in Marfan syndrome, the common finger deformities of camptodactyly, clinodactyly, syndactyly, hypoplasia of the limb generally and the presence of accessory digits). Clubbing of the fingers or cyanosis can be important in detecting a more generalized disorder.

The hand should be assessed for normal neurological function. In the young child, abnormalities of sensation may be difficult to elicit. It is useful to examine the sweat pattern of the hand as an indication of sensory loss. Movements of the fingers can be assessed. Like the wrist and elbow, the finger is a very sensitive measure of ligamentous laxity with hypermobility allowing hyperextension at the metacarpophalangeal joints.

Assess the movements of the elbow and measure flexion and extension. It is a good joint for assessing ligamentous laxity: hyperextension may occur and the elbow can extend beyond 0°. Then with the elbows flexed at a right angle, assess pronation and supination of the forearm. This may be completely absent in radio-ulnar synostosis, but remain undetected as a result of compensatory shoulder rotation.

Wrist

Observe the wrist for swelling, which may be localized (e.g. ganglia or localized swellings of bone such

FURTHER READING

Apley AG, Solomon L. Apley's *System of Orthopaedics and Fractures*, seventh edition. Butterworth Heinemann, Oxford, 1993.

Staheli LT, Corbett M, Wyss C, King H. Lower-extremity rotational problems in children. Normal values to guide management. *J Bone Joint Surg* 1985; **67**A: 39–47.

Chapter 2

General Approach to Paediatric Orthopaedics

Malcolm B Menelaus

Paediatric orthopaedics is one of the most interesting and satisfying subspecialities within medicine. Not only is it refreshing to be dealing with children, but it is also interesting because of the wide range of fascinating conditions encountered. Visible, and even dramatic, improvement in long-term appearance and function is commonly achieved by appropriate management.

It is unusual for the orthopaedic surgeon to carry out major surgery on children (somewhere between 1 in 15 and 1 in 20 patients require surgery and in only a small proportion of these is it major). Should major surgery be necessary or should the child be suffering from a chronic condition requiring repeated surgery, it is remarkable how well children stand up to the stresses involved; it is the parents who more commonly require support.

Many children present because of concern about self-correcting postural problems, and reassurance by describing the natural history of these conditions usually resolves the parents' concern.

Another rewarding feature of the management of orthopaedic conditions in childhood is that it provides the opportunity of influencing 70–80 years of future life, converting it from what might otherwise have been a restricted life into a normal life. As a corollary of this, there is the opportunity of long term follow-up.

CHRONIC DISORDERS

Some paediatric orthopaedic conditions require management over a prolonged period. Some (including congenital talipes equinovarus and late-presenting congenital dislocation of the hip) require one or several surgical procedures. Parents and children commonly accept all this provided they are given an adequate explanation. The best time to give a broad outline of the type of treatment necessary is at the first visit. Further detail can be given on subsequent visits when changing casts on club feet or adjusting the harness on children with developmental dysplasia of the hip. What is said at the initial consultation is commonly forgotten and requires repeating on at least one occasion.

When a child is born with talipes equinovarus the main concerns for the parents are:

- 'Will my child walk?'
- 'Will my child have a limp?'
- 'Will the foot look ugly?'
- 'Will he play games normally and lead a normal life?'

Often the parents do not verbalize these worries but it is clearly important that these worries are removed in the surgeon's opening comments and that a realistic account of the probable management is given, mentioning right at the start that surgery is likely to be necessary.

The complications of surgical management need not be mentioned early on, but should be mentioned when it has been decided to carry out surgery when the surgeon is explaining the expected duration of hospitalization, postoperative plaster immobilization and the subsequent management.

Children will accept multiple hospitalizations; it is the parents who require support, and they should be encouraged to ask questions and discuss their problems and their concerns. For some it is appropriate to suggest a further opinion.

THE CHILD WITH MULTIPLE DISABILITIES

Conditions such as cerebral palsy, spina bifida and osteogenesis imperfecta lead to lifelong disability and a life time of worry for the parents. All parents of disabled children have, at one time or another, feelings of disappointment, inadequacy, frustration, fear, guilt and anxiety. It is important that parents know that these feelings are nothing to be ashamed of, but are natural reactions. It is also important that parents realise that they should not hide these feelings from their spouse or others. Denial of the existence of these feelings may lead to less than adequate care of the child.

Children with multiple disabilities should be managed by a team of doctors who are working together, and the appropriate services can only be provided by a children's hospital. It is better, if one is not associated with such an institution, to refer the patient to a children's hospital where a coordinated service for the particular disability can be provided. If one is working in such a hospital, one should work closely with colleagues to ensure that the family has as few visits to the outpatient clinics as possible and gets the maximum support from ancillary services such as social workers, physiotherapists, orthotists and prosthetists. Surgery by different specialists should be planned and coordinated to ensure a minimum number of anaesthetics.

THE CONSULTATION AND EXAMINATION

The day of a particular child's consultation is not a big day in the life of the surgeon, but it will be the most important event in the day of the child and family, and for many will be the most important event of that month; it has frequently been awaited with a mixture of fear and hope. The orthopaedic surgeon should therefore behave as though he or she regards the occasion as important. This does not imply that a serious approach is necessary throughout; children and their parents may be put at ease with some light conversation appropriate to the age of the child.

It is important that the child should feel confident and secure in his relationship with the clinician, so that he or she is keen to relate some of the history and is cooperative in the examination. You cannot and should not ingratiate yourself to children—they cannot be hoodwinked; the most you can and should do is to show them that you are friendly.

Preliminary Conversation

Initial conversation may touch on a variety of topics according to the circumstances. If the general practitioner is well known to the orthopaedic surgeon this should be mentioned immediately to give everyone a friend in common. If the family have travelled a long way for the consultation, mention of their home town and a question about the trip to the hospital indicates that this as yet unknown doctor recognizes their place of origin and the difficulties that have been faced and overcome to obtain his opinion.

The History

The referring letter may provide useful information about the family as a whole and some of the history, but it is important that a full new history is taken. It is often appropriate for the consultant to start off with a comment such as 'I've read your doctor's letter, but I would like to hear from you about why you are here today?' Some member of the family (and it is seldom the patient) will then speak up, and it is generally best to let them speak on without interruption indicating that you have got plenty of time to listen and learn. It has frequently been previously decided by the parents who will do the talking. The consultant soon gets a feel for a particular family and how much of value is likely to be learned from various members of the family. If the mother, who commonly has the best grasp of the situation, does most of the early talking, it is wise to ask the father if he wants to add anything.

Clearly it is important to encourage the patient to talk and to feel confident about the relationship developing between themselves and the clinician. After about seven years of age the child is usually very good at describing a symptom in terms of pain, the position, type and exacerbating factors. Initially the questions should be clear with a straightforward answer such as:

- 'Is it painful?'
- 'Where does it hurt?'

Open-ended questions such as 'Tell me about the pain you have' are not helpful (*Figure 2.1*).

If the child is encouraged to talk he will gradually feel more confident and will elaborate more without being prompted. Younger children have most difficulty over the timing of events so questions about how long the pain has been present or when events took place should be reserved for the parent to add to the child's description of symptoms. Younger children should be directly questioned to indicate that

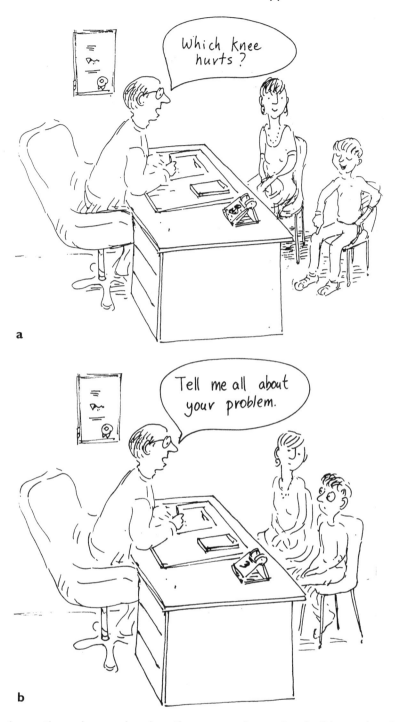

Figure 2.1 **a** A simple, easily understood and easily answered question builds up the child's confidence and encourages him to communicate. **b** Open-ended questions create fear and trepidation because the child is not sure what is expected of him.

they and their opinions are regarded as important. Even if the child's information is not immediately relevant, the clinician is able to assess the maturity of the child.

Adolescents are commonly shy, but become more talkative if they are included in the conversation with some warmth. Before asking for details of their symptoms it may be appropriate to ask them about the effect of their symptoms on sport and social events and this may open the door to more penetrating questions. Some adolescent girls will disagree entirely with everything their mother says. The clinician should listen to both stories and assess their relative values.

Clearly some questions have to be directed to the parents such as details about the pregnancy, delivery, birth weight, neonatal condition, duration of the child's hospitalization following delivery, the age of various milestones in the child's life and any relevant family history.

A Tentative Diagnosis

Generally a tentative diagnosis will have been made by the clinician within the first few minutes of the consultation and his questions are then directed to confirm this diagnosis. This does not imply that the tentative diagnosis is invariably correct, but questions should be succinct and to the point to confirm or refute it.

Ample time should always be allowed for the important discussion that is to follow the examination, and discussion about the possible treatment before the examination should be avoided.

Others Present at the Consultation

Sometimes a grandparent will come and may provide valuable support for the parents, particularly if the mother comes without the father and in one-parent families. The grandparent's presence is also valuable when the parents are young and have a child with a major disability such as cerebral palsy or spina bifida. The grandparent is less emotionally involved, more likely to provide useful information about the family history, and is frequently better able to listen to and recall aspects of the consultant's opinion than the parents because the parents have been managing the child or are too emotionally upset to hear what the doctor is saying.

If a physiotherapist attends with a child who has a long-term major disability it should be made clear to the parents that they are in no way excluded from contributing information by the presence of the physiotherapist. Such visits by the patient with their physiotherapist are of great value for children with major and generalized disability.

History Obtained in the Absence of the Child

Obtaining information in the absence of the child can readily be manoeuvred; it may involve getting the child back into the waiting room to play with toys and then asking the secretary to visit that room and take the parent away ostensibly to obtain an address or phone number, but in fact to enable further discussion. With older children more ingenuity is required. Such conversations are generally appropriate when there is a functional condition or when the child has a severe illness or requires major surgery. If it cannot be arranged smoothly then it is better to carry on further discussions over the telephone or at a separate consultation not attended by the child.

The Examination

As a result of the history-taking process, the clinician will have formed an opinion about how best to carry out the examination. Some children are clearly anxious and are likely to become uncooperative. In these circumstances, a great deal of sensitivity is needed whatever the age of the child. It may be appropriate to ask the child to remove only some portions of the clothing at a time. It is remarkable how many boys aged 5–10 years are embarrassed by the mere removal of their trousers; for these children, the statement 'I just want to see how long your legs are!' often removes the resistance.

Babies under six months of age can be easily examined on the couch. Reassuring words and looking directly into the child's eyes with a large smile can prevent some crying, but not invariably!

Over the age of six months, children have the ability to resist examination and frequently do. For infants and some toddlers and young children, the mother's lap is usually the most reassuring place for the examination, and if this is accomplished easily the child can be transferred to the couch or the floor by the parent to complete the examination.

Children over three years of age need to be examined on the couch. Lifting the child onto the couch is usually fiercely resisted, but confidence can be built up by asking the child to walk fully clothed towards or with a parent. This is an important part of the examination and when the child has achieved this he should be praised for doing it well. If asked 'Are you a good climber?' most children respond 'Yes'. The challenge is then issued, 'Do you think you could climb up onto the couch using these steps?' The challenge is rarely refused. Children are much more cooperative if they have climbed onto the couch themselves, but the sight of their parent close to their head to reassure them that all is well is often necessary.

Some children are frightened by loud voices, and talking in whispers is desirable. Big doctors are better on their knees when close to small children. They may require the help of a dummy or a bottle for the child to suck or keys for the child to play with. All handling should be gentle and begin with games. The clinician should play with the feet and legs before putting them through a range of movement. The clinician can then examine the relevant parts of the body, and this may require careful palpation to identify sites of tenderness that may indicate trauma or infection.

Children are commonly frightened that the doctor is going to give them an injection. It is wise to make it clear from an early stage that there are no needles in the room.

Examination of adolescent girls requires some sensitivity and repeat visits may be easier if they are instructed to come in a swim-suit for subsequent examinations.

THE DISCUSSION

Just how much of this discussion is directed towards the child and how much towards the parents will depend on the age and attitude of the child. Usually, whatever their age, some of the discussion will be directed to the child in terms that he or she can understand (babies can be exempt!).

As a result of the consultation so far it will have become clear who has the problem—the child, the mother, the father, the grandparents, the school teacher or a neighbour—and the clinician's comments should be skewed in an appropriate direction.

By this stage of the consultation the clinician will have some idea about the type of people he or she is dealing with, their preconceived ideas about the condition, their theory as to the cause of the condition, and the most appropriate type of explanation for them. Clearly it is necessary to use non-medical terms.

For those children who have postural variations the orthopaedic surgeon needs to describe the natural history of the condition and the expected time frame during which improvement may occur. It is useless to state merely 'it will get better;' it is necessary to make it clear that for the child who presents with bow legs at the age of one year, it may be two further years before the bowing is completely corrected. The offer of a further check in one year's time if there has been no improvement is often reassuring and rarely taken up.

It is necessary for the orthopaedic surgeon to answer not only those questions that the parents verbalize, but also their unspoken doubts; an anticipation of these questions usually results from experience of life and medicine. It is always wise to suggest that if there are any further questions that occur to

the parents later then they should phone up for the answers.

In some circumstances it will be clear that the parents are still in doubt and dissatisfied. In these circumstances it may be wise to involve others in the management of the child; it may be that an appropriate children's physiotherapist should be employed or a second opinion suggested.

It is no use saying to parents 'there is nothing wrong, or 'do not worry' or using similar general reassuring phrases. In order to reassure the parents sufficient empathy is needed to see the problem from their point of view, and from their point of view there is something wrong. What you can do as a consultant is to point out that 'the something wrong' will get better by itself or require recurrent observation, or to make some statement that implies a knowledge of the future for this condition and its appropriate management.

The discussion generally involves an outline of the prognosis of the condition both with or without treatment, and this enables rational decision-making. For complex or chronic problems and for problems requiring surgical management a follow-up letter should be sent to the parents, recapitulating the discussion and the aims, nature of, possible complications, and expected outcome of surgery.

FUNCTIONAL DISORDERS

Functional disorders are not uncommon, particularly in adolescent girls. Common presenting features of a functional disorder are:

- A limp without significant pain.
- Major pain following minor injury.
- A bizarre limp.
- Symptoms described by a smiling patient.

The management of these disorders presents a great challenge. A confrontational approach is usually disastrous. The consultation should be handled with sensitivity, agreeing with both the patient and parent, gaining their confidence and encouraging them to describe the symptoms in details. One should avoid denying there is a problem—clearly there is one. At some point, when confidence has been gained by a careful examination and possibly further radiological investigation, the explanation that there is nothing seriously wrong should be given. Listing the parental fears, such as bone tumours, osteomyelitis and arthritis, then saying that none of these are present is very reassuring. It is usually better if a specific explanation of the symptoms can be given even if it is as vague as 'the nerves in the limb are acting inappropriately (or misbehaving) and are misinterpreting what is happening in the limb.' A plan of action should then be outlined, which usually involves an empathic physiotherapist.

The clear statement that there is no serious organic pathology, that there is an explanation for the symptoms, and that there is a plan of action for therapy is very reassuring to parents. However the successful management of this type of patient remains a great challenge and sometimes involves the help of colleagues such as rheumatologists or pain clinics where available.

FAMILIES WHO BELIEVE IN VARIOUS FORMS OF MAGIC

Many families find it rewarding to seek treatment from chiropractors, podiatrists, iridologists, naturopaths, osteopaths and various others who have not had scientific training. On the one hand it is important not to be derisive of such forms of management; we are in no position to be derisive unless we can demonstrate that we have more to offer. On the other hand the families should not be allowed to believe that treatment from these workers is scientifically based. It can be gently suggested that this management may affect the spirit of man, but does not have any direct beneficial effects on the musculoskeletal system.

THE SECOND OPINION

A second opinion may have been requested by the parents after consulting another orthopaedic surgeon or may have been suggested by the other orthopaedic surgeon. If you are the person giving the second opinion you are in a position of advantage; by the time the parents see you they have had a chance to think about the whole situation and its management. If you make any statements about the condition that the previous doctor did not make (and he may not have made these statements for very good reasons) the patients are likely to side with you and wonder why the previous doctor did not make this point. Furthermore the parents who request a further opinion have an opportunity of justifying this decision by liking you and disliking the original specialist. Clearly medical ethics demand that you should not exploit this situation, but should send the patient back to the original doctor. Many parents will request you to carry out the management, but this

suggestion should be strenuously opposed. If they comment that they will not go back to the original orthopaedic surgeon, then the appropriate action is to refer them back to their own general practitioner and tell them that he will guide them as to the best action. Of course this will probably mean that the patient will be sent back to you, but you can then feel, and it will be evident to the parents and the members of the medical profession involved, that the demands of appropriate ethical behaviour have been met.

THE INJURED CHILD

Children who have suffered what may appear to be a simple fracture should never be regarded as having a simple problem. A constant awareness of the possibility of complications including vascular complications and redisplacement of the fracture is essential. Invariably the patient should be seen the day following the injury whatever treatment has been appropriate on the day of injury. Parents must be made aware of in writing those situations that are to be regarded as warnings of possible complications so that they can take appropriate and immediate action.

Children who have had multiple injuries and more severe injuries, as in motor vehicle accidents, should be encouraged to talk about their injury once their condition allows it. This may avoid hidden fears and nightmares and adds to their store of experience. The child's mother may need to stay in hospital with the child for a few days for added reassurance.

HOSPITALS AND CHILDREN

A hospital admission is a traumatic experience at any age. For children it may be devastating, and requires preparation, sensitivity and the provision of adequate information to the child and parents. A detailed explanation is only necessary for older children. Younger children require reassurance and encouragement to ask both the parents and the doctor questions. Live-in facilities and feeding facilities for a baby should be discussed with the parents. Handouts about the hospital should be provided, and a preliminary visit to the ward is a good idea.

If multiple hospitalizations or prolonged periods of hospitalization are necessary, occupational therapists are important, and it may be possible to arrange for the child to do some school work during the period of hospitalization.

CONCLUSION

Paediatric orthopaedics gives the clinician a unique opportunity to influence the growth and physical development of children. It is a branch of orthopaedic surgery demanding not only great sensitivity to the expectations of the parents, but also skill in relating to the child to gain their confidence in their treatment. Ultimately this can prove very rewarding for the clinician.

FURTHER READING

Wenger DR, Rang M. *The Art and Practice of Children's Orthopaedics*. Raven Press, New York. 1993

Chapter 3
Normal and Pathological Gait

H Kerr Graham and Donnchadha G Gallagher

The study of gait is an integral part of paediatric orthopaedic practice. Many acute and chronic orthopaedic problems present as a limp or some other disturbance of gait. The limp may be acute and painful due to an acute disease process such as osteoarticular infection or injury. A chronic limp may be due to a neurological disorder, which is usually painless. Clinical gait analysis is the study of these disturbances of walking.

NORMAL GAIT

Normal gait is a complex integration of neuromuscular events, both central and peripheral, which allows the individual to move smoothly and efficiently, keeping the deviations of the centre of mass to a minimum. The prerequisites of normal gait as described by Perry (1985) are stability in stance, a means of progression and the need to conserve energy. Table 3.1 documents the normal parameters of gait.

Table 3.1 Normal time–distance parameters

Velocity (distance per unit time)	90 ± 12 m min^{-1}
Cadence (steps per unit time)	116 ± 10 steps min^{-1}
Step length	0.78 ± 0.065 m
Stride length	1.56 ± 0.13 m
Step width	0.08 ± 0.01 m

The gait cycle is defined as the interval and events between successive contacts of the same foot and is divided into stance and swing phases.

- Stance phase is subdivided into initial contact, loading response, mid-stance, terminal stance and pre-swing.
- Swing phase is subdivided into initial swing, mid-swing and terminal swing (*Figure 3.1*).

There are three planes in which motion can be defined and studied: sagittal, coronal, and transverse.

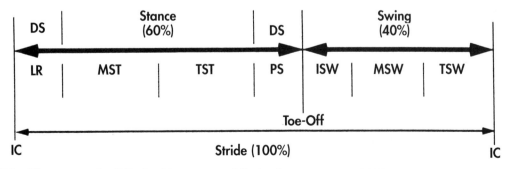

Figure 3.1 The gait cycle. DS, double support; LR, loading response; MST, mid-stance; TST, terminal stance; PS, pre-swing; ISW, initial swing; MSW, mid-swing; TSW, terminal swing. (Reproduced from Gage (1990) *Gait Analysis in Cerebral Palsy* with permission.)

Observational gait analysis is what all physicians practice when watching patients walk. Much can be gained from careful observation. However, even the most experienced eye cannot detect the nuances of disordered gait at the three levels of hip, knee and ankle in both lower limbs and in all three planes. Watching patients walk in real time or recording it on video will provide some information about the kinematics of the subject's gait, but reveals nothing about kinetics.

KINEMATICS

Kinematics is the study of motion in terms of displacement, angles and velocities, without regard to the forces behind the events. When normal motion is plotted as angular displacement against time, characteristic plots are generated at each joint level and in each plane. Kinematic data can be measured in various ways, but the most practical is by a photographic system, which tracks markers attached directly to the walking child (*Figure 3.2*).

KINETICS

Kinetics is the study of the forces that cause motion and the environmental reaction to them. A moment is defined as a force–couple, or a force acting at a distance about an axis of rotation. This creates an angular acceleration about that axis (e.g. a child on a see-saw). The units are force (newtons) × distance from the centre of rotation (metres) (i.e. newton metres). These units are then standardized by dividing by the subject's body weight (i.e. $Nm\ kg^{-1}$) (*Figure 3.3*).

Kinetic data are measured by asking the child to walk on a pressure sensitive 'force plate,' which is usually set into the floor of the gait laboratory. Kinematic and kinetic data are usually recorded simultaneously.

Joint power is the rate of generating or absorbing energy and is the product of the net joint moment and the net angular velocity. The unit of measurement is watts kg^{-1}.

Power generation results from concentric muscle contraction and feeds energy into the gait cycle at key points. The joint moment and angular velocity are in the same direction (e.g. the ankle plantar flexors in terminal stance).

Power absorption results from eccentric muscle contraction to smooth gait and acts as a braking mechanism. The joint moment and angular velocity are in opposite directions (e.g. the ankle plantar flexors in loading response and early stance).

ELECTROMYOGRAPHY

Electromyography (EMG) is the study of the electrical signal emanating from muscle during contraction and provides precise information about the timing of muscle activity, and to a lesser degree, the intensity of that activity. Recordings can be made from the surface of muscles by recording the signal from a large area through the skin or using fine-wire electrodes inserted into the muscle. Surface EMG has a problem with interference from signals detected from adjacent large muscle groups. Fine-wire EMG is limited because of the discomfort.

ENERGY STUDIES

Energy is required for walking and is provided by the oxidation of sugars in skeletal muscle. Normal walking conserves energy as a result of a constant interplay between storing potential energy as the centre of mass is elevated with each step, followed by conversion to kinetic energy as the centre of mass undergoes a controlled fall. The vertical and horizontal displacements of the centre of mass of the body follow a sinusoidal curve and are equal and opposite. If we walked with stiff limbs our centre of mass would have to rise and fall 9.5 cm with each step. By using coordinated pelvic, knee and ankle motions this can be reduced to 4.4 cm, and is important in conserving energy.

Abnormal gait is frequently characterized by a relative failure of these mechanisms and uses excessive energy. The stiff knee gait in cerebral palsy and the Trendelenburg gait in lumbar level myelomeningocoele are characterized by large centre of mass oscillations, which greatly increase energy consumption. Many teenagers are unable to sustain these increased demands without becoming excessively tired. Despite successful walking as younger children, some will increasingly need to use a wheelchair in secondary school.

Measurement of the energy cost of walking may therefore be the single most important parameter in assessing the efficiency of pathological gait. Various direct and indirect methods are used. The simplest is to measure the heart rate and velocity of walking and to derive the PCI or 'physiological cost index' (*Table 3.2*). This calculation has been used because heart rate and oxygen uptake may be linearly related.

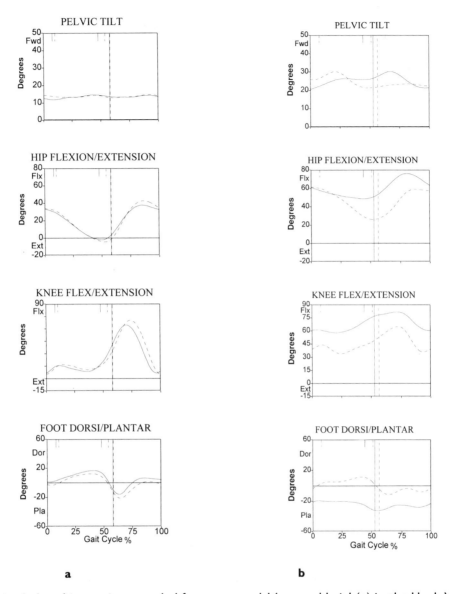

Figure 3.2   Sagittal plane kinematics recorded from a normal 14-year-old girl (**a**) in the Hugh Williamson Gait Analysis Laboratory, Royal Children's Hospital, Melbourne. Compare these traces with those from a 12-year-old boy (**b**) with severe asymmetric spastic diplegia before multilevel surgery. There are major differences between the normal girl and the boy with cerebral palsy, and between the right and left limbs of the boy. In particular note the equinus at the ankle on one side only, the flexed knees, which do not extend in stance, and the incomplete hip extension in late stance.

The oxygen used during walking can be measured directly by various means. Until recently the equipment was cumbersome and better suited to normal subjects in controlled laboratory conditions. Portable, light-weight telemetric systems are now available, which are capable of giving reproducible results in children with motor disorders using their normal aids and orthoses.

The energy efficiency of a car can be expressed as the number of kilometres travelled per litre of fuel. The pilot of a jet may be more concerned with the number of hours flying time left for a certain volume

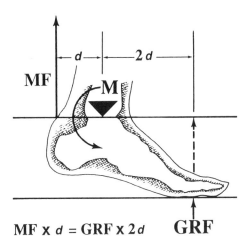

$$MF \times d = GRF \times 2d$$

Figure 3.3 Ankle kinetics. The ground reaction force (GRF) creates an anticlockwise torque (moment, M) at the centre of rotation or fulcrum. This is balanced by an internal clockwise torque (moment) provided by the muscle force (MF). If MF × distance = GRF × 2d, no motion takes place. When MF × d is slightly less than GRF × 2d, then the heel lowers slowly down to produce an eccentric action of the plantar flexors. When MF × d is more than GRF × 2d, the heel rises to produce a concentric action of the plantar flexors.

Table 3.2 Calculation of the physiological cost index (PCI)

PCI = (HW − HR)/S

(HW, heart rate on walking (beats min^{-1}); HR, heart rate at rest (beats min^{-1}); S, velocity (m min^{-1})

of fuel. By measuring oxygen uptake during walking, two values can be derived to describe the efficiency of gait. These are:

- Oxygen rate (ml of oxygen kg^{-1} min^{-1}).
- Oxygen cost (ml of oxygen kg^{-1} m^{-1}).

Many children with a motor disorder and an inefficient gait simply slow down to keep their oxygen rate within normal limits, but their oxygen cost remains markedly elevated compared to that of children with efficient gaits (*Figure 3.4*).

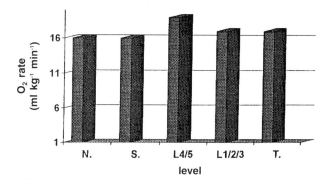

a

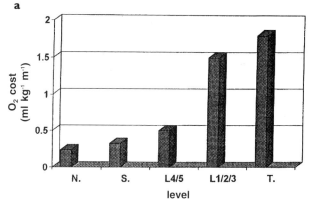

b

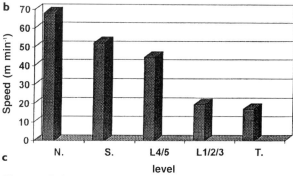

c

Figure 3.4 Oxygen rate (**a**), oxygen cost (**b**) and walking velocity (**c**) in normal children and children with spina bifida, subdivided according to neurological level. Oxygen rate is not affected by the neurological level, but walking velocity and oxygen cost are directly related to it. The children with spina bifida slow their walking speed to maintain a comfortable oxygen rate and in doing so incur a high oxgen cost, which few are able to sustain as walking adults. (N, normal; S, sacral; T, thoracic.)

In a study of oxygen consumption in children with spina bifida, it was found that the oxygen rate was not elevated in comparison to that of normal children, nor was it related to neurological level. However the oxygen cost was elevated in all children with spina bifida and directly related to neurological level. The explanation for this paradox is found in a comparison of walking velocity. The high neurological level spina bifida children simply slowed down to keep their oxygen rate at a comfortable level, incurring a very high oxygen cost. This very slow walking is not an effective means of walking for older children and is the main reason why many opt for a wheelchair as they get older.

Modern gait analysis techniques are used to study normal and abnormal gait, and to evaluate interventions in children with motor disorders such as spina bifida and cerebral palsy. The study of groups of children with specific disorders can yield useful information, which can help in the classification of the disorder and in understanding the pathomechanics. This is often the first step in planning logical management strategies.

CEREBRAL PALSY

A study of children with hemiplegia by Gage (1990) has resulted in a simple four group classification and suggested management plans. This is an example of the application of gait analysis to describe and define the pathomechanics of gait for those managing children with this condition.

Three-dimensional gait analysis can also be used as a tool for analysis and decision-making in individual patients. Children with abnormal gait are studied in the laboratory, and after a consideration of all the data (history, static clinical examination, radiographs, video, kinematics, kinetics, EMG and energy studies) a plan of management is made. The sagittal-plane kinematics are the main guide in planning tendon-lengthening surgery because the muscles that are most frequently spastic and contracted work mainly in this plane (i.e. iliopsoas, rectus femoris, hamstrings, and gastrosoleus). The transverse-plane kinematics help in the evaluation of bone torsional problems and may guide in decisions about femoral and tibial osteotomies as well as foot stabilization.

The management plan may include multilevel soft tissue surgery, osteotomies, arthrodeses, orthotic prescription and a carefully planned rehabilitation programme. After the child has gone through the full rehabilitation programme and the new gait pattern has stabilized, a repeat study can be performed. By comparing the pre- and post-intervention studies it is possible to judge the success or otherwise of the management. In this way it is possible to learn from each patient's surgery and to dramatically shorten the 'feedback loop' by which the surgeon evaluates his programme of care.

MYELOMENINGOCOELE

Gait analysis studies in children with myelomeningocoele have improved understanding of the patterns of gait disturbance and evaluation of interventions. For example the posterolateral iliopsoas transfer described by Sharrard in 1964 was designed to stabilize the hip in these patients, but it was expected that it would also help the gait by acting as an extensor and abductor of the hip during stance. However, gait analysis studies in which children with iliopsoas transfers were compared to those without a transfer, showed that the kinematics were worse in the group with the tendon transfer (Duffy et al., 1996). The transferred muscle was still working in swing phase and had not 'learned' to work in stance phase. This objective evidence replaces the subjective assessment of observational gait analysis.

ORTHOTICS AND PROSTHETICS

Orthotic and prosthetic devices are designed with specific aims in mind. Testing of the device in the gait laboratory can provide objective data, and help in the fine-tuning of the development of a new orthosis or prosthesis.

The reciprocal gait orthosis (RGO) has been widely used as a mobility aid for children with thoracic and high lumbar level spina bifida. Energy studies have confirmed that reciprocal gait with this type of device is less energy expensive than 'swing through' gait with traditional hip–knee–ankle–foot orthoses (HKAFOs).

Gait analysis has been very helpful in the assessment of the 'crouch gait.' In normal mid and late stance little activity is required in the quadriceps because the ankle plantar flexors direct the ground reaction force (GRF) anterior to the knee joint. This produces an extensor moment and forces the knee into extension. This is the normal function of the 'plantar flexion–knee extension' couple. This force couple fails in children with sacral level myelomeningocoele and in cerebral palsy children with an overlengthened tendo Achillis. The gait pattern in these children is characterized by 'crouch' or flexion at the hips and knees. This is energy expensive because the quadriceps must act continually throughout stance to keep the child upright. Although there is no surgical solution to this problem (except to avoid overlengthening of the tendo Achillis) a floor reaction ankle–foot orthosis

(AFO) can be a considerable help. This type of AFO mechanically blocks excessive dorsiflexion of the ankle in mid and late stance and helps control the direction of the GRF vector.

A new prosthesis for below-knee amputees in which a carbon fibre composite spring was tuned to store energy in early stance phase and to release the stored energy at terminal stance, just before push off, has been designed to replace the absent gastro-soleus. The characteristics of the spring have been studied by kinematic, kinetic and force plate data in the gait laboratory setting and showed that the aims had been achieved. The final assessment was by energy studies, which showed that the energy cost of running with the 'sports' prosthesis was signifi-cantly lower than with a regular below-knee pros-thesis.

REFERENCES AND FURTHER READING

Butler P, Engelbrecht M, Major RE, Taft JH, Stallard S, Patrick JH. Physiological cost index of walking for normal children and its use as an indicator of physical handicap. *Develop Med Child Neurol* 1986; **26**: 607–612.

Duffy CM, Hill AE, Cosgrove AP, Corry IS, Graham HK. Energy consumption in children with spina bifida and cerebral palsy: a comparative study. *Develop Med Child Neurol* 1996; **38**: 238–243.

Gage JR. *Gait Analysis in Cerebral Palsy*. MacKeith Press, Oxford, 1990.

Inman VT, Ralston HJ, Todd F. *Human Walking*. Williams and Wilkins, Baltimore, 1981.

Perry J. Normal and pathological gait. In: *Atlas of Orthotics*, edited by WH Bunch, second edition. pp. 76–111. CV Mosby, St. Louis, 1985.

Sharrard WJW. Posterior iliopsoas transplantation in the treatment of paralytic dislocation of the hip. *J Bone Joint Surg* 1964; **46B**: 426–444.

Chapter 4
Lower Limb Deficiencies

Ian P Torode

The incidence of congenital limb deficiencies is relatively low (1 in 2000 live births). The first contact doctor is often the obstetrician who will have little expertise in this field. It is important that the child is referred to a centre of expertise early to allow early discussion of appropriate treatment. If suggestions are made to the family as to what might or might not be done for their child without due regard for a complete management plan, it is highly likely that confusion will result, which will only serve to make the management more difficult.

Most parents will at some stage ask questions about aetiological agents. It is important to impress on the families that there is no evidence that anything they might have done has led to the child having a limb deficiency. There is enough emotional disruption associated with the child being born with a limb deficiency without adding to the guilt or anxiety. The exception is tibial hemimelia which can show autosomal dominant inheritance.

Management should be undertaken in a centre of expertise where a multidisciplinary team can be involved. There should include genetic counselling, consideration of the effect on the rest of the family, and prosthetic, orthotic and physiotherapy involvement. Children with limb deficiencies often have associated abnormalities in other systems, which may modify management.

Where amputations form a positive part of the child's management, it is advisable to arrange for parents to see other children functioning well in their prostheses. Where limb lengthening is considered, the family should understand that a limb lengthening of 6 or 8 cm may occupy 12 months of their life and will result in a major disruption of their normal day-to-day affairs.

CONGENITAL FEMORAL DEFICIENCIES

The more commonly used radiological classifications of these conditions are those of Aitken and Amstutz. The more recent review by Hamanishi illustrates that on radiographic criteria the number of categories is limited only by the number of cases seen.

However, although there is a spectrum of radiographic abnormalities, in terms of clinical signs and in terms of management, the femoral deficiencies fall into two groups – (i) the congenital short femur and (ii) the true proximal focal femoral deficiency (Gillespie and Torode, 1983).

Congenital Short Femur

The clinical picture is a child with a limb length discrepancy of up to 20–30%. The involved knee has a significant valgus deformity, which is often disguised by an external rotation deformity, and the foot lies approximately at the contralateral mid-tibial level (*Figure 4.1*).

The radiograph shows an intact femur, but about half its normal length. There may be significant coxa vara, although there is often delayed ossification of the proximal end of the femur up to the age of two years. Magnetic resonance imaging (MRI) may be helpful to identify the cartilage anlage. Coxa vara develops at the trochanteric or subtrochanteric level. There may also be lateral bowing of the diaphysis of the femur with sclerosis on the lateral cortex of the femur (*Figure 4.2*). Usually there is hypoplasia of the lateral femoral condyle producing valgus at the knee, and cruciate ligament deficiency which can be demonstrated by clinical examination.

The importance of this group of children is that if they possess a normal below-knee segment they have the potential to function without a prosthesis.

Management

The overall plan is to align the femur at an early stage and then correct the length of the femur later.

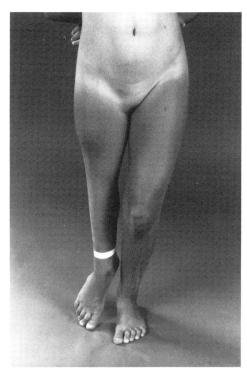

Figure 4.1   Photograph of a child with a right congenital short femur. The knee is featureless and there is external rotation. The femur is about 50% of the normal side.

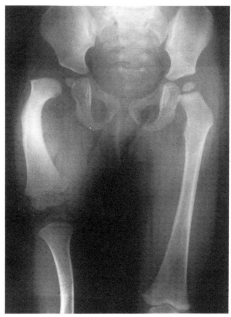

Figure 4.2   The femur is about half the length of the normal side. There is coxa vara and lateral bowing of the diaphysis with sclerosis on the lateral cortex of the femur. In this patient there is an associated congenital absence of the fibula.

Innominate osteotomy

These children often have a dysplastic acetabulum. A Salter innominate osteotomy, including a bone block to produce transiliac lengthening (Millis and Hall, 1979) will gain some length and also protect the hip joint from subluxation in later femoral lengthening.

Proximal femoral osteotomy

If coxa vara is present this osteotomy can gain length and correct the external rotation deformity. Care must be taken not to uncover the femoral head and put the joint at risk during later lengthening of the femur.

Distal femoral osteotomy

The valgus of the knee from hypoplasia of the lateral femoral condyle is best corrected before five years of age. This correction is obtained by an inverted dome osteotomy performed through a stab incision at the suprapatellar level in the femoral metaphysis.

Limb lengthening

Once the congenital short femur has been reconstructed into an aligned short femur, the femoral lengthening procedure can take place during the child's primary school years. This timing is optimal as the relative success of the femoral lengthening will dictate the need for a second femoral lengthening or contralateral epiphyseodesis of the femur.

It should be expected a child with a congenital deficiency of the femur will also have a cruciate ligament deficiency. Femoral and tibial lengthening around the knee joint with a deficient cruciate mechanism is associated with a significant incidence of subluxation or dislocation of the knee. While it is important to maintain flexion in the knee during lengthening, any loss of extension during lengthening should alert the surgeon to the possibility of posterior subluxation of the tibia on the femur. Lateral and anterior subluxation of the tibia on the femur can also occur. Joint deformities that arise during lengthening should be treated aggressively by the use of additional fixation points on the lengthening frame, soft tissue releases and serial casts. When the knee is grossly unstable, it may be necessary to connect the femoral and tibial frames with hinges.

Previously it has been recommended that lengthening be limited to 20% of the femur. With a better understanding of the physiology of lengthening, it is possible to achieve much greater gains than previously thought possible. This has the advantage of aiming for normal limb function rather than obligatory prosthetic use.

Epiphyseodesis

Although most families would not wish their child's 'good limb' to be subjected to any surgery, morbidity from such a procedure is minimal. Every centimetre gained in reducing limb length discrepancy will save the child approximately six weeks in a limb-lengthening device.

Proximal Focal Femoral Deficiency

These children have a very short thigh with a leg length discrepancy of 35–50% (*Figure 4.3*). They have fixed hip and knee flexion contractures, and the limb lies with the involved ankle at approximately the level of the contralateral knee. There is a variable deficiency of the proximal femur, and often a pseudarthrosis in the subtrochanteric region. Sometimes complete ossification may take place with marked varus in the classical 'Shepherd's crook' deformity. The associated soft tissue deficiencies around the proximal femur can be demonstrated by CT or MRI scans. The lateral femoral condyle is

hypoplastic, although the valgus knee deformity may be disguised by a flexion contracture (*Figure 4.4*).

Occasionally the opposite limb is involved and there is an associated congenital absence of the fibula in 50–80%. The instability from the cruciate ligament deficiency may be disguised by the knee flexion contracture.

Management

Surgery for children with unilateral proximal focal femoral deficiency should be aimed at providing optimal function. These children will always require some sort of prosthesis, and although lengthening procedures have been performed, the time these major lengthenings take is a deterrent to their use. Furthermore, the end-result of a long limb with stiff joints may not be a functional improvement over a child with a well-fitting prosthesis.

Fixation of the pseudarthrosis

This is not an immediate priority and correction where necessary can be incorporated into the knee fusion or the rotationplasty. Stabilization is achieved with an intramedullary rod across the pseudarthrosis

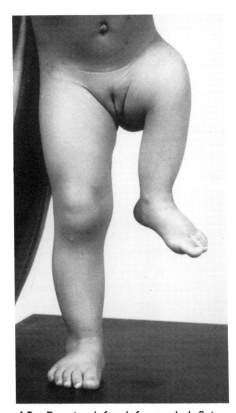

Figure 4.3 Proximal focal femoral deficiency. The femur is very short and there is a flexion deformity of the knee and an external rotation deformity of the leg. The foot lies at about the level of the opposite knee. In this child the below-knee segment is normal.

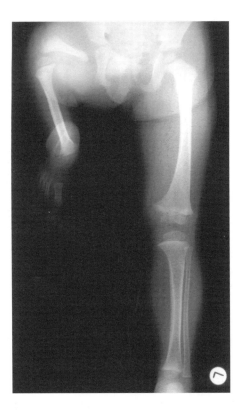

Figure 4.4 Proximal focal femoral deficiency with a reasonable acetabulum and a femoral head. This was associated with congenital absence of the fibula and an unstable ankle.

or by excision of the distal femoral fragment and fixation to the tibia. Although this may improve the radiological appearance of the proximal femur, the soft tissue deficiencies around the hip means that the child's Trendelenburg gait may not be improved.

Knee fusion

Knee fusion is recommended as mobility and deformity of that joint adds to the instability of the limb in a prosthesis and puts the weight-bearing line anterior to the trunk. The fusion is usually done by intramedullary rodding. Preoperative assessment of the desired length at maturity will dictate the need for retention of the distal femoral or proximal tibial growth plates. The use of a smooth rod across the growth plates will allow continued growth.

Syme amputation

Amputation of the foot is recommended where the foot itself is deficient and not contributing to function, or when a decision has been made not to proceed with rotationplasty in the case of a normal foot. The amputation can be performed at the same time as the knee fusion.

Van Nes rotationplasty

Where there is normal foot and ankle function, the leg can be turned round and the ankle used as a 'knee' in a hinged prosthesis. This is achieved by lateral rotation through the knee joint. The neurovascular structures come to lie anterior and a knee fusion is performed over a smooth intramedullary rod with care to avoid premature growth plate arrest of the epiphyseal plates. This has become increasingly popular recently as these children demonstrate improved function. Extensive preoperative consultation is recommended and the opportunity to meet with children who have undergone rotationplasty is valuable (*Figure 4.5*).

Iliofemoral fusion

This has been advocated in some circumstances to produce hip stability, and the knee acts as a pseudo-hip joint.

Summary

A unilateral proximal focal femoral deficiency presents the problem of a gross limb length discrepancy that will require prosthetic management. Judicious use of the surgical procedures outlined will enhance function, prosthetic fitting and cosmesis. The surgi-

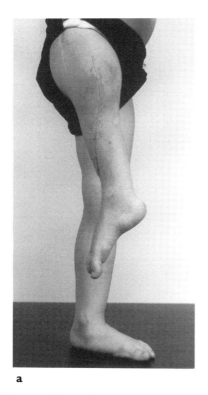
a

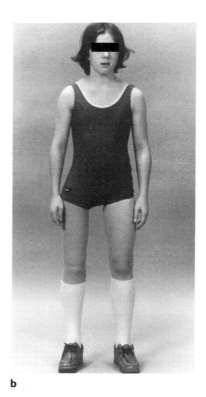
b

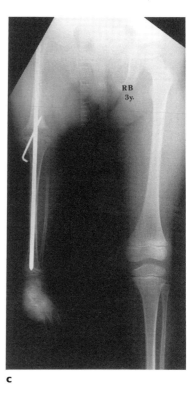
c

Figure 4.5 **a** Clinical picture showing results after a successful Van Nes rotationplasty. **b** Photograph of different child with Van Nes rotationplasty in her prosthesis. **c** Radiograph of successful Van Nes rotationplasty. Note that the deficient fibula now lies on the medial side.

cal plan should be discussed with the families and put in motion in early life. Patients with bilateral deficiencies must be individualized.

CONGENITAL DEFICIENCIES OF THE FIBULA

Congenital deficiency of the fibula is rare, but is the most common long bone congenital deficiency. Anteroposterior instability of the knee early in life will give the examining surgeon a clue to the presence of a congenital deficiency in a limb even when the foot is normal. In those patients in whom there is an associated deficiency of the femur, the management of the distal deficiency may be dictated by the severity of the proximal deficiency.

Classification

Coventry and Johnson (1952) subdivided the condition into three types.

Type 1 is the mildest type, with a range of deficiency from a shortened fibula to partial absence of the upper portion. It is unilateral and the tibial segment is slightly shortened. There is usually no foot deformity. Achterman and Kalamchi (1979) have divided them into:

- Type 1A where the ankle is stable although it may be a ball and socket joint.
- Type 1B where the deficient fibula allows an equinovalgus deformity at the ankle.

Type 2 is complete absence of the fibula and is unilateral. The foot is usually abnormal with lateral ray deficiencies, tarsal coalitions and abnormalities in shape of the talus and os calcis. The foot is usually in equinovalgus. The tibia is moderately short and usually bowed anteriorly. There is often a dimple in the skin over the kyphosis (*Figure 4.6*).

Type 3 is the most severe deficiency. It is bilateral and associated with other malformations such as proximal focal femoral deficiency or upper limb deformities.

Most type 2 and type 3 patients will be treated by some form of amputation and prosthetic fitting. Sometimes the foot is reasonable and the parents reject amputation so that reconstruction may be undertaken. This will involve correction of the equinovalgus deformity of the foot and correction of the tibial kyphosis.

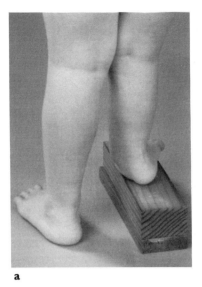 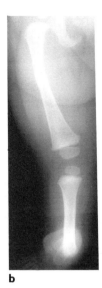

a   b

Figure 4.6 a Congenital deficiency of the fibula type 2. The heel lies in valgus and the tibia is short. **b** Radiograph of congenital deficiency of the fibula showing the foot in valgus with deficiency of the lateral ray of the foot.

Management

Ankle disarticulation

Ankle disarticulation was described by James Syme in 1843. It is a predictable procedure in terms of recovery, outcome and fitting of a prosthesis. Heel pad migration can be a problem with Syme amputation and can be avoided by fixing the remnant of the os calcis to the distal tibia as described by Boyd in 1939. We prefer to perform this procedure around the time of walking as the morbidity at this age is minimal, the hospital stay is short, the rehabilitation is simple, and the patient does not have the sense of loss that accompanies amputation in older children. The tibial kyphosis can be corrected by osteotomy and intramedullary rod fixation at the same operation.

The indications for a Syme's amputation are:

- A severely deficient foot that will not serve any useful purpose even if retained in a stable relationship to the tibia. Note that a three-ray foot may be quite functional and a useful foot.
- Gross deformity or instability of the ankle joint itself.
- Associated tibial deficiency such that the leg length discrepancy and ankle instability preclude limb lengthening.
- Associated femoral deficiency (i.e. proximal focal femoral deficiency), where the family elect for Syme's amputation with knee fusion or where the

foot deficiency is such that a rotationplasty is contraindicated.

Posterolateral release

In children with an unstable ankle and an equino-valgus deformity there is lateral subluxation of the talus on the tibia. If there is a useful foot and a reasonable tibia, a posterolateral release of the ankle will allow placement of the talus under the tibia. The release is extensive and involves the Achilles tendon, posterior and lateral capsules of the ankle, and lengthening or division of the peroneals and fibular anlage when present.

Occasionally in congenital fibular deficiency, the foot is in equinovarus. In these children the release should also include a lengthening of the tibialis posterior and a complete release of the ankle joint from its medial to lateral extent.

Ankle stabilization procedures with bone

Although these have been advocated in the past, they do not address the long-term problems and by necessity compromise the growth of the distal tibia because of damage to the distal tibial epiphysis. The Gruca procedure is an oblique osteotomy of the distal tibia allowing the medial portion to slide proximally to create a lateral buttress from the lateral portion of the tibial epiphysis and metaphysis (Thomas and Williams, 1987).

Limb reconstruction in bilateral cases

In bilateral cases the length of the legs is a secondary issue and it may be reasonable to consider retention of the feet with correction of the tibial kyphosis and soft tissue release of the equinovalgus deformity. The tibial kyphosis is corrected with the use of an Ilizarov frame and a tibial osteotomy at the level of the deformity. The frame is extended to the foot after a radical posterior release of the ankle. Gradual distraction across both the tibial osteotomy and the ankle joint permits correction of the gross equinus deformity to produce plantargrade feet.

CONGENITAL DEFICIENCIES OF THE TIBIA

Congenital deficiency of the tibia (tibial hemimelia) is the least common congenital deficiency of the lower limb. The deficiency may be complete or partial and is commonly associated with instability and varus deformity of the knee joint. There is usually equino-varus of the foot. Associated skeletal anomalies have included hips, feet, hands, femurs and spine in descending order of frequency. The fibula is usually intact and the involved leg is bowed and shortened. Many have a significant family history.

Classification is based on the severity of the deficiency (Jones *et al.*, 1978; Kalamchi and Dawe, 1985). Ossification of the proximal tibia may not be evident at birth so ultrasound or MRI should be used to look for a cartilage analogue to define the type.

Unilateral Complete Absence of the Tibia (type 1)

In this type there is no cartilage remnant of the tibia. There are severe deformities at birth with a marked fixed flexion deformity of the knee, and often a popliteal web. There are commonly foot abnormalities and the fibula is larger than expected. The distal femur is hypoplastic and its ossific nucleus, which is normally present at birth, may be absent. The proximal tibia, patella and patellar tendon are not palpable and the knee is grossly unstable.

Management

In these children a through-knee amputation is the recommended procedure. It is advisable to undertake this surgery early in life otherwise proximal migration of the fibula may take place.

Within this group there may be a small number of patients in whom the deformity at the knee level is less marked with a better development of the distal femur and without a popliteal web. These children may have demonstrable flexion and extension of the knee. Transposition of the fibula under the central part of the distal femur as described by Brown, 1965, may be useful.

Unilateral Partial Hemimelia (type 2)

The upper end of the tibia is present, but may be slow to ossify and should be identified by ultrasound or MRI. A well-developed lower femur should alert the surgeon to this possibility. The knee is well developed and worth preserving.

Management

The limb can be stabilized by creating a synostosis between the fibula and the tibial remnant. This surgery should be carried out early in life once satisfactory ossification has occurred to prevent proximal migration of the fibula. Approximately one-third of the fibula is resected, allowing the distal two-thirds of the fibula to be translated and fixed to the distal aspect of the remnant of the tibia. The resected fibula can be used as a bone graft.

These children also have limb length discrepancy, and foot and ankle problems. One approach is to stabilize the fibula into either the talus or the os calcis to provide a stable platform on which to walk. Recurrent deformity after centralization of the foot on the fibula is common, and the limb length discrepancy has to be addressed. A more attractive option may be ankle disarticulation and prosthetic use.

Distal Tibial Dysplasia–Deficiency (type 3)

The tibia is short and there is a diastasis between the tibia and fibula distally. With marked tibial deficiency the calcaneus articulates with the fibula but in less severe cases the equinovarus deformity may resemble a congenital club foot.

Management

If the tibia is too short to support the talus a synostosis of the fibula to the tibia will control the proximal portion of the leg. If the foot deformity is such that it can serve no useful purpose, a Syme amputation is indicated or alternatively a calcaneofibular fusion and Boyd amputation.

In some patients, however, the deficiency is not great and may present as a relapsing talipes equinovarus deformity. There is a varus deformity at the ankle and a relatively short tibia, but the distal tibial growth plate is present. The problem can be addressed by tibial lengthening and appropriate epiphyseodesis of the ipsilateral distal fibula and the contralateral limb. The foot is corrected by medial release and lateral column shortening.

Bilateral Deficiencies

Management

In children with bilateral total absence of the tibias the usual procedure of choice would be bilateral knee disarticulation. If, however, there are major abnormalities in the upper limbs and where there are features as described above that may favour reconstruction, then attempts could be made to stabilize the knees and retain the feet.

MALALIGNMENT PROBLEMS

Malalignment of the limb in children with limb deficiencies and amputations can significantly reduce the efficiency of gait and the comfort of the prosthesis. It is easy to overlook abnormalities in alignment and gait problems may be inappropriately attributed to the fit of the prosthesis. Often the prosthesis has been made of the components prescribed but failure to recognize an angular or rotatory malalignment may compromise its use.

If there is an external rotational malalignment of the femur the prosthetist faces the dilemma of whether to align the foot in the direction the patient is facing or in the plane of the knee joint. The latter produces a toe-out gait and the former looks ungainly.

The distal lateral femoral metaphyseal angle (LFMA) of the normal adult femur measures 81°. In the congenital short femur the LFMA usually measures approximately 75°. Often the valgus attitude of the leg may invite correction of the tibia, but the deformity is in the distal femur and should be corrected at this site.

Although a limb may be short or missing a foot the usual principles of assessment of the mechanical and anatomical axes are still valid. A radiograph of the complete limb in the prosthesis shows the weight-bearing line of the limb. If there is malalignment, the patient has to compensate by a lateral trunk shift in gait. This is inefficient, tiring and unsightly. Correction of the rotatory and angular deformities will improve the patient's comfort and function with the prosthesis and may increase the longevity of the knee and patellofemoral joint.

CONGENITAL PSEUDARTHROSIS OF THE TIBIA

Congenital pseudarthrosis of the tibia affects about one child in two hundred thousand. The deformity of the tibia extends from an anterolateral bow to frank pseudarthrosis. There is associated neurofibromatosis type 1 (NF1) in more than 50% of cases. The stigmata of this disease may not appear until later in life.

Despite the name the condition may not be obvious, nor the tibia fractured at birth and is rarely a true pseudarthrosis, but rather a fibrous nonunion of a pathological fracture.

The radiological classification by Crawford is:

- Type I (nondysplastic) – anterolateral bowing, dense medullary canal.
- Type IIA (dysplastic) – anterolateral bowing, widened abnormal medullary canal.
- Type IIB (dysplastic) – anterolateral bowing, cystic postfracture lesion.
- Type IIC (dysplastic) – anterolateral bowing, fracture, cysts and pseudarthrosis.

Classifications may not be easy to apply and the appearance may change with age and attempts at healing by the bone.

Prognosis

Outcome in this condition must take into consideration the patient's health and function and not only bone union. A short, stiff, scarred limb prone to refracture may be a less satisfactory outcome than a Syme amputation. Patients with NF1 have a greater than 25% risk of developing an intracranial tumour which may override the importance of the tibial lesion.

Management

Prophylactic

Bracing is the accepted management of anterolateral bowing without fracture. This is continued until fracture supervenes or the bone becomes mature. In neurofibromatosis it is estimated that the majority of bowed tibias will fracture by two years of age. Tibial bypass grafting has been used prophylactically in the prepseudarthrotic tibia of neurofibromatosis with moderate success.

Surgical Management

Intramedullary rodding and bone grafting A combination of resection of the pseudarthrosis, intramedullary fixation, bone grafting, external supports and electrical stimulation is the most commonly used approach in the management of congenital pseudarthrosis. Where technically possible dual intramedullary rodding may be preferable. The William's rod traversing the subtalar joint, ankle joint and tibia has the advantage of improved stability although the Sheffield 'growing rod' has the

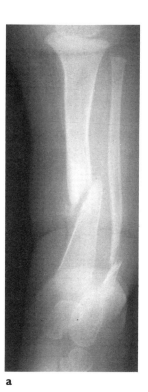
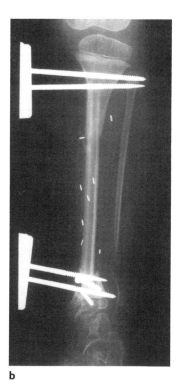
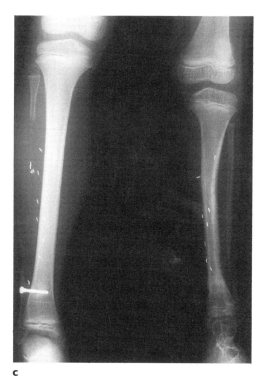

a   b   c

Figure 4.7 a Tibial pseudarthrosis. **b** This has been treated by excision of the defect and a vascularized fibular graft and then stabilized with an external fixator. **c** Two years following the procedure the fibular graft has hypertrophied. The distal end of the fibula, which has been resected, has been stabilized with a screw to prevent any valgus deformation of the normal ankle. (b,c are reproduced with permission from Williams PF, Cole WG. *Orthopaedic Management in Childhood.* Chapman & Hall, London.)

advantage of extension. Success rates in obtaining union vary from 40% to 80%.

Vascularized fibular grafts Free vascularized fibular grafting allows for extensive resection of all abnormal tissue although any donor site morbidity from the 'normal' limb is an obvious disadvantage. The most frequent problem is ankle valgus. Fixation by either an external frame (Ilizarov or similar) or internal fixation and cast is necessary.

Reported union rates are usually in excess of 80%, however long-term protection of the limb for maturation of the graft is necessary (*Figure 4.7*).

In the unusual situation that the fibula is intact an ipsilateral fibula graft on its vascular pedicle may be utilized thus avoiding morbidity in the opposite limb.

Ilizarov ring fixators The Ilizarov apparatus can be used to gain length and to correct deformity prior to the use of a free vascularized fibular graft or used for bone transport after excision of the lesion. This latter technique avoids the need for a donor limb but does require a prolonged period in the frame. The incidence of complications is significant and includes pin tract infections, nerve and vascular injuries, joint stiffness and subluxation.

As with other techniques, long term protection of the leg even after successful bone union is necessary.

Amputation Amputation should not be the operation of first resort nor the operation of last resort in this condition. Patients with Boyd or Syme amputations have excellent function and broad participation in sporting and other activities. This level of amputation is preferable in a child to avoid the problems of diaphyseal amputations with growth. Amputation should not be considered as a failure but as a positive decision to avoid repeated unsuccessful attempts at limb salvage.

The optimal age for surgical intervention is controversial. Some support an early age for intervention in the more radiologically aggressive lesions. The experience of the authors' hospital, however is that the union rate is higher and refracture lower in the older child. Consequently protection in an orthosis is preferred to early attempts at bone grafting.

POSTEROMEDIAL BOWING OF THE TIBIA

This presents at birth with a shortened limb with posteromedial bowing and a grossly calcaneus foot. It looks quite dramatic, but fortunately the condition is benign and improves in the first year or two of life, with the foot position improving in advance of the bowing. Radiographically the tibia and fibula are intact and the bow is most pronounced in their distal half. There is commonly shortening of the affected tibia and fibula and the amount of tibial shortening appears related to the angulation. The proportionate difference in lengths remains stable throughout childhood (*Figure 4.8*).

Management

In mild cases no active intervention is needed, however with severe foot deformity and marked bowing, serial casts have been advocated. For severe residual bowing after the age of three years corrective osteotomy should be considered. The limb length discrepancy in most cases can be managed by epiphyseodesis although some cases may require tibial lengthening.

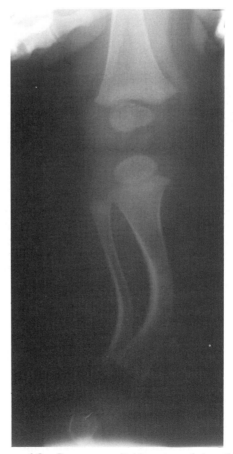

Figure 4.8 Posteromedial bowing of the tibia.

INFANTILE COXA VARA

This condition was first described by Fiorani in 1881 and the term congenital coxa vara presented by Hofmeister in 1894. The term 'infantile' has been used here as the condition is not evident until the child starts walking. However the condition has been reported at 18 months of age and in hindsight clinical signs may have been present at an earlier age.

Clinical Features

The patients are typically of short stature often with hyperlordosis of the lumbar spine. The child walks with a waddling gait and has a positive Trendelenburg sign. The affected hip has a decreased range of abduction and internal rotation, the greater trochanter is prominent and the thigh appears short. The inheritance pattern appears to be autosomal dominant with incomplete penetrance.

Radiology

The affected femoral neck is in varus with the proximal femoral epiphyseal plate being more vertical than normal. The neck-shaft angle in an infant is expected to be approximately 150° but in infantile coxa vara the angle is 120° or less. This is in contradistinction to the varus seen in congenital short femur where the deformity is more distal. If the femur is positioned appropriately a triangular fragment of bone is noted on the inferior aspect of the neck adjacent to the growth plate (Fairbank triangle).

Differential Diagnosis

The condition must be distinguished from coxa vara arising secondary to other causes, including Morquio osteochondrodystrophy, cleidocranial dysostosis, metaphyseal dysostosis, multiple epiphyseal dysplasia, achondroplasia and epiphyseal injury or fracture due to trauma or infection.

Management

The Hilgenreiner epiphyseal angle is useful when deciding on treatment. This is defined as the angle between the Hilgenreiner line (a horizontal line through both triradiate cartilages) and a line drawn along the capital femoral growth plate (*Figure 4.9a*). Normal values are about 25°. Where the angle is less than 45° resolution can be expected. When the angle is above 60° progression is to be expected and

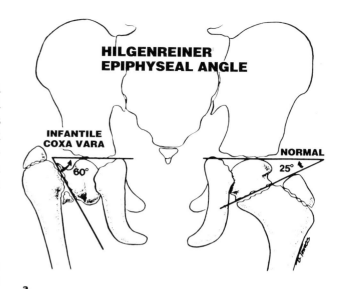

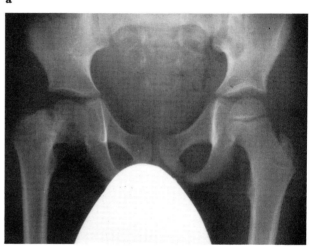

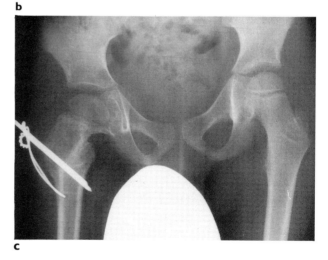

Figure 4.9 **a** The use of Hilgenreiner epiphyseal angle in the management of infantile coxa vara. **b** A case of infantile coxa vara in an otherwise normal child. **c** This has been treated by a Pauwels' osteotomy. (**a** reproduced with permission from Bennett GC. *Congenital Abnormalities of the Femur in Paediatric Hip Disorders.* Blackwell Science, Oxford, 1987.)

surgical correction should be undertaken. If the angle is between 45° and 60° the condition should be observed.

Surgery

Treatment is by upper femoral osteotomy to realign the neck into a valgus orientation of at least 140° to encourage healing. The Pauwels technique is popular for this (Cordes *et al.*, 1991) (*Figure 4.9c*). In the neglected case trochanteric transfer may be necessary. Any discrepancy in limb length is likely to be minor or within the realms of epiphyseodesis.

REFERENCES AND FURTHER READING

Achterman C, Kalamchi A. Congenital deficiency of the fibula. *J Bone Joint Surg* 1979; **61B**: 133–137.

Amstutz HC, Wilson PDJ. Dysgenesis of the proximal femur (coxa vara) and its surgical management. *J Bone Joint Surg* 1962; **44A**: 1–23.

Boyd HB. Amputation of the foot with calcaneotibial arthrodesis. *J Bone Joint Surg* 1939; **21**: 997–1000.

Boyd HB. Pathology and natural history of congenital pseudarthrosis of the tibia. *Clin Orthop Rel Research* 1982; **166**: 5.

Brown FW. Construction of a knee joint in congenital absence of the tibia (paraxial hemimelia tibia). A preliminary report. *J Bone Joint Surg* 1965; **47A**: 695–704.

Cordes S, Dickens DRV, Cole WG. Correction of coxa vara in childhood. The use of Pauwels' Y-shaped osteotomy. *J Bone Joint Surg* 1991; **73B**: 3–6.

Coventry MB, Johnson EWJ. Congenital absence of the fibula. *J Bone Joint Surg* 1952; **34A**: 941–945.

Eilert RE, Jayakumar SS. Boyd and Syme amputations in children. *J Bone Joint Surg* 1976; **58A**: 1138–1141.

Friskia DA, Moseley CF, Oppenheim WI. Rotational osteotomy for proximal femoral focal deficiency. *J Bone Joint Surg* 1989; **71A**: 1386–1392.

Gillespie R, Torode IP. Classification and management of congenital abnormalities of the femur. *J Bone Joint Surg* 1983; **65B**: 557–568.

Jones D, Barnes J, Lloyd–Roberts GC. Congenital aplasia and dysplasia of the tibia with intact fibula. Classification and management. *J Bone Joint Surg* 1978; **60B**: 31–39.

Kalamchi A, Dawe RV. Congenital deficiency of the tibia. *J Bone Joint Surg* 1985; **67B**: 581–584.

Millis MB, Hall JE. Transiliac lengthening of the lower extremity. *J Bone Joint Surg* 1979; **61A**: 1182–1194.

Panting AL, Williams PF. Proximal femoral focal deficiency. *J Bone Joint Surg* 1978; **60B**: 46–52.

Pappas AM. Congenital posteromedial bowing of the tibia and fibula. *J Pediatr Orthop* 1984; **4**: 525–531.

Paterson DC, Simonis RB. Electrical stimulation in the treatment of congenital pseudarthrosis of the tibia. *J Bone Joint Surg* 1985; **67B**: 454–462.

Pauwels F. *Biomechanics of the Normal and Diseased Hip*. Springer, New York, 1976.

Pho RWH, Levack B, Satku K, Patradul A. Free vascularised fibular graft in the treatment of congenital pseudarthrosis of the tibia. *J Bone Joint Surg* 1985; **67B**: 64–70.

Syme J. Surgical cases and observations. *Lond Edin Monthly J Med Sci* 1843; **26**: 93–96.

Thomas IH, Williams PF. The Gruca operation for congenital absence of the fibula. *J Bone Joint Surg* 1987; **69B**: 587–592.

Torode IP, Gillespie R. Rotationplasty of the lower limb for congenital defects of the femur. *J Bone Joint Surg* 1983; **65B**: 569–573.

Weinstein JN, Kuo KN, Millar EA. Congenital coxa vara. A retrospective review. *J Pediatr Orthop* 1984; **4**: 70–77.

Chapter 5
Skeletal Dysplasias

Virginia J Saxton and Mark D O'Sullivan

The skeletal dysplasias are a group of generalized disorders of bone and cartilage causing abnormalities of the skull, spine or limbs. They are a heterogeneous group and are mainly inherited. Most dysplasias tend to be rare, but because there are so many dysplasias, as a group they are reasonably common. They are characterized by clinical, genetic, biochemical and radiographic criteria. Classification is difficult because in the past the conditions were named without an overall view of skeletal dysplasias. They were named by the clinician who first described them (e.g. Ollier disease, Maffucci syndrome) or by descriptive terms (e.g. osteopoikilosis) or by the area of involved bone (e.g. multiple epiphyseal dysplasia). The classification used in this chapter is largely dependent on the area of the bone primarily involved (e.g. epiphyseal, metaphyseal, diaphyseal), but there is a large miscellaneous section at the end (*Table 5.1*).

Diagnosis

History
Most of the dysplasias are associated with a positive family history. However, some arise from new genetic mutations so the individual may be the first case in the family.

Examination
Complete examination is vital. Head size, facial features (e.g. frontal bossing, nasal bridge), the presence or absence of body parts, range of motion of all joints and spine, and any hand or foot abnormalities must be documented. The ratio of the length of segments of the limbs is also important. Blue sclerae may indicate osteogenesis imperfecta. Joint laxity is a feature of many diseases including Marfan syndrome, Ehlers–Danlos syndrome and Morquio syndrome.

Stature
A height of less than 1.25 m is considered to be short stature. These can be divided into:

- Proportional short stature in which the trunk and limbs are equally affected. Possible diagnoses include hypophosphatasia, hypophosphataemia and the severe forms of osteogenesis imperfecta and osteopetrosis.
- Short-limbed short stature with a normal or near-normal spine. Possible diagnoses include achondroplasia, hypochondroplasia, diastrophic dysplasia and chondroectodermal dysplasia.
- Short-limbed short stature with spinal involvement as occurs in spondyloepiphyseal dysplasia, metatropic dysplasia, and Morquio syndrome.

Radiology

Anatomic site
Radiographs demonstrate the site of the disorder (e.g. epiphyseal, metaphyseal) and spine or skull involvement. They also help determine which segment of the bone is short for example whether it is:

- Rhizomelic (proximal segment shortening).
- Mesomelic (middle segment shortening).
- Acromelic (distal segment shortening).

Bone density
Osteoporosis is a feature of some conditions such as osteogenesis imperfecta. Increased density is seen in osteopetrosis and Engelmann disease.

Computer Software

Computer software developed at the Royal Children's Hospital in Melbourne, called Possum and Ossum, allows a rapid identification of most genetic conditions.

Table 5.1 Classification of skeletal dysplasias

Disorders of the growth plate
Achondroplasia
Hypochondroplasia
Pseudoachondroplasia
Other short limb disorders
   Metatropic dysplasia
   Asphyxiating thoracic dysplasia (Jeune syndrome)
   Diastrophic dysplasia
   Chondroectodermal dysplasia (Ellis–Van Creveld
     syndrome)
	Storage disorders
	Mucopolysaccharidoses (Hunter, Hurler and
	   Morquio syndromes)
	Gaucher syndrome
	
	Connective tissue dysplasias
	Marfan syndrome
	Larsen syndrome
	Ehlers-Danlos syndrome

Disorders of the epiphyses Multiple epiphyseal dysplasia Spondyloepiphyseal dysplasia Punctate epiphyseal dysplasia Hemimelica epiphyseal dysplasia (Trevor disease)	**Miscellaneous** Cleidocranial dysplasia Nail–patella syndrome Neurofibromatosis Fibrodysplasia ossificans progressiva Klippel-Feil syndrome Dyschondrosteosis
Disorders of the metaphyses Metaphyseal chondrodysplasia Spondylometaphyseal dysplasia Metaphyseal dysplasia (Pyle disease)	Hereditary multiple exostoses Enchondromatosis (Ollier disease) Maffucci syndrome Osteopoikilosis Osteopathia striata (striated bone) Melorheostosis
Disorders of the diaphyses *With decreased bone density* Osteogenesis imperfecta *With increased bone density* Osteopetrosis Pyknodysostosis Diaphyseal dysplasia (Engelmann disease) Pachydermoperiostitis (familial hypertrophic osteoarthropathy)	Fibrous dysplasia **Chromosomal abnormalities** Trisomy 21 (Down syndrome) Turner syndrome Edward syndrome

DISORDERS OF THE GROWTH PLATE

Achondroplasia

This is the most common form of short-limbed stature (*Figure 5.1*). About 80% of cases are caused by a genetic mutation; the rest result from autosomal dominant inheritance. The primary problem is defective endochondral ossification and these children present at birth with short limbs, but the trunk is normal in length. They have a characteristic facial appearance with a bulging forehead and low nasal bridge. Approximately 50% have a non-rigid thoracolumbar kyphosis in infancy. Progression to a rapid structural kyphosis is prevented by delayed upright posturing. All develop a lumbar lordosis later.

The extremities show a rhizomelic pattern with the proximal segments more severely involved than the middle or distal segments ('rhizo-' refers to the root of the limb). The limbs are therefore short and the hands do not reach the buttocks. A trident hand is common (50%) and is characterized by a persistent space between the middle and ring fingers. In the lower limbs, genu varum commonly results from the deformity of the proximal tibia. Spinal canal stenosis and increasing spinal deformity can lead to neurological complications. Virtually all patients experience symptomatic sleep apnoea and about 50% need treatment.

Radiology

The bones are short in length, but normal in girth so they look 'stubby.' The central growth plate is more

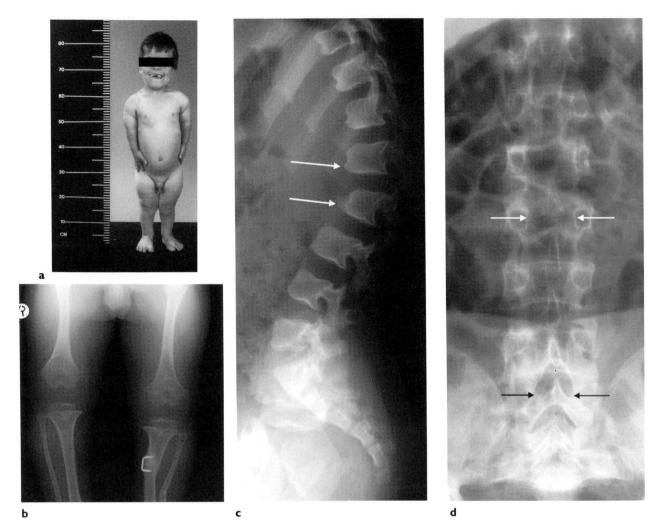

Figure 5.1 **a** This young boy with achondroplasia has frontal bossing, a flattened nasal bridge, rhizomelic shortening of his upper and lower limbs, and short stumpy hands and feet, but normal trunk height. **b** Lower limbs of a six-year-old with achondroplasia. The physes around the knee have a ball and socket or notched appearance because the central part of the growth plate is affected more than the periphery. A left tibial osteotomy has been performed to manage the severe tibial varus deformity. **c** Lateral spine of a two-year-old boy with achondroplasia. He has a marked thoracolumbar kyphosis with vertebral body flattening and disc space widening. Note the antero-inferior beaking of the vertebral bodies at the thoracolumbar junction (arrows). The sagittal diameter of the spinal canal is short and there is posterior scalloping of the vertebral bodies. **d** Anteroposterior radiograph of the spine of a seven-year-old girl with achondroplasia showing narrowing of the interpedicular distance from L1 to L5 (arrows). This causes spinal canal stenosis.

affected than the periphery in some joints such as the knee, giving a ball and socket epiphyseal/metaphyseal junction. Spinal changes are characteristic. The interpedicular distance narrows progressively from L1–L5 or remains the same, whereas it normally increases. On the lateral radiograph the vertebral bodies are flattened in the neonate (bullet-shaped rather than the normal oval shape) and the disc space is widened. There is often an antero-inferior vertebral body beak at T12, L1 and L2 (*Table 5.2*). The sagittal diameter of the spinal canal is decreased due to short pedicles and later there is scalloping of the vertebrae posteriorly. The pelvic radiograph has characteristic changes. The sacrum is set low on the ilia and it angles sharply backwards. The iliac bones are square with horizontal acetabular roofs. The sciatic notch is narrow and the femoral neck is shortened. The skull is large with a small face and a small foramen magnum. There may be associated hydrocephalus.

Table 5.2   Causes of anterior vertebral body beak

Lower third
Achondroplasia
Hurler syndrome
Down syndrome
Hypothyroidism
Neuromuscular disorders

Central
Morquio syndrome
Pseudoachondroplasia
Spondylometaphyseal dysplasia of Kozlowski

Hypochondroplasia

The inheritance of hypochondroplasia is autosomal dominant. It is a less severe condition than achondroplasia being characterized by a mild short-limbed short stature that involves all segments of the limbs rather than the rhizomelic pattern of achondroplasia (*Figure 5.2*). The skull is normal and there is mild limb shortening. The spine shows some shortening of the pedicles with mild caudal narrowing of the lumbar interpedicular distance. The fibula may be relatively long. Apart from lumbar spinal canal stenosis, the skeletal abnormalities rarely require treatment.

Pseudoachondroplasia

Pseudoachondroplasia is one of the less common skeletal dysplasias and is sometimes known as pseudoachondroplastic type of spondyloepiphyseal dysplasia (*Figure 5.3*). Most cases are sporadic. It is similar to achondroplasia, but with a normal head and a short trunk, so the sitting height is short. The major difference is the marked epiphyseal and metaphyseal involvement. The long bones are very short with flared metaphyses. The epiphyses are delayed, small, irregular and fragmented. The vertebral bodies range from normal, to biconvex with a central anterior tongue, to platyspondyly.

Other Short Limb Disorders

Metatropic Dysplasia

This condition is characterized by a changing pattern of body proportions. Initially the long bones are

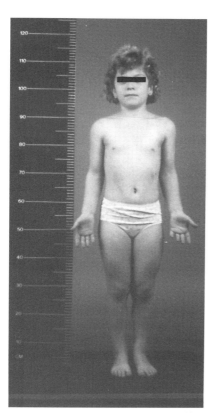

Figure 5.2   Hypochondroplasia in a young girl who has a mild short stature with shortening of her entire limbs. Her facial appearance is normal.

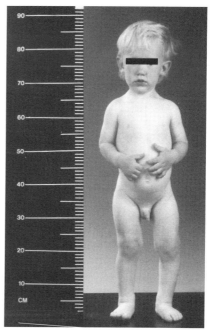

Figure 5.3   Pseudoachondroplasia is characterized by a short stature with short limbs, normal intelligence and a normal facial appearance.

Table 5.3   Platyspondyly in childhood

Congenital platyspondyly
Metatropic dysplasia
Osteogenesis imperfecta (type 2)

Platyspondyly in later childhood
Morquio syndrome
Spondyloepiphyseal dysplasia congenita
Spondyloepiphyseal dysplasia tarda

Acquired platyspondyly
Osteoporosis
Trauma
Neoplastic disease (e.g. leukaemia)
Histiocytosis X
Scheuermann disease
Infection
Sickle cell anaemia (central endplate depression)

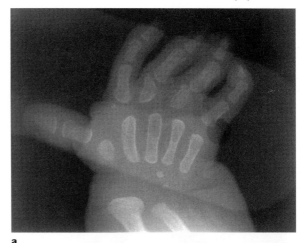
a

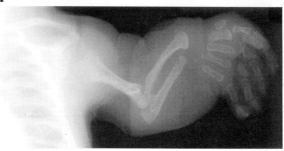
b

Figure 5.4   a The hand of a 10-week-old baby with diastrophic dysplasia. The proximal location of the thumb (hitch-hiker thumb) is one of the classical features.   **b** Upper limb of the same baby showing marked shortening of the long bones with severe joint contractures.

grossly short with marked metaphyseal flaring and straight diaphyses. The trunk is normal length at birth, but in the first 1–2 years rapidly progressive kyphosis develops, which if untreated leads to apparent shortening of the trunk (hence the name). There is marked platyspondyly in infancy (*Table 5.3*).

Asphyxiating Thoracic Dysplasia (Jeune Syndrome)

The inheritance of this condition is autosomal recessive. Severe cases die and mild cases may never be detected. The thorax is long and bell-shaped with short horizontal ribs. The limbs are short and postaxial polydactyly is found in some patients. Renal failure may occur later in childhood.

Diastrophic Dysplasia

This short limbed disorder is characterized by multiple joint contractures, equinus or equinovarus foot deformities, and progressive severe kyphoscoliosis (*Figure 5.4*). Transmission is autosomal recessive. The thumbs are proximally located (hitch-hiker deformity) and there is often swelling of the ear at birth due to a haematoma, which is easily treated by aspiration. There is a high incidence of cleft palate and hearing impairment. Scoliosis and joint contractures are the main problems in older children.

Chondroectodermal Dysplasia (Ellis-van Creveld Syndrome)

The inheritance of this condition is autosomal recessive. The limbs are short and there is polydactyly of the fingers and occasionally the toes. The nails, hair and teeth are dysplastic, and congenital heart disease is common.

DISORDERS OF THE EPIPHYSES

Disorders of the epiphyses form a large group of conditions. Multiple epiphyseal dysplasia (MED) primarily affects long bone epiphyses. Spondyloepiphyseal dysplasia (SED) is associated with changes in both the long bone epiphyses and the spine. The diseases have their maximal effect at different sites, but are similar in other regards and show some overlap.

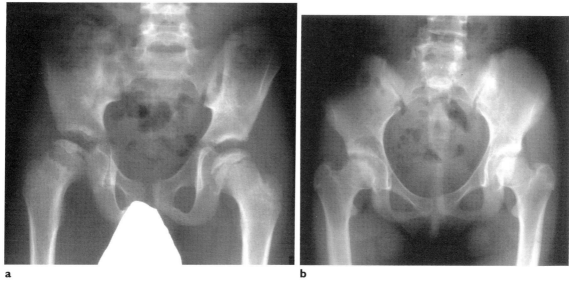

a   b

Figure 5.5 **a** Pelvis of a seven-year-old boy with multiple epiphyseal dysplasia. The upper femoral epiphyses are fragmented and irregular. The differential diagnosis would be bilateral Perthes disease, but other joints were involved. **b** Pelvis of a 14-year-old with multiple epiphyseal dysplasia. Ossification is now complete and the femoral heads are aspherical and uncovered, particularly on the left. Premature osteoarthritis is common. The knees and shoulders are commonly involved.

Multiple Epiphyseal Dysplasia

Multiple epiphyseal dysplasia is one of the commonest skeletal dysplasias and shows an autosomal dominant inheritance. Disordered epiphyseal growth affects most of the long bones symmetrically, ultimately leading to premature osteoarthritis (*Figure 5.5*). There is a wide range of severity and the diagnosis is radiological.

Clinical Features

The most common clinical presentation is with joint pain, stiffness or a limp. The hips, knees and ankles are the most commonly involved joints, but the disease may be restricted to the hips. Angular deformities, including coxa vara, genu valgum and genu varum may be present. Symptoms may develop in late childhood, adolescence or early adult life, and progress due to the development of secondary osteoarthritis. Individuals with the condition are usually slightly shorter than normal; the face and spine are normal. There are many different MED syndromes. Some are associated with specific features such as corneal dystrophy, deafness, club-feet and diabetes mellitus.

Radiology

The epiphyseal ossification centres appear late and are often fragmented and irregular. Ossification tends to be incomplete, leaving an excess of articular cartilage and therefore a widening of the radiographic joint space. The upper femoral epiphyses are nearly always involved and show some flattening of the femoral head, occasionally with poor coverage. Joint involvement is symmetrical and has the same pattern within families. There is a general delay in bone maturation. The spine is not involved apart from some end-plate irregularity in the lower dorsal spine.

Spondyloepiphyseal Dysplasia

The changes of SED arise from reduced physeal activity at the vertebral body growth plates producing platyspondyly. There may be a central tongue in the vertebral bodies (as in Morquio syndrome) due to delayed ossification of the ring apophyses. There are many subgroups of SED. The most common include:

- SED congenita with coxa vara, which is characterized by a short stature and a short trunk. Inheritance is usually autosomal dominant. Radiographs show platyspondyly and end-plate irregularity with coxa vara (*Figure 5.6*). Progressive kyphoscoliosis may occur. There is a high frequency of C1/C2 dislocation. Repeated screening is necessary because sudden death or postoperative quadriplegia has been reported. Fusion

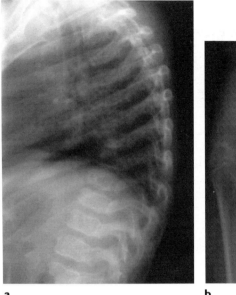
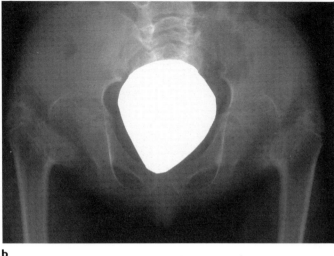

a   b

Figure 5.6 a Thoracolumbar spine of a three-year-old girl with a spondyloepiphyseal dysplasia congenita. Mild platyspondyly is evident throughout the spine. **b** Pelvis at 12 years of age in a child with spondyloepiphyseal dysplasia congenita. Severe changes are evident within the hips with gross coxa vara. The high location of the greater trochanters is typical.

should be carried out in patients with a pathological degree of C1/C2 mobility.

- SED tarda with coxa vara. The epiphyses and metaphyses range from normal to severely fragmented and delayed in appearance. The metaphyses are disordered and irregular. Coxa vara is mild.

Punctate Epiphyseal Dysplasia

Punctate epiphyseal dysplasia is a rare disorder and ranges from a severe form (autosomal recessive, death in infancy) to a moderately severe disorder with asymmetrical limb shortening (Conradi–Hünermann syndrome, X-linked dominant). The mildest form of the disorder (Sheffield type) is also inherited as an X-linked dominant condition and is associated with a high frequency of cervical vertebral dysplasias. The asymmetrical limb shortening presents after infancy with limb inequality or scoliosis. The diagnostic features are punctate stippling of the epiphyses (which are dysplastic) and extracartilaginous calcification (frequently around the vertebral bodies or pelvis) (*Figure 5.7*). The stippling usually disappears by four years of age, but epiphyseal abnormalities persist. Vertebral anomalies with scoliosis are commonly seen in the Conradi–Hünermann form. The skull is normal.

Hemimelica Epiphyseal Dysplasia (Trevor Disease)

This is a very rare disorder affecting either the medial or lateral half of the epiphysis in one limb (*Figure 5.8*). The affected half is either overgrown or has an additional ossification centre and presents clinically as an exostosis. Usually the lower limb (commonly the distal femur, distal tibia and tarsus) is involved, with deformity of the affected joint, restricted movement, and occasionally pain and locking. Limb length inequality may develop.

DISORDERS OF THE METAPHYSES

Metaphyseal Chondrodysplasia

This term covers a group of generalized metaphyseal disorders characterized by mild limb shortening with disordered metaphyseal ossification and variations in tubulation (*Figure 5.9*). The groups are distinguished by other associated changes:

- Schmid type is the most common form and has autosomal dominant inheritance. The limbs are short (especially the lower limbs). There is coxa vara with irregular, flared femoral metaphyses.

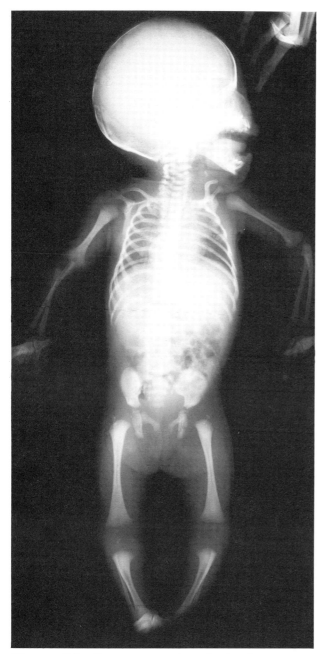

Figure 5.7 Punctate epiphyseal dysplasia in a newborn.

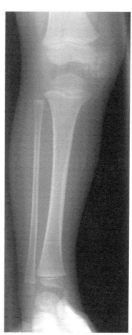

Figure 5.8 Hemimelica epiphyseal dysplasia. There are osteocartilaginous outgrowths from the medial femoral epiphysis and the distal tibial epiphysis. The medial involvement and multiple sites are typical.

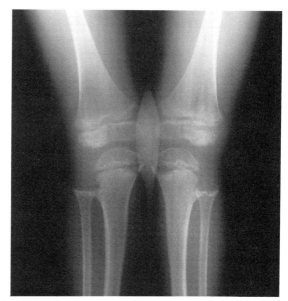

Figure 5.9 Lower limbs of a four-year-old with metaphyseal chondrodysplasia (Schmid type). The metaphyses are flared and irregular with widened growth plates. This is particularly severe in the metaphyses of the upper fibulas.

The limb metaphyses are irregular and expanded, and occasionally cupped, simulating rickets.

- McKusick type shows autosomal recessive inheritance. The children are of short stature and have short limbs, fine sparse hair and lax joints. The skull is normal, but the limb bones are short with an irregular shape and mineralization of the metaphyses, especially the knee.
- Jansen type is the rarest and most severe type. Inheritance is autosomal dominant. It is characterized by short stature and expanded metaphyses, which are markedly irregular in both shape and mineralization, mimicking rickets. The serum biochemistry is helpful in differentiating this from rickets, particularly as the serum calcium is raised in this group of children.

Other types are described in association with malabsorption and neutropenia.

Spondylometaphyseal Dysplasia

This is an heterogeneous group of disorders in which both the spine and metaphyses are involved, with the spine usually showing marked platyspondyly. Bone age (i.e. epiphyseal development) is normal for the chronological age.

The best known type is the Kozlowski type, which shows autosomal dominant inheritance. There is generalized platyspondyly and abnormal upper femoral metaphyses in particular. Coxa vara is common.

Metaphyseal Dysplasia (Pyle Disease)

This sclerosing bone dysplasia affects the metaphyses and skull and has autosomal recessive inheritance. It is usually found incidentally on radiography. There is poor modelling of all the long bones (including the hands) associated with expanded metaphyses and a cylindrical shape to the shafts of the bone (Erlenmeyer flask deformity). This may cause genu varum.

DISORDERS OF THE DIAPHYSES

These disorders commonly present as a result of complications arising from decreased or increased density of the long bones and spine. There are frequently abnormalities in submetaphyseal modelling associated with over- or under-tubulation of long and short tubular bones.

Disorders with Decreased Bone Density: Osteogenesis Imperfecta

Osteogenesis imperfecta (OI) is a connective tissue disorder that affects bone, teeth and soft tissues (*Figures 5.10* and *5.11*). The clinical features are variable depending on the type, but they all include a degree of osteopenia and increased bone fragility. The common biochemical defect is in the synthesis of type 1 collagen. This disorder has in the past been divided into two groups: congenita and tarda. However, four distinct groups are now recognized, according to clinical and genetic factors (Sillence *et al.*, 1979) (*Table 5.4*).

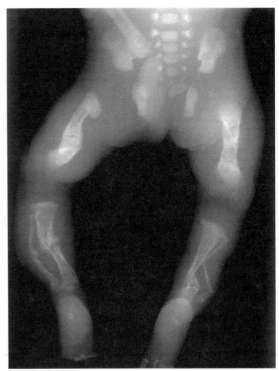

Figure 5.10 Pelvis and lower limbs of a newborn with type 2 osteogenesis. There are multiple fractures in the lower limbs. The bones are markedly short and deformed. Type 2 OI is usually fatal.

Clinical Features

The colour of the sclerae varies as shown in Table 5.4. The skin is thin and bruises easily. The head is large with a triangular face and approximately 30% of cases have abnormal teeth. Conductive deafness, and rarely sensorineural deafness, are found in up to 20%. Peripheral joints are lax and patients are short due to fractures, bowing, growth plate dysfunction from repeated trauma and a primary defect in growth.

Children with type 2 OI are born with crumpled long bones and multiple rib fractures, and the condition is lethal. This group was previously referred to as the congenita group. Children with other forms of OI may be expected to survive.

In general prenatal humeral fractures are accompanied by shortening and angular deformity of the limb bones and are a bad prognostic sign. In the later-onset forms, fractures vary in their frequency and age of occurrence. The lower limbs are more commonly involved. The fractures may heal well, but some heal with abundant callus formation and others lead to pseudoarthrosis. Joint abnormalities are common due to fracture, deformity and joint laxity. Genu valgum and coxa vara are common and

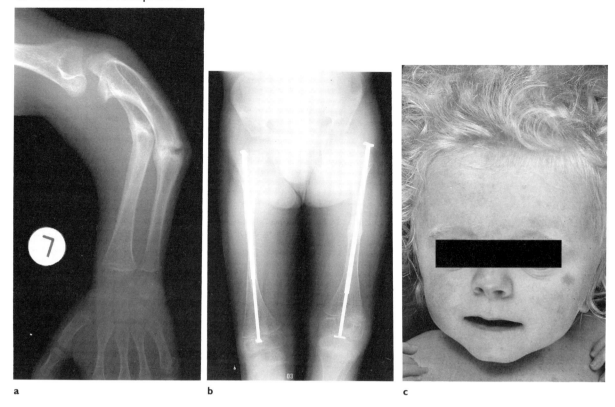

a   b   c

Figure 5.11 a Upper limbs of a child with type 4 osteogenesis imperfecta. Multiple fractures and increasing deformity are typical throughout growth. Both forearm bones have suffered recent fractures and there is marked bowing of the forearm secondary to previous fractures. **b** Lower limbs of a six-year-old with type 4 osteogenesis imperfecta. Multiple fractures and deformity in the long bones can be controlled with intramedullary rodding. **c** Child with type 3 osteogenesis imperfecta showing the classical features of an enlarged cranium and a small triangular face.

Table 5.4 Classification of osteogenesis imperfecta (Sillence *et al.*, 1979)

Type	Inheritance	Clinical features
1	Autosomal dominant	Blue sclerae, presenile deafness, most common group, comprises most of tarda group, fracture incidence and severity vary; approximately 10% have fractures at birth. A, normal teeth; B, dentinogenesis imperfecta
2	Autosomal recessive	Dark blue sclerae, high incidence of perinatal death or still birth, intrauterine fractures are characterized by the appearance of beaded healing fractures and crumpled long bones
3	Mostly sporadic, but also autosomal recessive and dominant	Fractures at birth, progressive deformity, white sclerae, normal hearing, ± dental abnormalities
4	Autosomal dominant	Osteoporosis and fractures, normal sclerae, normal hearing. A, normal teeth; B, dentinogenesis imperfecta

progressive. Acetabular protrusion occurs in 30% of those with severe disease.

Radiology

The radiological findings vary depending on the number and site of prenatal fractures. In OI types 1 and 4 the overall shape and modelling of limb bones is usually normal, although the thigh and leg bones may bow with or without fractures. Osteopenia is common and the bone cortices are thin. In OI type 3 there are characteristically wide metaphyses and overtubulation of the shafts of the long bones with decreased density and impaired ossification of the cranial vault. In the most severe cases of OI type 3 (and sometimes 1B and 4B) cystic (so-called 'popcorn') changes develop in the metaphyses and progress from the second year of life. Multiple wormian bones may be visualized radiographically after 12 months of age (*Table 5.5*). Skull ossification is markedly decreased with multiple wormian bones. In all types of OI spinal osteoporosis leads to severe biconcave compression of the vertebral bodies. Platyspondyly is not usually present at birth in non-lethal cases, but develops rapidly, depending on the severity of the osteopenia. Progressive scoliosis often begins in infancy. A basilar impression with upward deformation of the base of the skull characteristically occurs in OI type 4B, but may be found in other types of OI. It may lead to hydrocephalus or brain stem compression (resulting in quadriplegia or sudden death).

Diagnosis

This is not difficult in patients with multiple fractures, blue sclerae, abnormal dentition and a positive family history. However, it can be difficult in those patients with normal sclerae, no positive family history and a history of increased fractures. The diagnosis of OI has both legal and social implications if child abuse is suspected. The presence of wormian bones is helpful.

Management

Infants with OI must be handled gently to prevent fractures. When fractures do occur they tend to unite rapidly and usually require splintage until healed. It is very important to try to prevent worsening osteoporosis, which will occur with disuse following recurrent fractures. Intramedullary nailing has become vital in the management of osteogenesis imperfecta to prevent recurrent fractures and correct deformity. Multiple osteotomies are performed to straighten the deformity, and recently telescoping rods have been developed, which increase in size as the child grows. Scoliosis may be difficult to treat as bracing is ineffective, and severe deformity can develop easily.

Disorders with Increased Bone Density

This group is characterized by abnormal bone modelling, and in some cases, an increase in bone density. All show changes that can be related to varying degrees of osteoclastic failure in endochondral bone growth.

Osteopetrosis

Osteopetrosis consists of generalized osteosclerosis, bone fragility and failure of modelling (*Figure 5.12*). The severe congenital form has autosomal recessive inheritance and presents in infancy with failure to thrive, multiple fractures, anaemia, thrombocytopenia, delayed dentition, hepatosplenomegaly and lymphadenopathy. Death occurs before 20 years of age from overwhelming infection or haemorrhage. The form with a later onset has autosomal dominant inheritance and may be found incidentally or present as a result of a pathological fracture.

Radiology

The long bones are osteosclerotic with no distinction between cortical and cancellous bone. The metaphyses are expanded (conical) in shape. The small bones of the hands and feet, the ilia and the vertebral bodies show alternate bands of dense and normal bone due to fluctuations in disease activity. The ribs and clavicles are thick, undermodelled and sclerotic. The skull base is thickened and the cranial foramina

Table 5.5 Causes of wormian bones

Osteogenesis imperfecta
Hypothyroidism
Cleidocranial dysostosis
Pyknodysostosis
Hypophosphatasia
Down syndrome

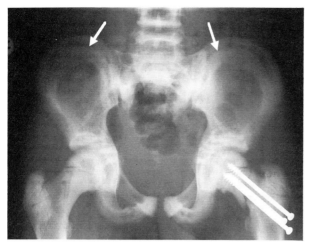

Figure 5.12 Pelvis of a 14-year-old boy with osteopetrosis. A pathological fracture in the left neck of femur has been fixed with cancellous screws. There is marked osteosclerosis and the ilia (arrows) show alternate bands of dense and normal bone due to fluctuations in disease activity.

may occlude, leading to deafness and blindness. In severe cases encroachment on the bone marrow gives rise to anaemia.

Pyknodysostosis

Pyknodysostosis is a rare condition characterized by a short-limbed, short stature. It is characterized by persistent open fontanelles, osteosclerosis with fragile bones and modelling defects, dysplastic facial bones and mandible, and hypoplastic clavicles and terminal phalanges. Inheritance is autosomal recessive. The diagnosis is usually made after a pathological fracture or because of short stature in infancy. Mild cases may be discovered incidentally. The skull shows wormian bones as well as open fontanelles and widened suture lines.

Diaphyseal Dysplasia (Engelmann Disease)

This is a rare congenital dystrophy of bone resulting in bilateral symmetrical diaphyseal sclerosis of the long bones. It affects endosteal and periosteal new bone. There is sclerosis of the skull base. The metaphyses and epiphyses are normal. Inheritance is autosomal dominant with variable penetrance. Patients present with limb pain, weakness, hypotonia or a waddling gait.

Pachydermoperiostosis (Familial Hypertrophic Osteoarthropathy)

The adult form presents in adolescence with a slowly progressive sclerosis of the long bones in addition to seborrhoeic skin hyperplasia and clubbing of the fingers and toes. Periosteal new bone affecting the tubular bones in the distal legs, forearms and extremities as well as clubbing of the fingers and toes are features of the infant form. Inheritance is autosomal dominant.

STORAGE DISORDERS

Mucopolysaccharidoses

These are a group of genetically-determined storage diseases in which mucopolysaccharides (glycosaminoglycans) are stored in tissue abnormally and excreted in the urine. The mucopolysaccharides (MPSs) principally involved are heparan sulphate, dermatan sulphate and keratan sulphate. They result from a deficiency of specific lysosomal enzymes involved in the degradation of MPSs. The incomplete degradation of MPSs results in their accumulation in tissues such as the growth plate cartilages, tendons, ligaments, brain, viscera, eyes, heart and lungs. The process is progressive. Six main groups comprising ten distinct enzymatic defects are recognized (*Table 5.6*). All have autosomal recessive inheritance apart from the Hunter syndrome which is X-linked. All groups show similar skeletal abnormalities (called dysostosis multiplex) although some are much more severely affected than others.

Clinical Features

These include coarse facies with frontal bossing and a protruding tongue (*Figure 5.13*), stiff joints (except MPS IV), hernias, hepatosplenomegaly, corneal opacities, short stature and mental retardation (except MPS IV and VI). Thoracolumbar kyphosis is common.

Radiology

The vertebral bodies are oval with ossification defects, especially of the superior ring apophysis. This is most marked at L1 or L2 giving a 'hooked' appearance. There is also a thoracolumbar kyphosis at this level due to posterior slip of the vertebra above (*Figure 5.13*). The skull is enlarged with a thick calvarium and J-shaped sella. Hydrocephalus

Table 5.6 The six groups of mucopolysaccharidoses

Group	Inheritance
Hurler syndrome (MPS1H), Scheie (MPS IS)	Autosomal recessive
Hunter syndrome (MPS II)	X-linked
Sanfilippo syndrome (four types; MPS IIIA, IIIB, IIIC, IIID)	Autosomal recessive
Morquio syndrome (two types; MPS IVA and IVB)	Autosomal recessive
Maroteaux-Lamy syndrome (MPS V)	Autosomal recessive
Sly syndrome (MPS VI)	Autosomal recessive

may develop due to obstruction and thickened meninges. The ribs are narrowed posteriorly and widened anteriorly ('paddle-shaped'). The inferior ilium is hypoplastic and the acetabula are steeply angled. There is coxa valga with dysplasia of the capital epiphyses. In the long bones the bony trabeculae and modelling are coarse, often resulting in shafts that are wider than the metaphyses. The phalanges are short and stubby, and the metacarpals are pointed proximally. Bone maturation is delayed,

and when the epiphyses do appear they are small and irregular.

Bone changes are less marked in the Hunter syndrome, and in the other groups they are mild (other than in Morquio syndrome).

Diagnosis

The syndromes are diagnosed by clinical findings and laboratory investigations. Urine analysis will demon-

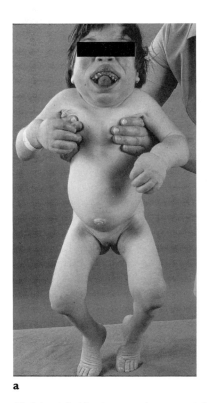
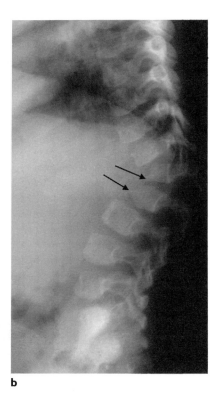

Figure 5.13 **a** Child with Hurler syndrome with coarse facial features, a protruding tongue, short stature, distended abdomen and umbilical hernia. **b** Lateral spine of a four-year-old with Hurler syndrome. Note the marked kyphosis at the thoracolumbar junction due to hypoplasia of L1 and L2. Hurler syndrome is another cause for an antero-inferior beak in the vertebral bodies at this level (arrows).

strate the affected glycosaminoglycan. Specific enzyme assays can be carried out on blood, skin fibroblast culture, amniotic fluid culture and chorionic villi.

Treatment

There is no specific therapy for MPS syndromes. Bone marrow transplantation has been used to correct organomegaly and airway obstruction, but it does not prevent progression in skeletal abnormalities (i.e. transplanted MPS I patients have all the problems of MPS IV and MPS VI patients).

Morquio Syndrome

Children with Morquio syndrome can be differentiated both clinically and radiologically (*Figure 5.14*). They have increased joint laxity, which may give rise to genu valgum and contributes to C1/C2 hypermobility. All patients with MPS IVA require elective fusion of their cervical spine. Their IQ is normal, they have a short neck and a protuberant sternum.

Radiology

The skull is normal, but the odontoid peg is dysplastic or absent, resulting in atlantoaxial instability. A thoracolumbar kyphosis and hook vertebra are present. There is platyspondyly with a central anterior tongue. Epiphyseal dysplasia is common, especially in the hips where severe disability from coxa vara can result. Long bone changes are less marked than in Hurler syndrome.

Gaucher Syndrome

This is an uncommon disease in which cells of the reticuloendothelial system accumulate glucocerebroside, which is a complex lipid (*Figure 5.15*). It is transmitted as an autosomal recessive and there is a high incidence among the Ashkenazi Jews.

Clinical Features

Patients tend to present in childhood with skeletal problems. Avascular necrosis of the femoral head is the most common symptomatic lesion. The distal

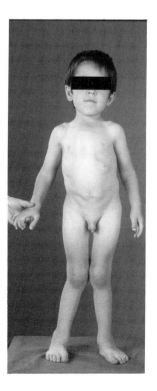 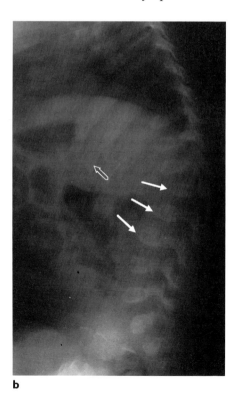

b

Figure 5.14 a This child with Morquio syndrome is short with a normal face and head. There is genu valgum and a protuberant sternum. **b** Lateral spine in Morquio syndrome, showing thoracolumbar kyphosis with hypoplasia of L1. Note the platyspondyly, the central beaking in the vertebral bodies (closed arrows) and the broadened ends of the ribs anteriorly (open arrows).

femur is also often involved with failure of modelling producing fusiform enlargement of the distal metaphyseal area (Erlenmeyer flask deformity). Bone crises similar to those seen in sickle cell anaemia are also common. Gaucher syndrome predisposes to osteomyelitis and it may be difficult to differentiate this from a bone crisis. It may or may not affect the central nervous system and there may be hepatosplenomegaly, lymphadenopathy and weight loss.

Diagnosis

Bone lesions with associated hepatosplenomegaly suggest the diagnosis. This may be confirmed by aspiration biopsy of typical Gaucher's cells from the bone marrow.

Management

Secondary joint problems and pathological fractures are treated conservatively because of the problems of bleeding and secondary infection. Enzyme replacement therapy with purified glucocerebrosidase is a particularly effective but expensive therapy.

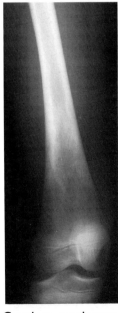

Figure 5.15 Gaucher syndrome. There is some failure of modelling in the distal femur producing a mild fusiform enlargement of the distal metaphyses (Erlenmeyer flask deformity). Note the patchy area of sclerosis in the distal medulla resulting from areas of bone infarction.

CONNECTIVE TISSUE DISORDERS

Marfan Syndrome (Arachnodactyly)

Marfan syndrome has autosomal dominant inheritance. Patients are tall with long slender bones and digits (arachnodactyly) and joint laxity (*Figure 5.16*). They have a generalized abnormality of collagen, so it is a multisystem disorder. Clinical features include arched palates, dislocated lenses, herniae, and cardiac abnormalities (aortic regurgitation, aortic dilatation, aneurysms and mitral valve prolapse). Orthopaedic surgeons may be involved because of the problems associated with the long and narrow hypermobile flat feet and the progressive kyphoscoliosis, which develops in about 50% of the patients (*Figure 5.16*). The arm span is greater than the height. The diagnosis can be made on radiological grounds by the metacarpal index: the ratio of metacarpal length to breadth (at midpoint) is averaged for the four finger digits and a ratio over 8.4 is diagnostic of Marfan syndrome.

Larsen Syndrome

Larsen syndrome is characterized by lax joints together with a depressed nasal bridge, bulging forehead and hypertelorism (*Figure 5.17*). There are often bilateral congenital hip and knee dislocations. Inheritance is both autosomal dominant and recessive. Radial head dislocations are associated with cubitus varus and loss of extension. Talipes equinovarus, cervical vertebral anomalies and hydrocephalus may be present. A double ossification centre in the calcaneus is diagnostic.

Ehlers-Danlos Syndrome

This rare disorder is characterized by excessive elasticity of the skin and friability of the skin and blood vessels due to collagen defects. The skin is loose, scarred and bruised. The joints are hyperextensible, resulting in local soft tissue damage, which tends to calcify on healing. Inheritance may be autosomal dominant, recessive or X-linked. The syndrome has now been divided into ten subgroups. Subluxation and dislocation of the joints are the striking features radiologically. Calcification of the subcutaneous fat occurs in some subtypes.

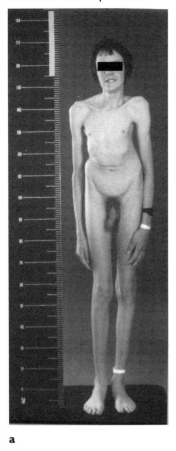
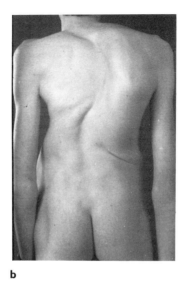
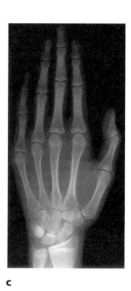

a   b   c

Figure 5.16 **a** This boy with Marfan syndrome is tall with long limbs, arachnodactyly and generalized ligament laxity. **b** Severe scoliosis may also be a feature of Marfan syndrome. **c** The hand of a 15-year-old with Marfan syndrome. Note the long fingers (arachnodactyly). The metacarpal index (see text) is helpful in the diagnosis.

MISCELLANEOUS

Cleidocranial Dysplasia

This disorder principally affects membranous bone and has autosomal dominant inheritance. The clavicles, skull vault, symphysis pubis and terminal phalanges are the main affected sites involved (*Figure 5.18*).

Clinical Features

Patients are short and have a large head with midface hypoplasia. Excessive shoulder mobility occurs because of the absence of part or all of the clavicles. When the clavicles are absent the shoulders may be brought together anteriorly. Scoliosis may also develop. Dental abnormalities include delayed dentition and defective formation.

Radiology

The clavicles are partially or totally absent. The symphysis pubis is wide with hypoplastic pubic rami and sometimes coxa vara. The skull contains wormian bones and the fontanelles close late. The terminal and middle phalanges of the index and little fingers are short.

Nail–Patella Syndrome (Osteo-Onychodysplasia)

This condition is characterized by dysplastic nails, subluxed radial heads, absent patellae and iliac horns (*Figure 5.19*). Inheritance is autosomal dominant. Renal dysplasia can occur.

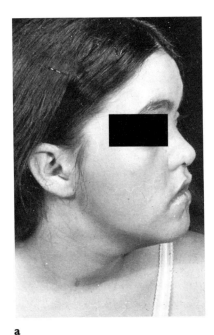 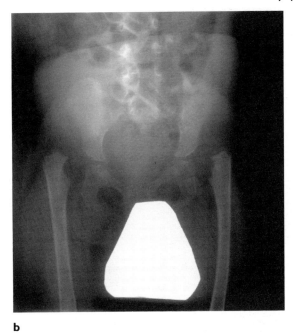

a   b

Figure 5.17 **a** Clinical features of Larsen syndrome. The depressed nasal bridge and bulging forehead are typical. **b** Pelvis in a 15-month-old child with Larsen syndrome. Note the bilateral hip dislocations.

Radiology

Radiologically the patellae are absent or hypoplastic. The capitellum is hypoplastic and the radial head dislocated, producing cubitus valgus. The iliac crests droop due to hypoplasia of the anterior half of the ilia and there are symmetrical exostoses arising from the posterior surface of the ilia (iliac horns). Specific orthopaedic complications include club-feet and scoliosis.

Neurofibromatosis

Neurofibromatosis (NF) is a congenital hamartomatous dysplasia affecting all three germ layers. It is now divided into two forms.

- NF1 (which used to be known as peripheral neurofibromatosis or Von Recklinghausen disease) is the most common with an incidence of about 1 in 4000. It has autosomal dominant inheritance due to a mutant gene on chromosome 17. About 50% are new mutations. It is characterized by café au lait spots and multiple neurofibromas. Axillary and groin freckling, short stature, learning disabilities and seizures are common. Disease expression varies from mild to severe, disfiguring and lethal.

- NF2 (which used to be known as central neurofibromatosis) is much less common with an incidence of 1 in 50,000. It also has autosomal dominant inheritance and is due to a mutant gene on chromosome 22.

Diagnosis

The diagnosis of NF1 is based on the presence of two or more of the following features (*Figure 5.20*):

- Six or more café au lait spots larger than 5 mm in prepubertal children and larger than 15 mm if postpubertal.
- Two neurofibromas of any type or one plexiform neurofibroma.
- Freckling in the axillary or inguinal regions.
- Optic glioma.
- Two or more Lisch nodules (iris hamartomas).
- A distinctive osseous lesion, such as sphenoid dysplasia or thinning of long bone cortex without pseudarthrosis.
- A first degree relative with NF1 identified by the above criteria.

Tumours of the central nervous system develop in NF2. These include acoustic neuroma and brain tumours such as astrocytomas, medulloblastomas and optic gliomas. Tumours can also occur along the spinal nerves and in the spinal canal.

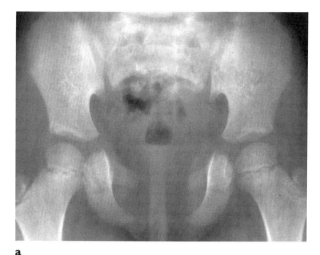

a

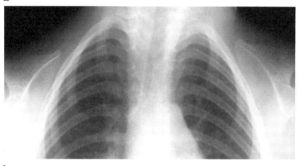

b

Figure 5.18 **a** Pelvis of a five-year-old child with cleidocranial dysplasia. Note the widening of the symphysis pubis and the hypoplastic pubic rami. **b** Chest of a five-year-old child with cleidocranial dysplasia. The clavicles are absent so the shoulders droop.

Radiology

Spine

Approximately 30% of patients have a scoliosis. Most look like an idiopathic curve, but they may have a short, sharply-angled curve with kyphosis and rib dysplasias. Approximately 40% of those with scoliosis have cervical spine anomalies. The vertebral bodies may show anterior, lateral or posterior scalloping. The first two are thought to be due to intrinsic developmental dysplasia, although magnetic resonance imaging (MRI) may show abnormal tissue here. Posterior scalloping is usually due to dural sheath ectasia, but an intradural mass can also be the cause. Nerve root fibromas give rise to pressure widening of the exit foramina as the neoplasm expands (dumb-bell tumour). MRI is the method of choice for imaging the intraspinal and paraspinal areas.

Thorax

The ribs may be thinned and twisted (ribbon ribs) and may be splayed by pressure from intercostal nerve tumours. Smaller tumours cause rib notching.

Extremities

The bones in the limbs may be overgrown. Approximately 10% of patients have a pseudarthrosis. This is most common in the tibia, but can occur in the forearm or even the humerus. The pseudarthrosis may rarely be present at birth or the tibia may be bowed anteriorly and sclerotic and subsequently

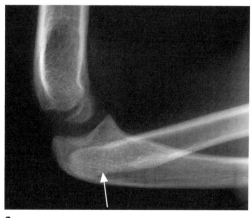

a

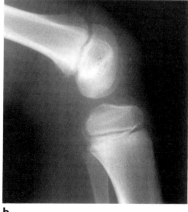

b

Figure 5.19 **a** Lateral elbow in an eight-year-old child with nail–patella syndrome. Note the dislocated and hypoplastic radial head (arrow). **b** Lateral knee in an eight-year-old child with nail–patella syndrome. The patella is absent.

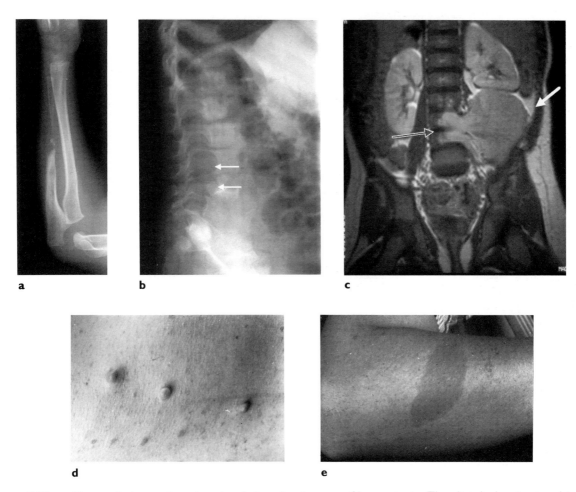

Figure 5.20 **a** Congenital pseudoarthrosis of the ulna in neurofibromatosis. The distal ulna is atrophic with thinning of the proximal end of the distal fragment. Posterior scalloping of the vertebral bodies due to tumour mass in neurofibromatosis. **b** Lateral view of the lumbar spine shows severe posterior scalloping of the vertebral bodies (arrows). **c** Coronal TI-weighted scan with gadolinium showing a large mass on the left (open arrow) displacing the kidney superiorly. There is tumour extending through the intervertebral foramina into the spinal canal (closed arrow). **d** Multiple neurofibromas are common in neurofibromatosis. **e** A large café au lait spot on the forearm of a patient with neurofibromatosis. This is the most common skin mark in this condition.

break (see Chapter 4). Non-union is followed by bone atrophy and smooth tapering of the fractured ends. The dysplasia may also produce cystic lesions in the bones or an angular deformity with irregular cortical sclerosis and lucency.

Soft tissues
Soft tissue changes include overgrowth, renal artery dysplasia, phaeochromocytoma, pulmonary stenosis and pulmonary fibrosis. MRI demonstrates soft tissue plexiform neurofibromas well.

Skull
Macrocephaly may be a feature. Tumours include optic nerve gliomas, astrocytomas, ependymomas, meningiomas and trigeminal or acoustic neuromas.

Bilateral acoustic neuromas are diagnostic of neurofibromatosis and are well seen on MRI. The facial bones and the sphenoid wing may be dysplastic, and if the latter is aplastic can result in pulsating exophthalmos.

Complications

Bone growth may be disordered causing leg length discrepancy. Malignant change occurs in 5% of patients and most neoplasms are neurogenic in origin (e.g. phaeochromocytoma, neurofibrosarcoma). Other malignant tumours include leukaemia, Wilms tumour and urogenital rhabdomyosarcoma.

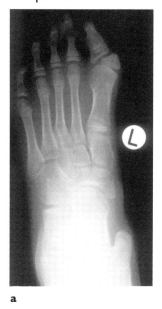
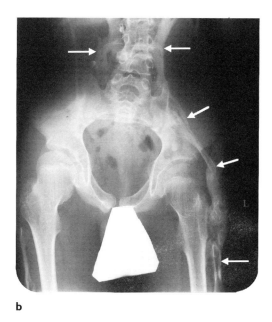

a   b

Figure 5.21 **a** The foot in fibrodysplasia ossificans progressiva. The great toe is short due to hypoplasia or absence of the proximal phalanx. **b** Abdomen in a 12-year-old boy with fibrodysplasia ossificans progressiva. There is widespread ossification in the soft tissues (arrows). The trunk and limbs are a common site for this.

Fibrodysplasia Ossificans Progressiva

This rare condition with an onset in the first decade is characterized by calcification and then ossification of fasciae, aponeuroses and tendons, and secondarily affects muscles (*Figure 5.21*). The first metatarsal is short. The condition was previously known as myositis ossificans progressiva. Inheritance may be autosomal dominant, but is usually sporadic with a male predominance. The cervical vertebrae may be small with thick pedicles and massive spinous processes, which later fuse. The hips show acetabular dysplasia with enlarged femoral heads and necks. The hallux is short due to fusion or absence of phalanges and the short first metatarsal. Calcified masses develop over the trunk, neck and proximal limbs. The process is progressive, and death is usually due to respiratory embarassment in adulthood.

Klippel–Feil Syndrome

Classically Klippel–Feil syndrome involves a clinical triad of a short neck, a low posterior neck line and decreased neck mobility (*Figure 5.22*). However this is only seen in 50% of patients and the term Klippel–Feil syndrome is used to indicate a congenital fusion of two or more cervical vertebrae. The congenital fusion in the cervical spine may involve the vertebral bodies and the posterior elements. If the fusion is partial, non-traumatic spontaneous dislocation may occur. Associated features include Sprengel shoulder, which may be either unilateral or bilateral,

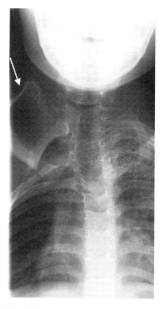

Figure 5.22 Klippel–Feil syndrome, showing multiple fusions in the proximal thoracic spine. Note the absence of some ribs on the right, and the high scapula (Sprengel anomaly) (arrow), which is often associated with Klippel–Feil syndrome.

a congenital scoliosis or kyphosis in the cervical region, deafness and congenital heart disease. There is a high incidence of associated renal anomalies such as unilateral renal agenesis. An ultrasound of the renal tract is advisable in patients with congenital cervical spine anomalies.

Dyschondrosteosis

This is a mesomelic shortening of the extremities with a wide range of severity and autosomal dominant inheritance. There is dysplasia of the distal radial epiphysis giving ulnar and volar tilting of the articular surfaces resulting in a Madelung deformity of the wrist bilaterally. The radius is short and bowed, with dorsal dislocation of the ulna and alteration of the carpal angle (*Table 5.7*). The tibia is short and the fibula may also be short at either end, disrupting the knee or ankle mortice.

Hereditary Multiple Exostoses

This is one of the most common skeletal dysplasias and consists of multiple osteochondromatous exostoses, which may arise at any site of endochondral bone growth. Other names include osteochondromatosis and diaphyseal aclasia. Inheritance is autosomal dominant. Lesions are typically found at the ends of long bones and in secondary apophyseal centres around the pelvis and shoulder girdles (*Figure 5.23*).

Clinical Features

Patients usually present with bony lumps, angular deformities, limb length discrepancies or symptoms due to pressure on adjacent structures. Most patients are slightly short. Exostoses are most commonly seen about the knee, shoulder girdle, wrist, hip and ankle. Upper limb involvement is common, particularly in the forearms (where shortening and angular defor-

Table 5.7 Causes of Madelung type deformity

Post-traumatic
Enchondromatosis
Hereditary multiple exostoses
Turner syndrome
Idiopathic
Dyschondrosteosis

mity are reasonably common) and in the shoulder girdle.

Radiology

As the bone grows, cartilage-capped exostoses migrate up the shaft of the long bone and tend to point towards the diaphysis. Lesions may be pedunculated or sessile. The latter may cause irregular expansion of the metaphysis, sometimes with severe

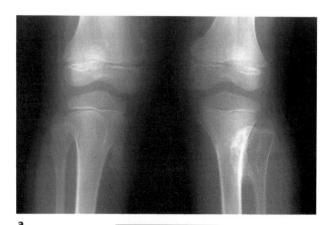

a

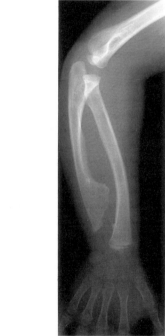

b

Figure 5.23 **a** Tibia and fibula in hereditary multiple exostoses. There are multiple osteochondromas affecting the distal femur and proximal tibia and fibula. **b** Deformity of the forearm is a common sequel in hereditary multiple exostoses. In this patient an osteochondroma of the distal ulna has resulted in a short forearm with bowing of the radius.

damage to the growth plate resulting in bowing, varus or valgus deformity, or inequality of paired bones, especially at the wrist where a Madelung type of deformity is frequent. Seen end on the cortex of the exostosis may produce a circular or oval density over the primary bone. The exostoses stop growing after skeletal maturation and new ones do not occur. They can compress nerves (e.g. lateral popliteal), arteries or tendons, and the exostoses themselves can fracture. Malignant change from sarcomatous degeneration of the cartilage cap occurs in probably around 2% of affected individuals over 20 years and is most likely in the pelvic or pectoral girdle exostoses. It is extremely rare in childhood.

Differential Diagnosis

This includes the trichorhinophalangeal syndrome, which may be associated with multiple exostoses, but the face is unusual, the hair is sparse and there are cone-shaped epiphyses. The forearm deformity of a short ulna and a curved radius is similar to that of enchondromatosis, but in enchondromatosis the disease is asymmetrical with enchondromas and there are no exostoses.

Management

Osteochondromas are generally left alone unless they are causing problems. Symptoms such as pain, interference with function, progressive deformity of the wrists or rapid growth are typical reasons to remove them.

Enchondromatosis (Ollier Disease)

This generalized disorder may occur at any site of enchondral bone formation and has no genetic inheritance. It is characterized by multiple enchondromas, located primarily within the metaphyses. It is produced by groups of cartilage cells, which escape replacement by bone and are left in the metaphysis as the physis continues to grow. The disorder is frequently confined to one limb or even one side of a limb (e.g. radial or ulnar). The range of severity is variable (*Figure 5.24*).

Clinical Features

The condition is generally recognized in childhood with the development of palpable masses, unilateral shortening of an extremity, or angular deformity. The enchondromas often affect the short tubular bones of the hands and the feet as well as the long

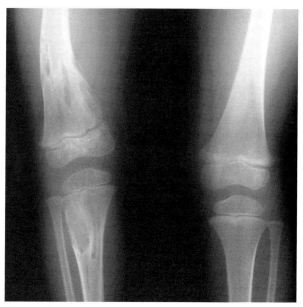

Figure 5.24 Enchondromatosis in this five-year-old girl is unilateral. It has caused some bowing of the distal right femur and therefore a little shortening of the leg.

bones of the upper and lower limbs. The lesions tend to be asymmetrical and may be unilateral. There is an increased risk of chondrosarcoma occurring in an enchondroma, but this is more common in Maffucci syndrome.

Radiology

Multiple irregular translucent areas in the metaphyses extend from the growth plate and end in a round or oval radiolucency, which may expand the bone and erode the cortex. The lucencies may contain scattered flecks of calcification. Any one individual lesion looks like a solitary enchondroma. The diaphyses are not involved. The effect of the lesions depends on their size. In some cases hand digits may be grotesquely expanded. As there is interference of long bone growth, paired bones may be unequal in length giving a Madelung type of wrist deformity and varus or valgus deformity of the elbow, knee or ankle. Lesions stop growing after bone maturation. The incidence of malignancy is very rare. Fractures may occur through the abnormal bone.

Differential Diagnosis

The forearm deformity of enchondromatosis is similar to that of severe cases of multiple exostoses, but exostoses elsewhere differentiate the latter.

Management

This is usually aimed at correcting the deformity or leg length discrepancy.

Mafucci Syndrome (Enchondromatosis with Haemangiomas)

This very rare disorder combines multiple enchondromatosis with multiple soft tissue haemangiomas. Inheritance is not genetic and the incidence is much less frequent than enchondromatosis. Malignant change in either the soft tissues or bone (chondrosarcoma) is reported in up to 20% of cases. Other malignancies, particularly of abdominal organs, are more likely to develop. Radiological appearances resemble those of enchondromatosis except that the soft tissues around the bony lesions are enlarged and contain multiple phleboliths (circular calcifications). Close follow-up is necessary because of the high risk of malignancy.

Osteopoikilosis

This radiological curiosity shows autosomal dominant inheritance. There are discrete round or oval sclerotic patches in the metaphyses and epiphyses of the long bones and hands. The pelvis may be involved, but the skull and spine are spared (*Figure 5.25*). There may be whitish spots in the skin (disseminated lenticular dermatofibrosis).

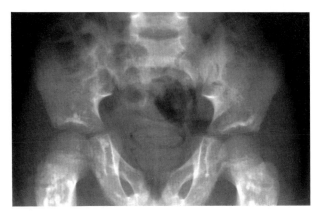

Figure 5.25 Osteopoikilosis. There are multiple small well defined sclerotic areas in the pelvis.

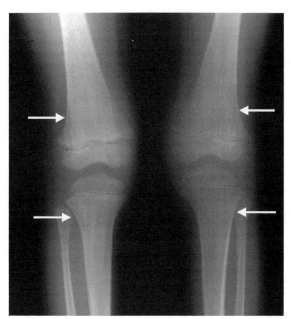

Figure 5.26 Osteopathia striata. There are linear 'streaks' in the distal femora and the proximal tibiae.

Osteopathia Striata

This rare bone disorder is characterized by dense striations in the metaphyses of long bones (*Figure 5.26*). The ilium and vertebral bodies may also be affected. The aetiology is unknown and the patient is asymptomatic.

Melorheostosis

This is characterized radiologically by dense, often linear, hyperostosis affecting mainly the periosteal, but also the endosteal surface of the bone. The appearance of the hyperostoses has been likened to dripping candle wax. The condition is mono- or polyostotic and is usually confined to a single limb, which is stiff, painful and sometimes deformed with soft tissue contractures and fibrosis. Inheritance is not genetic.

Fibrous Dysplasia

This mesodermal disorder shows patchy irregular replacement of medullary bone by fibro-osseous tissue and is sometimes associated with gross deformities and pathological fractures. Inheritance is not genetic. Presenting features are usually pain and

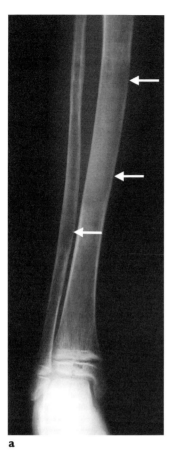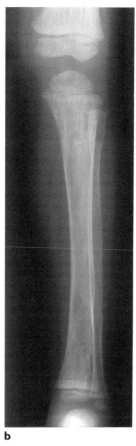

a   b

Figure 5.27 **a** In this eight-year-old girl the tibia and fibula are affected by fibrous dysplasia. Note the mild thinning of the cortex and the ground glass appearance (arrows). **b** The tibia in polyostotic fibrous dysplasia. Multiple areas of fibrous dysplasia affect the proximal and distal tibia and fibulas as well as the distal femur.

deformity from pathological fractures of the affected bone. The monostotic form is more common and typically involves the ribs, femurs, tibias, mandible, calvaria and humeri. Polyostotic involvement (*Figure 5.27*) occurs in 20–30% of patients and this is the form that produces most orthopaedic problems. It may be unilateral, and in addition to the extremities commonly involves the skull, face and pelvis. The association of polyostotic fibrous dysplasia with skin pigmentation and endocrine dysfunction (especially precocious puberty) is known as the McCune-Albright syndrome and is seen in 2–3% of cases (mainly female). Occasionally hyperthyroidism, hyperparathyroidism and hypophosphataemic rickets are associated with fibrous dysplasia. Unaffected bone is normal (i.e. this is a disease of multiple lesions rather than a generalized disorder). Epiphyses

are not usually involved. Malignant transformation (most frequently osteosarcoma) is very rare unless the patient has had previous radiotherapy.

Radiology

A typical area shows a radiolucency that looks cystic with a sclerotic margin in the metaphysis or diaphysis. The lesion is often of 'ground glass' density, possibly with internal septation and focal calcification. Lesions may cause local expansion and cortical thinning. Periosteal new bone does not occur. While this may describe typical lesions, the appearance can be purely lytic, patchy, sclerotic, expansile, mixed, or multiple, or simply trabecular streaking. Affected areas weaken easily, and repeat fractures with local bone softening may produce a severe varus deformity in the proximal femur (classical shepherd's crook deformity). The lesions enlarge and progress until the epiphyses close. Affected parts of the skull and face tend to show sclerotic rather than lucent bone. This may obliterate the sinuses. If sufficiently extensive there may be the grotesque facial swelling and asymmetry of 'leontiasis ossea.' Encroachment of the neural foramina may lead to blindness, deafness and vestibular disturbances. Vertebral lesions may be complicated by scoliosis.

On a bone scan the lesions are hot, and in polyostotic fibrous dysplasia the bone scan will show the full extent of the lesions. On MRI the areas of fibrous dysplasia show up as a low signal on T1-weighted scans and a low to high signal on T2-weighted scans.

In the lower limb confusion may arise with fibrocartilaginous dysplasia, which typically occurs in the anterior tibial cortex, producing a lytic expansile process with sclerotic demarcation. The histology, however, is completely different.

CHROMOSOMAL ABNORMALITIES

Down Syndrome (Trisomy 21)

This hereditary condition is caused by trisomy of chromosome 21. The incidence is 1 in 8000 live births. The clinical features include microcephaly, low-set ears, slanting eyes with epicanthic folds, a protruding tongue, a short neck, generalized ligamentous laxity, curved fifth fingers, transverse palmar creases, and hypotonia. Approximately 50% of these children have congenital heart disease. Mental retardation is mild to moderate. Atlanto–axial instability occurs in up to 20%, but only a small percentage require treatment. The distinctive radiological sign is flaring of the ilia with thin, rather hypoplastic pubic bones. There is an increase in the carpal angle, clinodactyly of the little finger (not specific), eleven pairs of ribs, and double ossification centres for the manubrium sterni.

Turner Syndrome (XO)

This is a rare condition in which there is absence of one X chromosome (45,X) or a structural abnormality of one X in a phenotypic girl. These females have short stature and 50% have webbing of the neck. The fourth metacarpal is short in 30%. They may have a Madelung deformity due to a carpal dysplasia, cubitus valgus and a small exostosis on the medial aspect of the upper tibial metaphyses. The medial femoral condyle may be overgrown with compensatory depression of the opposing tibial plateau. Cardiovascular and renal abnormalities and osteoporosis (best seen around the wrist) are common.

Treatment is oestrogen replacement at the time of puberty. Synthetic growth hormone advances skeletal maturation, increases bone density and advances bone density towards chronological age.

Edwards Syndrome (Trisomy 18)

This rare condition presents with multiple congenital malformations including bilateral severe talipes equinovarus. These children usually die before one year of age.

REFERENCES AND FURTHER READING

Basset GS, Scott CI. The osteochondrodysplasias. In: *Paediatric Orthopaedics*, edited by RT Morrisy, pp. 91–142. JB Lippincott, Philadelphia, 1990.

Blackston RD. Medical genetics for the orthopaedist. In: *Paediatric Orthopaedics*, edited by RT Morrisy, pp. 143–173. JB Lippincott, Philadelphia, 1990.

Certner JM, Root L. Osteogenesis imperfecta. *Orthop Clin North Am* 1990; **21**: 151–162.

Crawford AH Jr, Bagamery N. Osseous manifestations of neurofibromatosis in childhood. *J Paediatr Orthop* 1986; **6**: 72–88.

Crawford AH. Neurofibromatosis. In: *Paediatric Orthopaedics*, edited by RT Morrisy, pp. 175–201. JB Lippincott, Philadelphia, 1990.

Mulliken JB, Young AE. *Vascular Birthmarks: Haemangiomas and Malformations*. WB Saunders, Philadelphia, 1988.

Silence DO, Senn A, Danks DN. Genetic heterogeneity in osteogenesis imperfecta. *J Med Genet* 1979; **16**: 101–116.

Smith DW, Jones KL. *Smith's Recognisable Patterns of Human Malformation*, fourth edition. WB Saunders, Philadelphia, 1988.

Wynne–Davies R, Hall CM, Apley AG. *Atlas of Skeletal Dysplasias*. Churchill Livingstone, Edinburgh, 1985.

Chapter 6
Metabolic Bone Disease

Mark D O'Sullivan and Virginia J Saxton

Bone is a solid structure in a constant state of turnover, which is regulated by hormones which in turn respond to changes in mineral ion concentration. All changes to the bone structure are brought about by cellular activity. Osteoblasts create bone and osteoclasts resorb it. Metabolic bone diseases are generalized disorders caused by abnormalities of this system.

STRUCTURE

Bone is a complex structure made up of cells, matrix and mineral.

Bone Cells

The three types of bone cells are osteoblasts, osteocytes, and osteoclasts.

- Osteoblasts are derived from mesenchymal cells and produce all the components of the organic matrix, including collagen, and associated proteins. Osteoblasts respond to a number of hormones through surface receptors. They may become osteocytes when surrounded by bone and lying in lacunae.
- Osteocytes communicate with each other by extensions in the canaliculi. Their function is not clear, but they may respond to mechanical stimuli.
- Osteoclasts are derived from the haemopoietic system and are concerned with bone resorption. They are mainly controlled by osteoblasts, but also respond to calcitonin.

Bone Matrix

The main component of matrix is type I collagen within a mucopolysaccharide ground substance. Proteoglycans and other proteins add to the complex.

Bone Mineral

The mineral content of bone consists mainly of calcium and phosphate in the form of crystalline hydroxyapatite.

PHYSIOLOGY OF BONE

Bone Metabolism

Only 1% of the body's calcium is readily exchangeable, as 99% is stored in bone and the calcium stored in bone can be exchanged only very slowly. Calcium and phosphate concentrations depend on intestinal absorption and renal excretion. The turnover of bone calcium depends on the ratio between osteoclastic and osteoblastic activity and the factors that drive these cells. The complex balance of intestinal calcium absorption, renal tubular excretion and calcium turnover in bone is controlled by both systemic and local factors.

Parathyroid Hormone

Parathyroid hormone (PTH) is the fine regulator of calcium exchange and keeps extracellular calcium within very narrow limits. The production and release of PTH is stimulated by a fall in plasma calcium, while a rise in plasma calcium suppresses PTH production and release (*Figure 6.1*). The target organs are the renal tubules and the bone and indirectly the gut. PTH increases renal tubular reabsorption of calcium and increases phosphate excretion. It also stimulates osteoclastic bone resorption and increases plasma calcium by increasing vitamin D synthesis, which stimulates intestinal absorption.

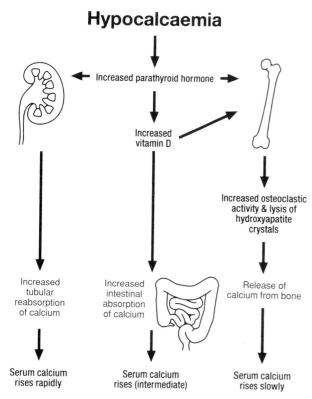

Hypocalcaemia

Figure 6.1   The effects of hypocalcaemia.

Vitamin D

Through its active metabolites, vitamin D is mainly concerned with bone remodelling and the mass movement of calcium. Vitamin D itself is inactive. Ergocalciferol is absorbed from the diet and ultraviolet light acting on the skin causes the production of cholecalciferol from its precursor 7-dehydrocholesterol. Ergocalciferol and cholecalciferol are then converted to active metabolites in the liver and kidney: 25-hydroxylation takes place in the liver, followed by 1-hydroxylation in the kidney.

Active vitamin D or 1,25-dihydroxycholecalciferol (or calcitriol) increases calcium uptake in the small intestine, thereby promoting bone deposition. Vitamin D acts directly on bone to promote resorption.

Other Hormones

Calcitonin

The action of calcitonin opposes that of PTH. It suppresses bone resorption and increases renal calcium excretion.

Oestrogen

It is thought that oestrogen stimulates calcium absorption and protects bone from the unrestrained action of PTH.

Adrenal Corticosteroids

These increase bone resorption, decrease bone formation and decrease intestinal calcium absorption.

PTH-Related Peptide

This hormone has actions very similar to PTH. It is secreted by some tumours and may be a fetal hormone.

RICKETS

Rickets is defined as inadequate mineralization of bone with an excess of osteoid on histology. In children this occurs in areas of active endochondral ossification.

Aetiology

There are multiple causes of rickets, which may affect the synthesis of vitamin D along its pathway (*Figure 6.2*).

Deficiencies in the amount or action of vitamin D

- *Nutritional rickets* remains the commonest form of rickets. Vitamin D is fat soluble and is present in margarine. Nutritional rickets is particularly seen in some ethnic communities where a poor intake is associated with inadequate exposure to sunlight. Malabsorption can prevent intestinal absorption of vitamin D, for example in coeliac disease and primary biliary cirrhosis
- *Deficiencies of 25-hydroxylation* can result from phenytoin ingestion, which can interfere with this process in the liver. However, a deficiency of the 25-hydroxylation is unusual, in severe chronic liver disease.
- *Deficiencies of 1-hydroxylation* can result from chronic renal disease, but often the picture is mixed with a secondary hyperparathyroidism. There is also a rare genetic abnormality with a selective deficiency of the enzyme responsible for 1-hydroxylation.
- *Abnormal receptors* are a rare cause and can be treated with large doses of calcitriol.

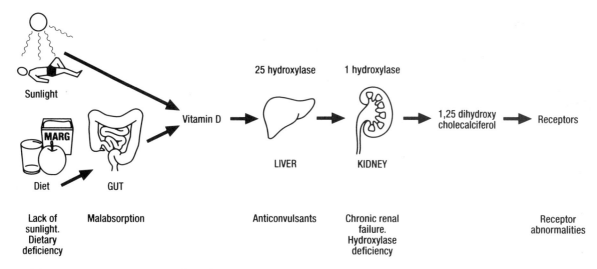

Figure 6.2 The causes of vitamin D deficiency.

Phosphate deficiency

- *Vitamin D-resistant rickets* is a familial condition with a selective defect in the reabsorption of phosphate in the renal tubules.
- *Fanconi syndrome* is associated with a more generalized aminoaciduria associated with the phosphate loss. The commonest form is in cystinosis or cystine storage disease, where cystine crystals are deposited in the kidney damaging the renal tubules.
- *Nutritional phosphate deficiency* can occur in neonates on total parenteral nutrition for many weeks because only a limited amount of phosphate can be added before the calcium and phosphate precipitate out of the solution.

Clinical Features

The most common presentation of rickets in an infant who has not started to walk is with softening of the occiput (otherwise known as craniotabes). In infants, rickets may also present with tetany or convulsions. The child is hypotonic, and muscular weakness may be an early symptom. The infant has a protuberant abdomen, delayed motor development, enlargement of the costochondral junctions (rickety rosary), and thickening of the metaphyses at the knees, ankles and wrists. Bones tend to have an accentuation of the normal curves, and this may be particularly seen with distal tibial bowing.

In older infants bow legs are the characteristic presenting feature. However, knock knees are also common. Stunting of growth may be obvious in severe rickets. Spinal curvature, coxa vara and bending or fractures of the long bones may occur.

Proximal myopathy is a striking feature and may delay motor development.

Laboratory Investigations

Biochemical changes occur in all forms of rickets. The exact changes depend on the type of rickets.

- If there are deficiencies in the amount or action of vitamin D there is a low serum calcium, a low serum phosphate and a raised PTH.
- If there is phosphate deficiency there is a low serum phosphate, a normal serum calcium and a normal PTH.

If the serum concentration of calcium multiplied by the concentration of phosphate is less then 2.4 this is diagnostic for rickets. A bone biopsy is not required, but there is an excess of unmineralized osteoid.

Radiology

Plain radiographs show widening of the growth plate with irregular metaphyseal margins (*Figure 6.3*). This is because the zone of provisional calcification is ill-defined due to defective mineralization. There is also splaying and cupping of the metaphyses as the hypertrophic zone continues to grow and protrude into the weakened metaphyseal region. The bone is osteopenic with an indistinct cortex produced by the uncalcified subperiosteal osteoid. The anterior ends of the ribs are cupped and there are large costochondral junctions, producing the 'rickety rosary.' The weakened bone may fracture and cause bowing of the extremities as well as scoliosis, triradiate configuration of the pelvis, basilar invagination of the skull

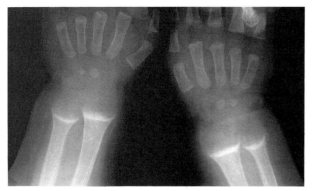

Figure 6.3 Rickets in an 11-month-old child. The wrists show classical changes of rickets. There is irregularity of the metaphyses with cupping and splaying.

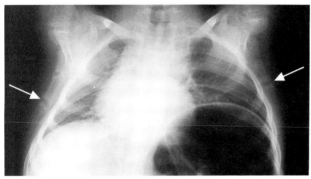

Figure 6.4 This 13-year-old girl with rickets shows classical Looser zones (arrows) in the scapulae due to underlying rickets.

and slipped upper femoral epiphyses. Looser zones are occasionally seen, but are less common than in the osteomalacia of adults (*Figure 6.4*).

Management

Nutritional rickets is prevented by exposing the skin to sunlight. If this is not possible oral vitamin D (up to 400 units per day) is given.

Treatment of nutritional rickets requires vitamin D 3000 U daily for a few weeks.

Differential Diagnosis

The radiology is distinctive so the diagnosis is usually not difficult. In osteogenesis imperfecta there is osteopenia and bowed limbs, but there are no metaphyseal changes. Early scurvy can mimic rickets, but the zone of provisional calcification is normally mineralized unlike in rickets and the cortical margins are well-defined in contrast to the indistinct margins seen in rickets. Metaphyseal chondrodysplasia and hypophosphatasia can mimic rickets, but the serum calcium and phosphate are normal in these conditions. In young gymnasts repetitive trauma to the growth plate may cause changes in the metaphysis that mimic early rickets.

TYPES OF RICKETS

Vitamin D-Resistant Rickets (Familial Hypophosphataemic Rickets)

This is an X-linked disorder that causes a defect in the renal tubules and limits phosphate reabsorption. It commences in infancy or soon after and causes severe bone deformity. The children are generally of short stature, boys more so than girls. There is no myopathy. The serum phosphate is very low.

Radiology

Radiographs show markedly bowed legs with widened growth plates, metaphyseal irregularity and flaring. Bone density is normal (*Figure 6.5*).

Management

Large doses of vitamin D and phosphate are used until growth ceases. This may cause nephrocalcinosis. The amount of oral phosphate needed to correct the low serum phosphate often causes nausea and

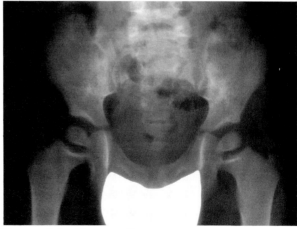

Figure 6.5 Vitamin D-resistant rickets in a child presenting at three years of age with apparent widening of the growth plate and some mild irregularity of the proximal femoral metaphyses.

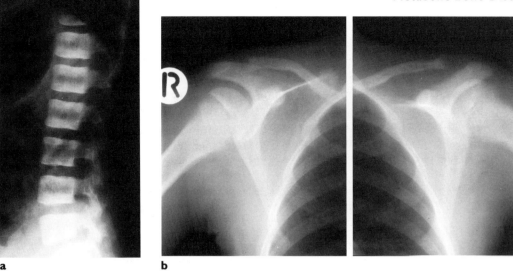

Figure 6.6 a Spinal changes of renal osteodystrophy. Note the sclerosis at the vertebral end-plates giving a 'rugger jersey' spine. **b** The irregularity and apparent destruction of the distal ends of the clavicles are features of renal osteodystrophy. Note the lack of clarity of the cortex in the proximal humeral shaft.

diarrhoea, so compliance is a problem. If the condition is discovered early, deformities can be avoided by medical treatment alone. Surgery is used when medical treatment has failed.

Differential Diagnosis

The radiological appearance should be differentiated from that of the various forms of metaphyseal chondrodysplasia (see Chapter 5), which although rare, can mimic vitamin D-resistant rickets, but the serum calcium and phosphate are normal.

Renal Osteodystrophy

Patients with chronic renal failure are liable to develop diffuse bone changes, which are produced by a combination of rickets, secondary hyperparathyroidism and osteosclerosis (*Figure 6.6*).

Clinical Features

Growth is stunted and knock knees are typical, particularly after two years of age. The complexion is sallow. Marked rachitic deformities develop with enlarged metaphyses. Myopathy is common.

Radiology

The radiological appearance of the rickets includes widened growth plates, splayed and irregular metaphyses, and coarse, fuzzy trabeculae with osteopenia.

Marked bone resorption may partly account for the overall osteopenia in these patients.

Secondary hyperparathyroidism gives rise to sub-periosteal resorption in the radial aspect of the middle phalanges of the second and third digits, and less commonly in the proximal tibia, humerus and femur. Secondary hyperparathyroidism may also give rise to brown tumours. These well-defined lytic lesions occur mainly in the mandible, pelvis, ribs and femur. Osteosclerosis (aetiology unknown) occurs in 15–20% of patients. In the spine it predominates near the end-plates producing a 'rugger jersey' spine. Soft tissue calcification occurs in the vessels and in a periarticular distribution (especially if the patient is on haemodialysis or after renal transplantation).

Laboratory Investigations

Serum calcium is low with a high serum phosphate and alkaline phosphatase. Urinary excretion of calcium and phosphate may be raised. PTH may be raised.

Management

This includes the management of the renal disease. Calcitriol and calcium carbonate are used to treat the osteodystrophy. Surgery is used to correct deformities and epiphyseodesis is occasionally required for epiphyseal slips.

Neonatal Rickets

This occurs in premature infants as a result of combined dietary deficiency (e.g. prolonged hyperalimentation) and impaired hepatic hydroxylation of vitamin D. Bone changes are visible around the second month and typically show osteopenia and multiple fractures. Metaphyseal changes (see above) do occur, but are much less marked.

HYPERPARATHYROIDISM

This is an uncommon primary disease in childhood, but the secondary disease may be associated with renal failure. The disease in childhood causes the same skeletal changes as in adults.

Radiology

The main feature is subperiosteal bone resorption. This is seen in 10% of patients in the radial aspects of the middle phalanges of the second and third digits (*Figure 6.7*). Bone resorption also occurs in other sites (intracortical, endosteal, subchondral, trabecular and subligamentous). The bones are osteopenic. Brown tumours (osteoclastomas) are focal lytic lesions in the metaphyses and diaphyses caused by collections of giant cells. They may be solitary or multiple.

SCURVY

Vitamin C deficiency is rare and results in an inability to manufacture normal intercellular collagen and organic bone matrix. The disease can develop in infants from six months of age.

Clinical Features

These include irritability, anorexia and failure to thrive. There is general tenderness in the limbs and swelling along the shafts of the long bones. Capillary fragility leads to haemorrhages in the gums and skin.

Radiology

There is widening and increased density in the zone of provisional calcification at the ends of the long bones (*Figure 6.8*). Similar changes occur around the epiphysis, resulting in a thin ring of increased density around the epiphysis. Behind the zone of provisional calcification there is a transverse band of radiolucency due to a suppression of osteoblastic activity. This area of weakened bone may fracture with subsequent subperiosteal haemorrhage, which may be florid and later calcify. The widening of the zone of provisional calcification results in periosteal elevation and marginal spur formation. Subepiphyseal

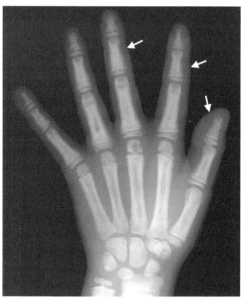

Figure 6.7 Severe changes of hyperparathyroidism in this eight-year-old girl with renal osteodystrophy. There is extensive subperiosteal resorption in the phalanges (arrows), and a more focal area of resorption in the epiphysis of the third metacarpal (early Brown tumour).

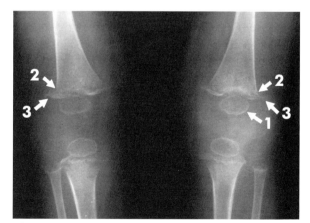

Figure 6.8 Severe changes of scurvy in this 10-month-old child. There is a pencil-like increased density around the epiphyses (1). The zone of provisional calcification is dense in part and behind this there has been fracturing through the transverse band of radiolucency (zone of Trummerfeld) (2). This has resulted in marginal spur formation (3).

infractions result in varying degrees of separation of the epiphysis from the metaphysis.

LEAD POISONING

This condition became uncommon after the reduction in the lead content of paint. The incidence increased with motor vehicle pollution, but recently catalytic converters in cars have reduced the lead levels in the air. It causes anaemia, constipation and myopathy.

Radiology

The most characteristic feature is a dense transverse band across the metaphyses of the long bones and along the margins of the flat bones (*Figure 6.9*). This can also be seen with other heavy metal poisoning such as bismuth.

VITAMIN A TOXICITY

This condition causes two main skeletal abnormalities:

- Cortical hyperostosis.
- Ectopic ossification of the ligaments, particularly of the spine.

In children, prolonged overdose with vitamin A causes pain and tenderness in the long bones with local swelling. The cortical density of the long bones is increased, but the bones are abnormally fragile and liable to fracture.

HYPOTHYROIDISM

Hypothyroidism from birth (cretinism) is rare and is usually apparent during the first year of life. Testing at birth has reduced the incidence. Most cases are now due to thyroid aplasia. The child becomes sluggish and sleepy and has noisy respirations and a large tongue. Nasal obstruction and a large abdomen gradually develop. Body temperature is low, the skin is dry and cold, there is difficulty feeding, and there is a marked delay in growth and skeletal age.

Radiology

There is a marked delay in the appearance of the ossification centres and of their subsequent growth. Centres that do ossify are often irregular and stippled. The capital femoral epiphyses may resemble those of Perthes disease (*Figure 6.10*). Other radiological changes include thickening of the cranial vault, brachycephaly, wormian bones and hypoplasia of the sinuses and mastoids. The vertebrae are a little flattened, and there may be kyphosis at the thoracolumbar junction with a hypoplastic body of L1 or L2 and an antero-inferior beak. Coxa vara with a short femoral neck also occurs, as can a slipped upper femoral epiphysis.

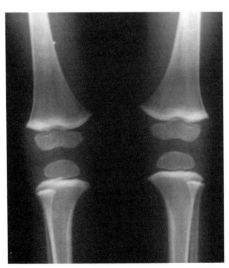

Figure 6.9 Lead poisoning in a two-year-old girl. There is a dense and widened zone of provisional calcification (including the fibulae).

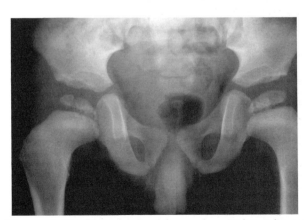

Figure 6.10 The proximal femoral capital epiphyses in this four-year-old boy with hypothyroidism are decreased in height and fragmented. In addition there is a dense transverse metaphyseal band. These appearances are classical of hypothyroidism. The differential diagnosis includes Perthes disease and multiple epiphyseal dysplasia.

Table 6.1   Causes of osteoporosis

Idiopathic	Idiopathic juvenile osteoporosis
Endocrine	Cushing
Disuse	
Iatrogenic	Steroids
Inflammatory	Juvenile chronic arthritis
Deficiency states	Scurvy
Congenital	Osteogenesis imperfecta, Turner syndrome, homocystinuria, hypophosphatasia
Tumour	Leukaemia

OSTEOPOROSIS

Osteoporosis is characterized by a decreased volume of otherwise normal bone on histological examination.

Aetiology

The causes of osteoporosis are listed in Table 6.1.

Radiology

There is generalized osteopenia (*Figure 6.11*) and the cortices are thinned and accentuated. The primary trabeculae are accentuated while the secondary ones are thinned. Fractures occur in the femoral neck and distal radius as a result of minor trauma. The vertebral bodies may show wedging or biconcave collapse (*Figure 6.12*).

IDIOPATHIC JUVENILE OSTEOPOROSIS

This condition of unknown aetiology is characterized by temporary osteoporosis of the long bones and spine. Fractures particularly occur in the metaphyses and spine. Children present before puberty with back pain, kyphosis, severe knock knees and pain around the joints of the lower limbs. Biochemistry is normal. The condition often begins to improve at puberty and the treatment is symptomatic.

Radiology

Osteoporosis is particularly marked in the thoracic and lumbar vertebrae (*Figure 6.12*). This may cause vertebral collapse with anterior wedging. Long bone fractures typically occur in the metaphyses, and slipped capital femoral epiphysis is a complication.

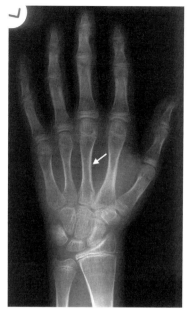

Figure 6.11   Hands of a 13-year-old boy with osteoporosis. Note that the cortical thickness is markedly decreased (arrow). In a normal patient the cortical thickness should be one-third to one-quarter of the metacarpal width. In this case it is clearly much less than this.

HOMOCYSTINURIA

This metabolic disorder has autosomal recessive inheritance and is due to lack of the enzyme cystathionine synthetase. Patients are tall, thin and may have joint laxity and dislocation of the lens. Scoliosis is common. The condition differs from Marfan syndrome because of the presence of marked osteoporosis, mental retardation and thromboembolic disease. Homocystine levels are raised in the blood and urine. Approximately 50% of the children can be cured by the administration of pyridoxine from early childhood.

HYPOPHOSPHATASIA

This rare familial deficiency of alkaline phosphatase causes defective ossification of bone. There is a wide spectrum of manifestations from the severe lethal perinatal form to the mild adult form. Serum calcium and phosphate are normal, but the serum alkaline phosphatase is low.

Radiological changes may mimic those of rickets or osteogenesis imperfecta depending on the form.

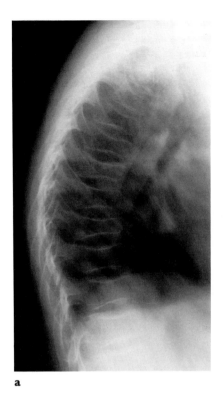 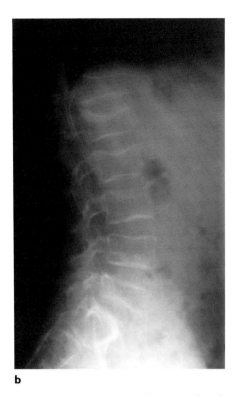

a   b

Figure 6.12 Idiopathic juvenile osteoporosis in this 11-year-old girl has caused generalized osteopenia throughout the spinal column with biconcave vertebral body collapse.

FURTHER READING

Boden SD, Kaplan FS. Calcium homeostasis. *Orthop Clin North Am* 1990; **21**: 31–42.

Campbell DE, Fleischman AR. Rickets of prematurity: controversies in causation and prevention. *Clin Perinatol* 1988; **15**: 879–890.

Grainger RG, Allison AJ. *Diagnostic Radiology*. Churchill Livingstone, Edinburgh, 1986.

Helms CA. *Fundamentals of Skeletal Radiology*. WB Saunders, Philadelphia, 1989.

Jaffe HL. *Metabolic, Degenerative and Inflammatory Diseases of Bone and Joints*. Lea and Febiger, Philadelphia, 1972.

Mankin HJ. Rickets, osteomalacia and renal osteodystrophy: an update. *Orthop Clin North Am* 1990; **21**: 81–96.

Ozonoff MB. *Paediatric Radiology*, second edition. WB Saunders, Philadelphia, 1992.

Smith R. Juvenile osteoporosis in the young. *J Bone Joint Surg* 1980 **62B**: 417–427.

Chapter 7

Bone and Soft Tissue Tumours

Mark D O'Sullivan and Virginia J Saxton

Tumours of bone and soft tissue in childhood are reasonably common. The vast majority are benign. Malignant bone and soft tissue tumours are uncommon, but when they occur are devastating to the patient and family and may be fatal. The classification of bone and soft tissue tumours is based on the predominant tissue in the lesion (*Tables 7.1, 7.2*).

Table 7.1   Bone Tumours

Benign	
Bone	Osteoid osteoma
	Osteoblastoma
	Osteochondroma
Cartilage	Enchondroma
	Chondromyxoid fibroma
	Chondroblastoma
Fibrous tissue	Fibrous cortical defect, non-ossifying fibroma
	Fibrous dysplasia
	Fibrocartilaginous dysplasia of the tibia
Miscellaneous	Simple bone cyst
	Aneurysmal bone cyst
	Giant cell tumour
	Langerhan cell histiocytosis
	Massive osteolysis
	Osteofibrous dysplasia
	Haemangioma of bone
	EOSINO PHLIC GRANULOMA.
Malignant	Osteosarcoma
	Ewing sarcoma
	Chondrosarcoma
	Fibrosarcoma
Metastatic disease	

Diagnosis

History

The diagnosis is usually suspected from the history. The child often presents with a history of pain or a lump and there is often an incidental history of trauma. If the pain has developed rapidly or involves night pain, one should be suspicious of tumour. A rapid increase in the size of a mass is also suggestive of a malignant tumour.

Examination

Examination of the child may be normal apart from the involved area. There may be an area of tenderness or a mass. The area involved may be warmer than surrounding tissues and may be painful when moved. The adjacent joint may have limited movement. Lymph nodes should be examined, as should the abdomen for liver or splenic enlargement.

Table 7.2   Soft Tissue Tumours

Benign	
Vascular	Haemangioma
Fibrous	Fibromatoses
Nerve	Neurofibroma
	Neurilemmoma
Fat	Lipoma
Synovial	Pigmented villonodular synovitis *PVNS*
	Synovial osteochondromatosis
Miscellaneous	Tumoral calcinosis
	Dermatomyositis
Malignant	
Muscle	Rhabdomyosarcoma
Fat	Liposarcoma
Synovial	Synovial sarcoma

Radiology

Plain films are the first test in the diagnosis of bone tumours. They may be diagnostic and they are most helpful in the differentiation of a benign from a malignant tumour. Four criteria are helpful in diagnosing the tumour: age, site, appearance, and whether it is benign or malignant.

Age

This is a very important consideration in the diagnosis of bone tumours. Most have a peak age of incidence and a range of common incidence; outside this range they are rare. For example primary malignant bone tumours are rare before five years of age so a permeative lesion in a two-year-old is most likely due to leukaemia or disseminated neuroblastoma. In contrast giant cell tumours are rare before epiphyseal closure.

Site

This is extremely helpful. The site of a lesion will often narrow down the differential diagnosis considerably. A well-defined lytic epiphyseal lesion is most likely to be a chondroblastoma, whereas a well-defined lytic lesion in the diaphysis of a phalanx is most likely to be an enchondroma.

Appearance

Some tumours have a classical appearance. Indeed they may be an Aunt Minnie (I know that's Aunt Minnie because she looks like Aunt Minnie!). For example a fibrous cortical defect is a lesion 2 cm or less with a well-defined, thin scalloped border that arises from the cortex of the metaphysis in a long bone, typically in the distal femur. An osteoid osteoma is a small lucency with an extensive area of surrounding sclerosis and well-defined periosteal reaction. However, although some tumours may have a classical appearance they do not always adhere to it.

Benign or malignant

In calling a lesion benign or malignant it is really being classified as having either non-aggressive or aggressive features. Benign and malignant are useful terms provided it is remembered that some benign processes may appear aggressive and some malignancies may look non-aggressive. The differentiation between benign and malignant may be straightforward or very difficult. Three criteria are helpful.

- The zone of transition is the most useful indicator of whether a lesion is benign or malignant. It is the border between the lesion and the normal bone. If

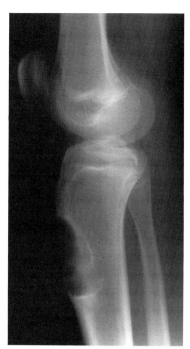

Figure 7.1   Benign bone tumour. The lesion is well-defined and has a very narrow zone of transition. There is a thin sclerotic rim and marked cortical thinning anteriorly. This was a chondromyxoid fibroma.

this is well-defined (such that it can be drawn with a pen) the zone of transition is said to be narrow and it is a benign lesion (*Figure 7.1*). If the lesion has a sclerotic border it has by definition a narrow zone of transition. If the zone of transition is wide and cannot be drawn with a pen, it is aggressive. An aggressive lesion is not necessarily malignant as similar zones of transition are seen in infection and eosinophilic granuloma. Permeative lesions, in which the border contains multiple small holes, have no clear border and therefore a very wide zone of transition. They indicate an aggressive process (*Figure 7.2*).

- Periostitis: a periosteal reaction can appear indolent and well-defined, or ill-defined. A slow-growing lesion produces a thick wavy uniform periosteal reaction (e.g. osteoid osteoma). A malignant tumour does not give the periosteum time to consolidate so it is amorphous lamellated (onion-skinned) or even sunburst (at right angles to the cortex) in appearance. The distinction is useful, but not infallible. Some benign lesions may cause an aggressive periostitis (e.g. infection and eosinophilic granuloma, *Figure 7.3*). However, malignant lesions do not generally cause benign-looking periostitis.

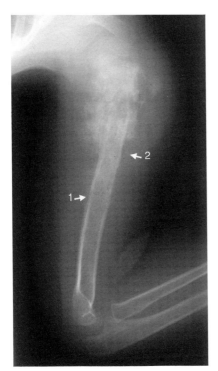

Figure 7.2 Malignant bone tumour. This lesion has all the hallmarks of a malignant bone tumour with destruction of the proximal humeral metaphysis and a permeative infiltration extending down the shaft of the humerus. The margins of the tumour are ill-defined. The periosteal reaction is aggressive with a Codman triangle (1), which indicates that the tumour is fast growing, has sunray spiculation (i.e. at right angles to the shaft, 2) and areas of ill-defined new bone formation. This tumour was a highly aggressive osteosarcoma.

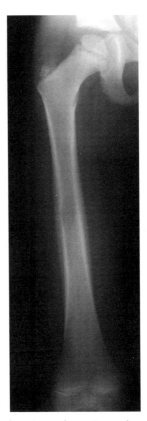

Figure 7.3 Laminated periosteal reaction. In the diaphysis with minor underlying bone destruction and no marked soft tissue swelling. This was an eosinophilic granuloma (i.e. a benign lesion) giving a more aggressive-looking periosteal reaction.

- Cortical destruction: malignant tumours cause cortical destruction but this can be mimicked by some benign processes such as infection and eosinophilic granuloma. A slow-growing benign lesion such as a simple bone cyst or an enchondroma will cause cortical thinning (see *Figure 7.1*) and endosteal scalloping. Difficulties in diagnosis can arise when some less aggressive tumours such as a giant cell tumour or an aneurysmal bone cyst cause so much cortical thinning that the thin rim of cortex left is invisible on plain films. These appearances suggest cortical destruction and malignancy. A computerized tomography (CT) scan will show the remaining thin cortex.

Bone scan

The primary tumour almost invariably shows increased uptake. However, the advantage of the bone scan is in the detection or exclusion of other lesions such as metastatic spread or multifocal primaries. If a tumour is purely osteolytic with no osteoblastic response in the surrounding bone (e.g. eosinophilic granuloma) then the bone scan may be cold.

Computerized tomography

This now has a secondary role to magnetic resonance imaging (MRI) in the evaluation of bone tumours. It is, however, the best modality for looking for tumour calcification, early cortical erosion and periosteal reaction, although the sensitivity and specificity of MRI for the latter two is improving to the point of approaching that of CT. CT is the technique of choice for detecting lung metastases.

Magnetic resonance imaging

This is the examination of choice for imaging bone tumours because of the excellent contrast between normal and pathological processes and the ability to distinguish normal from abnormal marrow. MRI shows the intraosseous extent of tumour spread as well as the soft tissue extent and any neurovascular or joint involvement. Other advantages include the lack of radiation and the ability to image in different planes and build up three-dimensional images of the tumour. MRI should always be carried out before the biopsy to avoid overestimating the tumour size as a result of post-biopsy haemorrhage. It is also helpful in deciding on the site of biopsy.

The cellular components of most tumours are seen as decreased or intermediate signal intensity on T1-weighted scans and bright on T2-weighted scans. However, other processes such as oedema and fluid (including tumour necrosis) can also show as a low signal on T1- and a high signal on T2-weighted scans. Chronic fibrosis and reactive bone show as a decreased signal on both T1- and T2-weighted scans. Acute haemorrhage shows as an intermediate signal intensity on T1 and as a decreased signal on T2. An area that is bright on both T1- and T2-weighted images may represent fat, subacute haemorrhage, mucus or contrast agents such as gadolinium.

For many tumours the MRI appearance is non-specific showing a low signal intensity on T1- and a high signal intensity on T2-weighted images. However, if there is evidence of blood, the possibility of a haemorrhage into a lesion, recent biopsy or a primary haemorrhagic tumour (e.g. telangiectatic osteogenic sarcoma) should be considered. If fat is present then a lipoma, liposarcoma and teratoma should be considered. The MRI appearance of each individual tumour will not be discussed in this chapter unless there are any particular distinguishing features.

Staging

The Enneking classification is the one most often used. It divides the tumours into high or low grade and into intra- or extra-compartmental sites (*Table 7.3*).

Table 7.3 The Enneking Classification

Stage	Grade	Site
IA	Low G I	Intracompartmental T I
IB	Low G I	Extracompartmental T2
2A	High G2	Intracompartmental T I
2B	High G2	Extracompartmental T2
3	Any G	Regional or distant metastases

Biopsy

Attention to detail is vital when biopsying a potentially malignant tumour. It should be carried out by the surgeon who will perform the definitive surgery and is the last investigation after radiological investigations are completed. The biopsy can be performed as an open procedure or by needle. Whichever way it is performed the biopsy tract must be excisable with the lesion at the time of definitive surgery. Longitudinal incisions are better than transverse and dissection is limited. No flaps are raised and the neurovascular bundle is not exposed. Dissection is straight through the muscle and not between. Tumour is taken from the periphery of the lesion. The biopsy is sharply cut and both the pseudocapsule and a portion of tumour are excised as a block and sent to pathology. A frozen section is needed to ensure an adequate specimen.

The use of a tourniquet is controversial because it potentially increases the risk of metastatic disease. If it is used, then an exsanguinating bandage is not used. The limb is elevated for three minutes before the tourniquet is applied. Haemostasis is secured before closing the wound and the tourniquet is deflated to ensure this. Drainage should be through the wound.

BENIGN BONE-FORMING TUMOURS

Osteoid Osteoma

Osteoid osteoma is a benign bone tumour that affects more boys than girls (ratio 3:1). The age range is 5–24 years. A typical patient presents with unrelenting aching pain, which is relieved by aspirin. Night pain is usually a feature. Any bone may be involved, but 50% affect the femur and tibia. It is also common in the spine, where osteoid osteomas affect the posterior elements and may present with a scoliosis and pain. The talus and calcaneum may also be involved.

Radiology

The classical appearance is of a cortically-based sclerotic lesion with a small central lucency (nidus) in the diaphysis of a long bone (*Figures 7.4, 7.5*). The nidus is the osteoid osteoma and the sclerosis is the reaction of the host bone. If the osteoid osteoma is medullary or within a joint capsule the sclerosis is much less reactive and the plain films may look normal. The nidus is usually lucent, but may par-

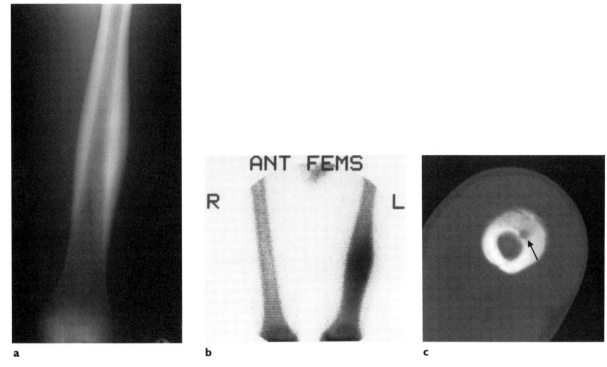

Figure 7.4 a Osteoid osteoma. The left femur shows extensive cortical sclerosis in the diaphysis. There is no obvious nidus. **b** Osteoid osteoma. A bone scan shows increased uptake in the same area. **c** A computerized tomographic scan through the area shows the lucent nidus (arrow) in the sclerotic area. The appearances of Figures 7.4a,b and c are typical of an osteoid osteoma.

tially or totally calcify. It may not be visible on plain films, but is shown well on a CT scan. The sclerosis is a combination of endosteal sclerosis and well-laminated periosteal new bone.

An osteoid osteoma may mimic osteomyelitis on plain films. Both are hot on bone scan. CT is helpful in demonstrating the nidus and for percutaneous removal of osteoid osteomas. There is no real role for MRI in the diagnosis of osteoid osteomas because the nidus may not be visible and the intramedullary oedema may give a misleading appearance of malignancy.

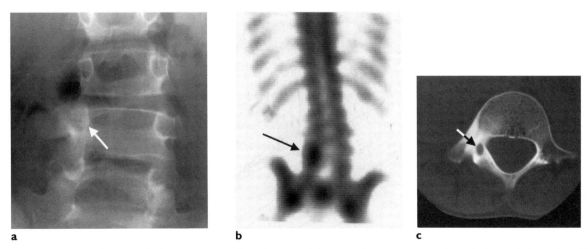

Figure 7.5 a This 13-year-old boy presented with a painful scoliosis due to osteoid osteoma of the spine. Plain radiographs show sclerosis and enlargement of the right L4 pedicle (arrow). Note the mild left-sided scoliosis. **b** Bone scan shows increased uptake in the right L4 pedicle (arrow). **c** Computerized tomographic scan shows a nidus (arrow) at the junction of the right L4 pedicle and lamina with surrounding sclerosis.

Pathology

The nidus is composed of numerous vascular channels, osteoblasts and thin lace-like osteoid seams.

Management

Treatment is by excision of the nidus. Once the nidus has been removed the surrounding sclerosis gradually resolves. The adequacy of the excision can be confirmed by radiology of the lesion showing the presence of the nidus. The excision can be guided by perioperative bone scan and the use of a hand-held radiation detection unit at surgery. Alternatively it can be carried out percutaneously with CT guidance. The choice of open or percutaneous removal depends on the site of the nidus and the expertise of the operators.

The natural history of the condition is for gradual resolution over time. If the symptoms are not severe and are relieved by aspirin one can wait for natural resolution. However significant pain usually demands excision.

Differential Diagnosis

This includes low-grade chronic osteomyelitis (Brodie's abscess).

Osteoblastoma

These lesions are histologically identical to osteoid osteomas, but are larger. A nidus greater than 1.5 cm is said to be an osteoblastoma. About 50% of the lesions occur in the spine and they usually involve the posterior elements.

Radiology

The lesion is predominantly radiolucent and well defined and approximately 50% show a variable amount of calcification in the matrix. Although the tumour is benign it may be expansile. An osteoblastoma may look like a very large osteoid osteoma (greater than 1.5 cm), particularly in the spine.

Management

This differs from the management of osteoid osteomas because these lesions must be excised completely or recurrences may occur.

Osteochondroma

These account for 50% of bone tumours. The cause is unknown, but is related to the periphery of the growth plate. There is an outgrowth of normal cartilage adjacent to the growth plate, which undergoes endochondral ossification to produce the bony component. The most commonly affected areas are the rapidly growing ends of the long bones. Clinically, patients usually present with a painless lump. Osteochondromas grow slowly, occasionally causing pain due to irritation of overlying muscle or trauma. Hereditary multiple exostoses are discussed in Chapter 5.

Radiology

The cortex of an osteochondroma is continuous with the normal bony cortex and presents as a bony outgrowth. Typical sites include the distal femur, proximal tibia, proximal humerus, pelvis and scapula. As it grows the marrow extends into the osteochondroma. The cartilage cap is not visible on plain radiographs until it ossifies with age. Lesions can measure up to 8–10 cm in length. The peripheral margin of the stalk is well defined and there is no bony destruction. The base of the tumour may be broad (sessile) or narrow (pedunculated). Osteochondromas typically point away from the adjacent joint.

Management

During childhood increased growth is expected, but excision is indicated only if the lesion is symptomatic. The risk of malignant degeneration is unknown, but very small. There is an increased risk in lesions of the spine, scapula and pelvis.

BENIGN CARTILAGINOUS TUMOURS

Enchondroma

This is an intramedullary cartilaginous lesion, which is usually located in the metaphysis. It occurs in bones that develop by endochondral ossification and is most common in the small tubular bones of the hand. The tumour often presents following a pathological fracture through the lesion or on routine radiographs. Approximately 40% occur in the bones of the hands and feet. The femur and proximal humerus are the next most common sites.

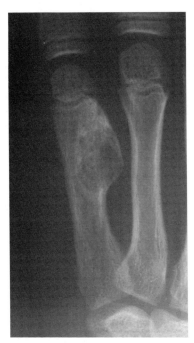

Figure 7.6 An enchondroma in the fifth metacarpal has expanded and thinned the cortex. This location in a tubular bone of the hand is a common site for an enchondroma.

Radiology

The classic appearance is of a solitary or multiple lytic lesions arising from the medulla in the diaphysis or metaphysis of a tubular hand bone in the immature skeleton (*Figure 7.6*). The tumour is well defined and causes thinning and displacement of the cortex with no periosteal reaction. Enchondromas tend to calcify and can be hard to distinguish radiologically from bone infarcts or chondrosarcomas. Bone infarcts do not expand the bone and chondrosarcomas are associated with pain, growth and poor definition of the lesion.

Management

Most enchondromas do not need treatment, unless they become painful or enlarge over time, when curettage and grafting are warranted. The recurrence rate is high, but malignant change is rare.

Chondromyxoid Fibroma

This uncommon tumour occurs in the second and third decades. Patients often complain of a dull steady pain, which is usually worse at night. The tumour may occur in any bone, but is most common in the lower limb, particularly in the proximal tibia.

Pathology

Chondromyxoid fibromas consist of myxomatous material, hyaline cartilage and fibrous tissue.

Radiology

The tumours typically show as an eccentric well-defined lytic lesion in the metaphysis of the proximal tibia involving the cortex and medulla. There is a sclerotic rim, thinning of the cortex and no periosteal reaction. The lesion may be trabeculated and somewhat expansile (*Figure 7.7, see also Figure 7.1*).

Management

Treatment is by curettage and bone grafting, but there is a considerable risk of recurrence.

Differential Diagnosis

This includes non-ossifying fibroma, aneurysmal bone cyst and fibrous dysplasia.

Chondroblastoma

These are epiphyseal lesions, most commonly occurring in the proximal humerus (20%). Approximately 50% occur in the lower limb. They affect patients with open growth plates.

Radiology

The appearances are diagnostic. The tumour is round, lytic and well-defined with a fine sclerotic margin and situated in the epiphysis (*Figure 7.8*). Occasionally they may extend a little into the metaphysis. About 50% calcify.

Management

Treatment is by thorough curettage, but the risk of recurrence is high.

Differential Diagnosis

The differential diagnosis is listed in *Table 7.4*.

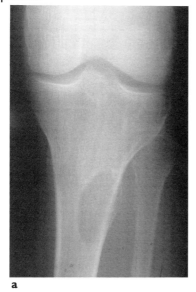 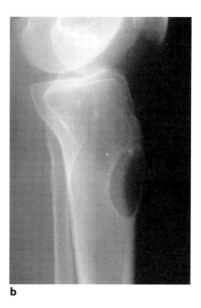

a   b

Figure 7.7 Chondromyxoid fibroma of the proximal tibia in a 17-year-old boy. **a,b** This is a typical lesion. It is an eccentric well-defined lytic lesion with a sclerotic rim, thinning of the cortex and no periosteal reaction (see also Figure 7.1).

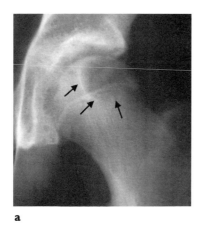 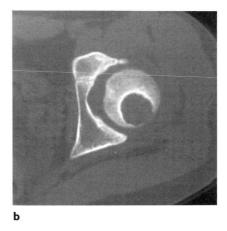

a   b

Figure 7.8 **a** Plain radiograph of a chondroblastoma of the left femoral capital epiphysis showing a well-defined lesion (arrows) within the left femoral capital epiphysis. There is a fine sclerotic margin and the lesion appears to extend into the metaphysis. **b** Computerized tomographic scan showing that the lesion is well-defined within the femoral capital epiphysis, with a fine sclerotic margin and no obvious extension into soft tissues.

Table 7.4 Differential diagnosis of chondroblastoma

Lytic epiphyseal lesions
Chondroblastoma
Infection
Subchondral cyst (e.g. post-traumatic, avascular)
Osteochondritis dissecans
Giant cell tumours (but very rare before growth
    plate closure)

Periosteal Chondroma (Juxtacortical Chondroma)

This tumour arises from the surface of the cortex, deep to the periosteum. More than 50% occur in the proximal humerus and the others occur throughout the long bones.

Radiology

A periosteal chondroma presents as a scalloped pit due to pressure erosion on the outer surface of the cortex with a mature periosteal reaction. A thin external shell of bone may be visible.

Management

Treatment is by a wide excision that includes the underlying cortex.

BENIGN TUMOURS OF FIBROUS ORIGIN

Fibrous Cortical Defect and Non-ossifying Fibroma

These are the most common lesions of bone, occurring in up to 40% of children with 90% in the distal femur. They are benign asymptomatic lesions and are usually discovered incidentally on radiographs. The term fibrous cortical defect is commonly used to refer to the lesion when it is small (2 cm or less) and non-ossifying fibroma when it is larger than 2 cm.

Radiology

Fibrous cortical defect and non-ossifying fibroma are histologically identical. They typically occur at the junction of the diaphysis and the metaphysis of a long bone and arise from the cortex. They are well-defined, lucent and oval-shaped with a thin sclerotic border (*Figure 7.9*). They are slightly expansile. Larger lesions have a lobulated 'soap bubble'

appearance and may present as a result of a fracture through the lesion.

Management

Treatment is usually unnecessary as most lesions resolve with time. If more than 50% of the diameter of a long bone is replaced by tumour, curettage and grafting are recommended to prevent a pathological fracture.

Differential Diagnosis

This includes chondromyxoid fibroma, and even an aneurysmal bone cyst if the lesion is large enough.

Fibrous Dysplasia

This is not a bone tumour as such but a developmental anomaly in which fibro-osseous tissue replaces normal bone. It may be monostotic or polyostotic and is discussed fully in Chapter 5. It often appears in the differential diagnosis of a number of bone tumours.

Fibrocartilaginous Dysplasia of the Tibia

This uncommon condition affects the medial portion of the proximal tibia, causing a varus deformity. Presentation is between six months and two years of

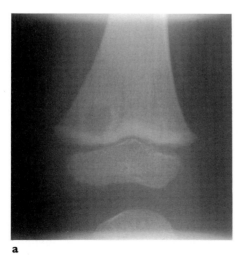
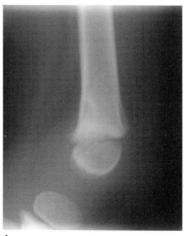

a   b

Figure 7.9 **a** Fibrous cortical defect producing an oval lucency in the distal left femur with minimal surrounding sclerosis. **b** A lateral view of Figure 7.9a shows the lesion is located posteriorly and the appearances are typical of a fibrous cortical defect.

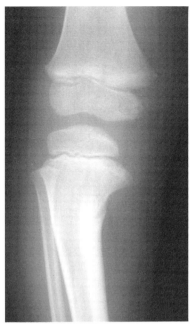

Figure 7.10 Fibrocartilaginous dysplasia. This two-year-old girl has severe bowing of the tibia due to an area of focal fibrocartilaginous dysplasia of the proximal tibia. This tends to be a progressive problem requiring an osteotomy.

age with unilateral bowing of the tibia. Radiographs show a radiolucency of the medial tibia at the site of the deformity (*Figure 7.10*).

Most children progress to severe deformity requiring a valgus osteotomy. Biopsies of the lesion demonstrate dense fibrous tissue, and in some, cartilaginous differentiation. There is no recurrence after surgical correction.

MISCELLANEOUS BENIGN BONE TUMOURS

Simple Bone Cyst (Unicameral Bone Cyst)

This is a common lesion. The aetiology is unclear, but it appears to arise from the growth plate and particularly affects the proximal femur and the proximal humerus (90%). It is rare around the knee. The calcaneus can also be affected. The lesion is initially metaphyseal, but grows away from the growth plate to be diaphyseal. It occurs in skeletally-immature individuals (male to female ratio is 2:1). Approximately 70% present between 4–10 years of age and disappear in adults. It is usually found after a pathological fracture or incidentally on radiology.

Radiology

The classical appearance is of a well-defined radiolucency in the proximal metaphysis of the humerus or femur (*Figure 7.11*). The cyst lies central in the shaft and causes thinning of the cortex and some expansion of the bone. There is no periosteal reaction unless there is a fracture. There is a narrow zone of transition with a sclerotic rim in parts. Occasionally a fragment of cortex may break off and 'fall' into the cyst ('falling fragment sign'). As the bone grows the tumour migrates slowly towards the diaphysis and disappears.

Management

The aim of treatment is to prevent pathological fractures. Injection of corticosteroid is the treatment of choice, and curettage and bone grafting is reserved for those lesions where injections are unsuccessful. Three injections can be tried. A fracture through the cyst may speed up its resolution. Reassurance that there is no risk of malignancy is often a large part of the management of the parents after advice from other clinicians who have not recognized the diagnosis.

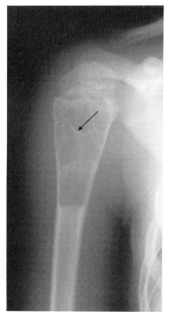

Figure 7.11 Simple bone cyst in the proximal humerus of a seven-year-old boy. This lesion arises from the growth plate of the proximal humerus and is particularly common in both this area and in the proximal femur. This is a well-defined central lucency in the metaphysis with some expansion of bone and cortical thinning. There is no periosteal reaction but there has been a pathological fracture with a 'falling fragment' sign (arrow).

Technique

Under general anaesthetic, a 19 gauge needle is inserted into the cyst. Clear yellow fluid is aspirated, which becomes stained after aspiration. A second needle is inserted and radiopaque dye is injected to confirm that the cyst is unicameral; 80 mg of depot methylprednisolone is then injected and the needles are removed. Radiographs are taken at three months. If there is no improvement a repeat injection is performed.

Differential Diagnosis

This includes a small aneurysmal bone cyst and fibrous dysplasia.

Aneurysmal Bone Cyst

This tumour occurs mainly in teenagers with 80% occurring between the ages of 10 and 20 years. However, it may occur at any age. Over 50% occur in large tubular bones and usually affect the metaphysis, while approximately 30% occur in the spine. They present with local pain and swelling.

Radiology

The name describes the appearance! Typically it is an eccentric, expansile lesion with a radiolucent (cystic) matrix located in the metaphysis of a bone. The cortex is very thin and may be invisible if the cystic space enlarges rapidly. The periosteum may be lifted at the margin with normal bone due to the rapid tumour expansion (a Codman triangle). The matrix is often trabeculated (*Figure 7.12*). The presence of multiple haemorrhagic and serous fluid levels on MRI is fairly characteristic.

Aneurysmal bone cysts are divided into two groups: primary and secondary.

- Primary have no known association with any other lesion.
- Secondary are found in association with other osseous lesions such as fibrous dysplasia or giant cell tumour and occasionally malignant lesions.

Differential Diagnosis

This depends on the site and includes giant cell tumour, telangiectatic osteosarcoma, osteoblastoma (in the spine), fibrous dysplasia and simple bone cyst.

Pathology

The lining is composed of haemosiderin-laden macrophages, multinucleated giant cells and a fibrous stroma, and usually small amounts of osteoid.

Management

The treatment of choice is curettage and grafting. There is a risk of recurrence and some aneurysmal bone cysts grow rapidly after surgery.

Giant Cell Tumour

This tumour is very rare in the skeletally immature. It mainly occurs in the late teens and the third and fourth decade. In skeletally immature children the tumour starts in the metaphysis and occasionally spreads to the epiphysis. In skeletally mature individuals, the tumour lies adjacent to subchondral bone. About 50% occur around the knee. The distal radius, proximal humerus and sacrum are also affected. In the spine, giant cell tumours affect the vertebral body.

Radiology

Four features are helpful in the diagnosis of a giant cell tumour (*Figure 7.13*):

- Giant cell tumours are rare before the epiphyses have fused.
- The tumour occurs at the end of the bone (i.e. it is subarticular). If it involves an apophysis it is subcortical.
- The tumour is eccentric, although when large it may extend across the medulla.
- The zone of transition is fairly sharp with no sclerosis.

Virtually all giant cell tumours fit these criteria. The tumour may thin and even breach the cortex with soft tissue extracortical extension. In these cases CT and especially MRI are helpful in showing the full extent of the lesion. Approximately 1% of giant cell tumours metastasize to lung. It is not possible to differentiate a malignant giant cell tumour from a benign one on radiological grounds, but metastases can occur after excisional curettage.

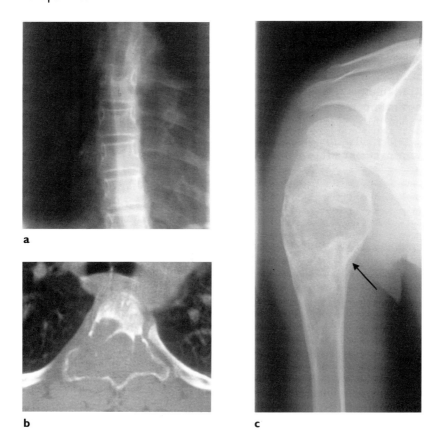

a

b

c

Figure 7.12 Aneurysmal bone cyst in the thoracic spine. **a** Plain radiograph of the thoracic spine showing loss of the normal architecture of T5. There is bony enlargement and loss of the normal outline of the pedicles, indicative of tumour. **b** Computerized tomographic scan at T5 shows an expansile tumour of mainly the posterior elements with loss of the normal posterior architecture and extension into the body of T5. The lesion is well defined, with a narrow sclerotic margin and osteopenic matrix. There are some bony septa running through the lesion and no obvious extension into soft tissues. This is typical of an aneurysmal bone cyst. **c** Aneurysmal bone cyst in the proximal humerus of a six-year-old boy. This lesion is markedly expansile (greater than a simple bone cyst, compare with Figure 7.11). The matrix is trabeculated and there is lifting of the periosteum (arrow) at the margin with normal bone due to rapid tumour expansion.

Pathology

The tumour consists of multinucleated giant cells in a background of fibrous tissue and small nucleated cells.

Management

In most instances curettage is used, often with adjuvant therapy (methylmethacrylate, phenol or liquid nitrogen). Resection is indicated for lesions in expendable bones such as the fibular head, for lesions that recur, and for lesions that destroy the bone beyond salvage.

Langerhans Cell Histiocytosis (Histiocytosis X)

This disease covers a broad spectrum of focal or systemic manifestations produced by the idiopathic proliferation of histiocytes. The cause and pathogenesis are uncertain. Males are affected more often than females (2:1) and the disease is rare in blacks. The spectrum can be divided into three overlapping groups.

- Eosinophilic granuloma (localized form, 70%). The disease is limited to bone and occurs in the 5–15-year age group. Patients present with local pain, tenderness and a mass or swelling. An associated low-grade fever, a raised erythrocyte

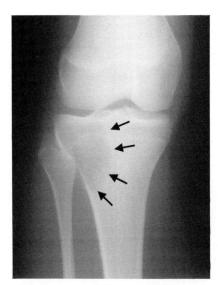

Figure 7.13 Plain radiograph showing a giant cell tumour of the proximal tibia in a 15-year-old girl. This tumour is rare in skeletally immature children, but when it occurs it starts in the metaphysis, occasionally spreading to the epiphysis. This lesion is well defined (arrows) without a sclerotic margin. There is thinning and expansion of the cortex.

sedimentation rate (ESR), mild leucocytosis and a normochromic anaemia mimic the features of osteomyelitis.

- Hand–Schüller–Christian disease (chronic recurring form, 20%). The bone lesions are multifocal and the reticuloendothelial system (RES) is involved. It predominantly affects 1–5-year-olds.
- Letterer–Siwe disease (fulminant form, 10%). There is disseminated involvement of bone and the RES with a fulminant clinical course. Affected children are less than two years of age.

Radiology

The skull, pelvis and long bones are frequently affected sites in children. In the skull and pelvis, the lesions are typically focal and punched-out with no periosteal reaction. A sclerotic rim appears with healing. In the long bones the lesion is diaphyseal or metaphyseal and the margins may be less well defined. The predominant associated new bone formation may mimic malignancy or osteomyelitis. In the spine the lesion classically produces a vertebra plana (*Table 7.5*) with total uniform collapse of the vertebral body (Calvé disease) (*Figure 7.14b*).

A bone scan shows increased uptake in the lesions with reactive bone formation and cold spots where

Table 7.5 Causes of vertebra plana

Eosinophilic granuloma
Infection (especially tuberculosis)
Ewing sarcoma
Metastatic tumour

there is pure osteolysis. The false negative rate can be up to 35%. MRI shows the lesions as low signal on T1, and high signal on T2 and enhancing with gadolinium. The adjacent soft tissue swelling and inflammatory change is well seen with MRI.

Management

This varies from observation or biopsy to curettage, total excision, injection with corticosteroids, radiotherapy or low-dose chemotherapy if the lesions are multiple. Children over two years of age with isolated or multifocal bony involvement have the most favourable prognosis.

Differential Diagnosis

This includes osteomyelitis and Ewing sarcoma.

Massive Osteolysis (Vanishing Bone Disease)

This very rare disorder occurs in children and young adults. There is progressive destruction and resorption of the bones, which are replaced by haemangiomatous tissue. There is no periosteal reaction. Pathological fractures occur and may be the presenting complaint, but there is no attempt at callus formation. The natural history is poor and there is no treatment available.

Osteofibrous Dysplasia

This disorder affects children up to five years of age and predominantly involves the tibia. In 20% the ipsilateral fibula is involved, and rarely the disease is bilateral. There is a lytic lesion in the anterior cortex of the mid-tibia causing bowing, and occasionally a fracture (*Figure 7.15*). The lesion heals spontaneously although pseudarthrosis and recurrence occasionally occur.

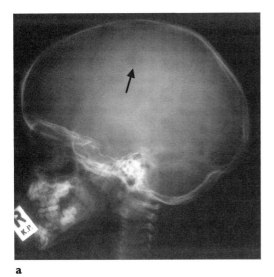

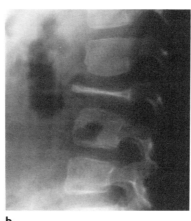

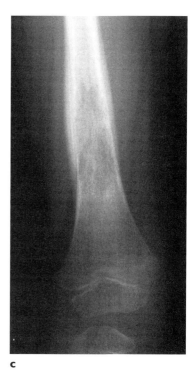

a   b   c

Figure 7.14   a Skull radiograph of a three-year-old boy with histiocytosis X. The skull is a frequently-affected site in this condition. The lesion (arrow) is punched out with no periosteal reaction and no sclerosis. A sclerotic rim may appear with healing.   **b** Lumbar spine in a three-year-old boy with histiocytosis X. Vertebra plana is a classical lesion in this condition. There is total uniform collapse of the vertebral body of L2 with maintenance of the adjacent discs. Bowel gas overlies L3. The differential diagnosis includes osteomyelitis and just occasionally a Ewing sarcoma will present with a vertebra plana.   **c** Distal femur in a three-year-old boy with histiocytosis X. This child presented with pain in the distal femur. There is an area of patchy destruction without well-defined margins and an associated laminated periosteal reaction. These appearances raise the possibility of an aggressive lesion, but note that there is no significant soft tissue mass. These appearances of histiocytosis X in the diaphysis can be quite misleading and at times appear quite aggressive, hence its notoriety as a great mimicker! (see also Figure 7.3).

Differential Diagnosis

This includes neurofibromatosis and fibrous dysplasia.

Haemangioma of Bone

This is rare in childhood.

Radiology

In vertebrae the classical appearance is of vertical striations with loss of secondary trabeculae. The vertebra may collapse producing neurological symptoms. In tubular bones the tumour is striated along the line of axis of the bone. In flat bones the tumour is well defined with a 'soap bubble' appearance. In the skull associated radiating spiculation gives a sunburst appearance. The mature nature of the bone distinguishes it from a malignant lesion.

MALIGNANT BONE TUMOURS

These are uncommon lesions.

Osteosarcoma

Osteosarcoma is defined as a primary malignant bone tumour characterized by the production of osteoid.

Most patients present in the second decade, although there is a smaller peak in the sixth decade secondary to Paget disease. The patients present with pain and swelling in the affected area. Occasionally they present following a pathological fracture. Systemic symptoms and lymphadenopathy are rare. The

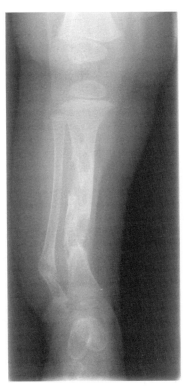

Figure 7.15 Osteofibrous dysplasia. In this seven-year-old girl there is bowing of the tibia with associated areas of osteopenia within the tibia and fibula.

tumours usually occur in the metaphyses of rapidly growing bones. About 50% of lesions occur around the knee, affecting the distal femoral and proximal tibial metaphyses. The proximal femur, proximal humerus and pelvis are also common sites.

Radiology

Plain films may be diagnostic. Initially destructive, the tumour has a permeative pattern with a wide zone of transition. Mineralization of the tumour osteoid combined with reactive new bone gives a sclerotic appearance (*Figure 7.16*). There is cortical destruction with an enlarging soft tissue mass, which may ossify irregularly (*Figures 7.17, 7.18*). There is an aggressive periosteal reaction; it is amorphous, irregular and perpendicular to the cortex (sunburst spicules). A Codman triangle may occur at the tumour margin. This is a reactive triangle of periosteal bone due to periosteal elevation by tumour deep to the periosteum. It signifies rapid soft tissue extension outside the cortex, and although often seen in osteosarcomas is not specific to this tumour. Some osteosarcomas may be extremely sclerotic and others much more lytic. CT will help identify the extent and location of the soft tissue mass and will clearly show the tumour mineralization. MRI will show the soft

tissue extent with neurovascular or joint involvement better than CT and is also useful for assessing the intramedullary spread. Intramedullary spread shows as a low signal on T1-weighted scans and a high signal on T2-weighted scans. The tumour will enhance with gadolinium. Telangiectatic osteosarcomas have a fairly characteristic appearance with high signal intensity on T1- and T2-weighted scans due to the large blood-filled cavities. Lung metastases can ossify and may be shown on a chest radiograph or with CT. A bone scan will detect any secondary spread to bone.

Pathology

There are five types: osteoblastic, chondroblastic, fibroblastic, mixed and telangiectatic. Most tumours are mixed. Some osteosarcomas may be multifocal.

Management

There have been many advances in the management of this tumour over the last 30 years. Resection is now the treatment of choice for the primary tumour and adjuvant chemotherapy is used pre- and post-operatively. These tumours are not radiosensitive. Amputation or limb-salvage resection is used depending on the spread of the tumour and ability to obtain a wide surgical margin. The five-year survival figures associated with amputation and limb-salvage resection are equal. The five-year disease-free state is approximately 55% using current chemotherapy protocols for those tumours without metastases. The effect of chemotherapy on the tumour is prognostic and the survival of patients with 90% tumour necrosis after preoperative chemotherapy is significantly better than that of those with less than 90%. Lung metastases are often resectable. Chemotherapy protocols are constantly under review and multi-centre trials have been very helpful in guiding decisions about the most appropriate regimes.

Differential Diagnosis

This includes osteomyelitis and trauma. Ewing sarcoma and occasionally post-traumatic myositis ossificans are also important differential diagnoses.

Juxtacortical Osteosarcoma

Parosteal and periosteal osteosarcomas behave differently to those of medullary origin. They are less locally aggressive, have less tendency to spread and

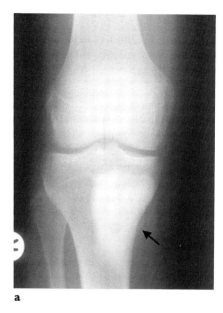

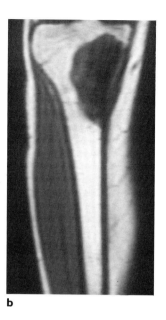

a   b

Figure 7.16 a Plain radiograph showing osteosarcoma of the proximal tibia in an 18-year-old boy. Osteosarcomas tend to arise in the metaphyses of the long bones around the knee. This is a sclerotic type of osteosarcoma, which is mainly intramedullary, but has extended outside the cortical margin with some aggressive periosteal reaction (arrow). **b** This T1-weighted magnetic resonance image (MRI) of the lesion shows it up clearly as low signal (i.e. 'dark') in the proximal tibia. MRI is vital in showing the full intramedullary extent.

are less common. They mainly occur in 20–30-year-olds. The distal femur is the most common site and symptoms are usually minimal.

- Parosteal osteosarcoma: the plain films are usually diagnostic. A dense mass of mature bone arises from the cortex and wraps around the shaft of the underlying bone. In the early stages a well-defined radiolucent line separates the tumour from normal cortex. Later, both cortex and medulla are involved. There is no or little associated soft tissue mass.
- Periosteal osteosarcoma: this rare and small tumour often arises from the anterior aspect of the tibia and tends to be diaphyseal. A typical lesion is hemispherical and closely applied to the bone cortex unlike parosteal osteosarcoma. The outside tumour margin may show radiating spicules.

Ewing Sarcoma

Ewing sarcoma typically presents in the 5–15 year age group with 75% occurring in under 20-year-olds. They usually present with pain and swelling, but occasionally mimic other conditions such as osteomyelitis. The male to female ratio is 3:2. Any bone can be affected, but the most common are the femur

(20%), pelvis (12%) and the humerus (11%). There is usually a palpable soft tissue mass.

Radiology

The classical appearance is of a permeative and destructive lesion in the diaphysis of a long bone (*Figure 7.19*). The tumour crosses the cortex, eroding it and spreading to form a large soft tissue mass. The classical Ewing sarcoma has a multilaminate (onion peel) periosteal reaction due to the periodic activity of the sarcoma. However, many have an amorphous or spiculated periosteal reaction. The tumour may have a mixed or sclerotic appearance, and this is more commonly seen when it occurs in a flat bone. The large soft tissue mass can be difficult to appreciate, especially when in a flat bone or an axial bone.

A CT scan or MRI is necessary to appreciate the full extent of the tumour. When arising from a rib, the tumour may cause a large pleural effusion. The bone destruction and soft tissue mass can be missed because of the effusion, but the CT scan will show the underlying tumour and its soft tissue extent. The tumour is hot on bone scan, and this will also pick up any bony metastases. MRI is invaluable for assessing the full intra- and extraosseous spread of the tumour. A chest radiograph and a CT scan of the lungs will show any lung metastases.

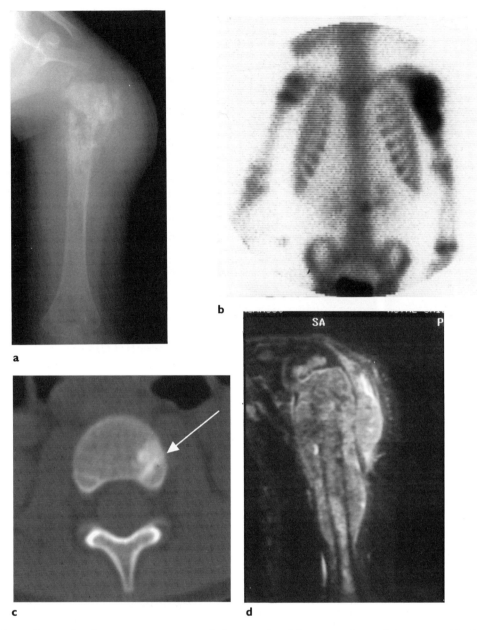

Figure 7.17 a Plain radiograph of an osteosarcoma of the proximal humerus in a three-year-old girl. This aggressive osteosarcoma is very unusual in a three-year-old as the highest incidence is during the second decade. The features shown are all of a highly malignant tumour (see Figure 7.2). **b** Bone scan shows marked uptake in the proximal humerus and in the left side of the L2 vertebral body. **c** Computerized tomographic scan of the lumbar spine showing a sclerotic lesion (arrow) in the left side of the L2 vertebral body with some soft tissue extension. Biopsy showed this to be osteosarcoma (metastatic spread). **d** Magnetic resonance image with gadolinium enhancement. The extent of the osteosarcoma in the humerus is clearly seen. There is a large soft tissue extension outside the original cortex of the bone and the tumour shows marked enhancement with gadolinium.

Differential Diagnosis

The main differential diagnosis is infection, which usually produces a smaller, less well-defined soft tissue mass, but this is not an infallible rule. The more sclerotic tumours may mimic an osteosarcoma, especially if they arise from a metaphysis. Ewing sarcoma is a very rare cause of a vertebra plana.

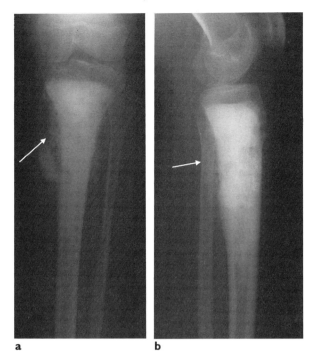

a   b

Figure 7.18   Osteosarcoma of the proximal tibia in a 13-year-old girl. **a,b** The plain films show the classical features of an osteosarcoma. There is dense sclerosis in the proximal tibial metaphysis extending right up to the growth plate and there is a highly aggressive periosteal reaction (arrows) along with patchy bony destruction.

Pathology

Ewing sarcoma is a small round cell tumour similar to lymphoma and secondary neuroblastoma. Approximately 90% of Ewing sarcomas stain positively with periodic acid–Schiff stain due to cytoplasmic glycogen, but this is not diagnostic; however, genetic studies showing an 11/22 gene translocation are diagnostic.

Management

The usual treatment is chemotherapy followed by surgical resection and then continuing chemotherapy for 12–18 months. Irradiation may be used in surgically-inaccessible areas. There is usually marked tumour shrinkage after initial chemotherapy. There is some debate as to the use of surgery versus radiotherapy for Ewing sarcoma, but there is no doubt that chemotherapy has greatly improved survival with both modalities. Surgical resection is used

whenever possible in our institution. Five-year survival is approximately 60%.

Chondrosarcoma

This malignant tumour originates from cartilage and is rare before 20 years of age. The tumour may arise from an enchondroma or an osteochondroma. Presentation is with pain of insidious onset or enlargement and pain in a benign lesion (e.g. an enchondroma or osteochondroma). The lesions are lytic and expansile on plain films, often with foci of ossification, and the cortex may be thinned, poorly defined or destroyed (*Figure 7.20*).

Management

Treatment is surgical excision. There is no role for adjuvant therapy.

Differential Diagnosis

This includes bone infarcts (rare in children) and enchondromas.

Fibrosarcoma

Fibrosarcoma presents with pain and swelling, and sometimes a pathological fracture through a long bone. The tumour consists of a fibrous proliferative matrix devoid of cartilage, osteoid or bone. It occurs in adults in the third and fourth decades, but in children it tends to occur in the first two years of life and has a better prognosis than in adults.

Radiology

Radiographs show osteolysis and moth-eaten destruction of bone with a wide zone of transition. There is cortical destruction, little periosteal reaction, a soft tissue mass, and occasionally mineralization. CT and MRI show the extent of the tumour.

Management

Treatment is surgical excision. There is no role for adjuvant therapy.

METASTATIC BONE TUMOURS

Bone metastases in children are much less common than in adults, and are most commonly associated

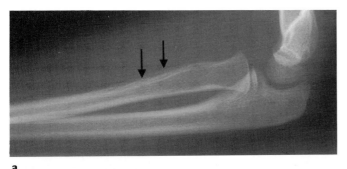

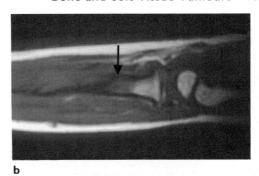

a

b

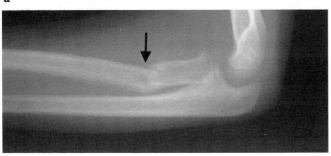

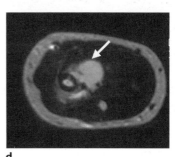

c

d

Figure 7.19   a Ewing sarcoma of the proximal radius in a six-year-old girl. Early films show subtle periosteal reaction (arrows) along the anterior surface of the proximal radius.   **b** One month later there has been further bony destruction of the radius and a pathological fracture has occurred (arrow).   **c** T1-weighted sagittal magnetic resonance image of the radius shows a low signal (arrow) at the site of the sarcoma in the proximal radius. Other images showed this extending down to the distal two-thirds.   **d** Axial T2-weighted MRI scan clearly shows the soft tissue extension of the tumour (high signal) (arrow).

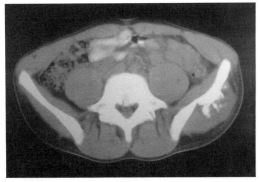

Figure 7.20 Chondrosarcoma in an 18-year-old. Computerized tomographic scan of the pelvis shows soft tissue calcification and an associated soft tissue mass of chondrosarcoma.

with neuroblastoma and leukaemia. Both usually occur in the under-five age group. A bone scan is the method of choice for screening the skeleton for metastases.

Leukaemia

Metastases may present as lytic transverse lines in the metaphyses, permeative infiltration of bone (some-

times with a periosteal reaction), focal destructive lesions, and occasionally a diffuse sclerosis (*Figure 7.21*).

Neuroblastoma

The metastases show as multiple destructive lytic areas involving any part of the skeleton. There may be associated areas of sclerosis. In the long bones the metastases may permeate the whole shaft or may be more focal and lytic in the metaphysis. They are often symmetrical and associated with periosteal new bone (*Figure 7.22*). Skull lesions are common. A bone scan shows the full extent of the metastatic spread.

Other Tumours

Other tumours metastasizing to bone include rhabdomyosarcoma, lymphoma, Wilms tumour and retinoblastoma (direct spread or bloodborne). Both osteosarcoma and Ewing sarcoma can metastasize to bone. In the former the metastases may resemble the primary tumour, in the latter they may resemble leukaemia or disseminated neuroblastoma.

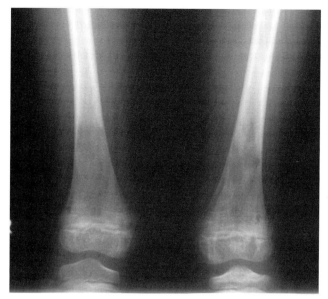

Figure 7.21 Leukaemia deposits in bone. There are widespread bony metastases from acute leukaemia in this five-year-old girl. There is extensive bony infiltration and destruction in the distal femora and the infiltration of leukaemic deposits throughout the pelvis causing osteopenia and patchy focal destruction.

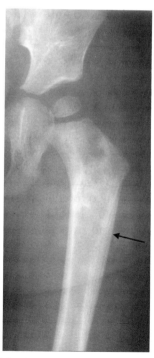

Figure 7.22 Metastatic neuroblastoma in a three-year-old boy who presented with a limp and feeling unwell. Plain films showed areas of sclerosis and some lucency in the proximal left femur associated with a laminated periosteal reaction laterally (arrow).

BENIGN VASCULAR TUMOURS

Haemangioma

These are the most common tumours of infancy. They are usually not seen at birth, but are characterized by rapid postnatal growth and slow involution. The proliferating phase occurs during the first year of life and is followed by the involution phase lasting several years. Haemangiomas rarely cause bony hypertrophy or distortion.

Vascular Malformations

In contrast to haemangiomas these are present at birth, although some may appear later. They can be separated into low-flow (capillary, venous, lymphatic or combined) and high-flow (arteriovenous) lesions. Low-flow vascular malformations are frequently associated with skeletal hypertrophy in the affected limb, distortion or limb inequality (*Figure 7.23*).

Radiology

Plain films may be normal. MRI and angiography are the investigations of choice for diagnosing and delineating the full extent of the lesion. Ultrasound may be of use for high-flow lesions.

Management

Embolization is occasionally used for deep extensive lesions with obvious large feeding vessels. Sclerotherapy may be used, but complications include necrosis of adjacent tissue and overlying skin. Excision is often very difficult to achieve and the lesion recurs if the excision is incomplete. However, resection may be indicated to reduce bulk and improve contour and function. Limited excision may also play a role in controlling chronically painful areas within a venous anomaly.

Combined Vascular Malformations and Hypertrophy Syndromes

- Klippel–Trénaunay syndrome: this is an association of a vascular anomaly with limb hypertrophy. The vascular lesion should be considered as a combined capillary/lymphatic/venous malformation. In 95% of patients the lower limb is involved, usually unilaterally.

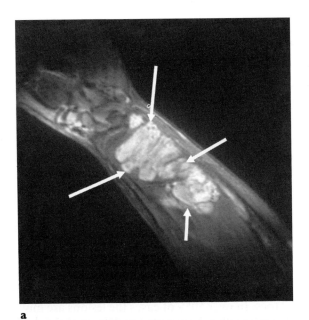

a

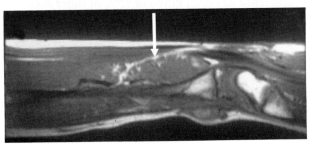

b

Figure 7.23 a Low-flow venous vascular malformation in a 14-year-old boy. T1-sagittal magnetic resonance image (MRI) shows an abnormal mass (arrows) around the distal radius. **b** T1-MRI with contrast enhancement (and fat suppression) shows clear enhancement of the vascular malformation. MRI is a good modality for showing the soft tissue extent of the vascular malformation.

- Parkes–Weber syndrome: this condition is less common than Klippel–Trénaunay syndrome. The differences are that the vascular lesion in this case is arteriovenous and the upper limb is more commonly affected than the lower.
- Maffuci syndrome: this condition is characterized by the coexistence of vascular malformations and enchondromatosis (Ollier disease). Complex vascular anomalies are present in the subcutaneous tissues. These are usually venous, but sometimes lymphatic in nature. Malignant tumours develop in approximately 20% of these patients.

BENIGN SOFT TISSUE TUMOURS OF FIBROUS ORIGIN (THE FIBROMATOSES)

These conditions are important in the differential diagnosis of soft tissue sarcomas of infancy and childhood. The fibromatoses are proliferative lesions composed of cells resembling fibroblasts associated with the production of a variable amount of collagen and ground substance. They have ill-defined margins and tend to recur locally. Some fibromatoses undergo spontaneous regression after a period of growth, while others continue to grow progressively. They are classified as shown in *Table 7.6*. Those that are commonly seen in orthopaedic practice are discussed below.

Juvenile Subcutaneous Fibromatosis (Fibrous Hamartoma of Infancy)

This lesion usually presents in the first decade with a subcutaneous nodule fixed to the skin and underlying fascia. The lesions tend to be multiple and may occur in any part of the body, but do show a predilection for the upper body and arms. The majority of these lesions resolve completely.

Aggressive Fibromatosis

This lesion is very uncommon. It is characterized by fibrous proliferation in deep tissues that shows continuous and relentless growth if untreated and tends to recur locally, infiltrating and destroying local structures. When the histology is bland, yet the behaviour aggressive, the term 'desmoid' has been applied. In other cases it is difficult to differentiate

Table 7.6 Classification of the fibromatoses

Juvenile subcutaneous fibromatosis (fibrous
  hamartoma of infancy)
Aggressive fibromatosis (desmoids)
Plantar and palmar fibromatosis
Fibromatosis colli
Juvenile aponeurotic fibroma
Congenital generalized fibromatosis
Nasopharyngeal angiofibroma
Recurring angiofibroma
Recurring digital fibroma of Reye
Fibromatoses of bone

these lesions from fibrosarcomas. Aggressive fibromatosis may occur anywhere.

The tumours usually present in children over ten years of age as a slowly enlarging mass. It may appear in the sole of the foot or as a thick cord in the subcutaneous tissues of the limbs or trunk. MRI is the best imaging modality.

Management

This lesion has a marked tendency to recur after simple excision. Although it is not a malignant lesion, it may be locally aggressive and tends to grow along muscle planes. Wide excision is essential as recurrences tend to be more invasive and may appear more proximally. Amputation may occasionally be required.

Plantar and Palmar Fibromatosis

Plantar fibromatosis can occur at any age between birth and 70 years, but is usually a disease of young adults. One or more nodules can be felt in the sole as hard round lesions, which are firmly attached to the plantar aponeurosis and cause discomfort on walking. Approximately 10% are bilateral. It rarely occurs in association with palmar fibromatosis.

Most of these lesions can be treated non-operatively and some regress spontaneously. The indications for operative treatment include pain and local aggression as demonstrated by clinical examination, evidence of invasion of neurovascular structures, and MRI. Predictable results are difficult to achieve and recurrence is common after local excision, often with a more aggressive rapidly growing form of the disease. The most reliable outcome has been after a wide radical excision including skin, with grafting of the defect. Methotrexate has been used as adjuvant treatment for the more aggressive lesions.

Plantar fibromatosis of the heel in childhood is a separate condition from plantar fibromatosis seen in young adults. It has also been referred to as benign fatty heel lumps, but the histology shows fibrous tissue. The lesion is on the plantar medial aspect of the heel in its anterior portion and may be bilateral. It does not usually require treatment as it does not behave in an aggressive fashion and usually resolves spontaneously.

Palmar fibromatosis has an unclear relationship with Dupuytren contracture. It is much less common than plantar fibromatosis. No contractures developed in the small group at our institution.

Congenital Generalized Fibromatosis

This is a rare form of fibromatosis in which multiple subcutaneous and visceral fibroblastic nodules present at or shortly after birth. Many of the reported cases have been fatal. Bone lesions may develop and present as radiolucent defects, typically in the metaphyses.

Recurring Digital Fibroma of Reye

These lesions tend to occur in children less than one year of age and present clinically as firm subcutaneous nodules on the dorsum or sides of the fingers or toes. In over 50% of cases the lesions are multiple. Recurrence has been noted in 75% of those excised.

Fibromatoses in Bone

Bone may be involved by:

- Fibromatoses that arise outside bone and invade it.
- Primary fibromatosis.

These primary lesions have been described at all ages, with most occurring in the metaphyseal ends of long bones.

BENIGN SOFT TISSUE TUMOURS OF NEURAL ORIGIN

Neurofibroma

This can be solitary or multiple (neurofibromatosis, see Chapter 5). They may arise in the skin or on a peripheral nerve. Most can be left, but if solitary and not involving a major nerve, they may be removed. If there is any increase in the size of the lesions in neurofibromatosis, the lesion must be biopsied because of the small chance of malignancy.

Neurilemmoma

This tumour arises from the nerve sheath. It is usually solitary and slow growing. It can arise from any nerve, but does not invade the nerve. The treatment is marginal excision of the tumour, leaving the nerve itself.

BENIGN FAT TUMOURS

Lipoma

These tumours are not common in children. They may be subcutaneous, intramuscular or occasionally subperiosteal, and are painless, non-tender and soft.

Radiology

Radiologically a lipoma appears as a clearly-defined radiolucent mass in the soft tissues. CT (very low attenuation) and MRI (high signal on T1- and T2-weighted images) images are also characteristic and will show the full extent, but are not usually indicated.

BENIGN SYNOVIAL TUMOURS

Pigmented Villonodular Synovitis

This is a rare chronic inflammatory process causing synovial proliferation. It is principally a disease of adolescents and young adults and affects mainly the knee and hips, but finger joints and tendon sheaths can be involved. It presents with a swollen painful joint and may be mistaken for monarticular juvenile chronic arthritis (see Chapter 12) or low-grade infection such as tuberculosis (see Chapter 11).

Radiology

The aberrant synovium produces large periarticular bony defects with fine sclerotic margins, giving a cystic appearance. Synovial thickening is visible as lobular soft tissue swelling around the joint. Matrix calcification and juxta-articular osteopenia are rare.

Pathology

The synovium is hyperplastic with both nodules within it and villi on its articular surface. It is brown or deep purple as a result of haemosiderin deposition. The synovium contains fibroblastic tissue with foamy histiocytes and multinucleate cells or giant cells.

Management

Surgical excision is the procedure of choice. In the knee the synovectomy should be as extensive as possible, including a posterior synovectomy, because recurrence is common. In the past radio-therapy has been used because of the rate of recurrence, but this is unwise in the growing child.

Synovial Osteochondromatosis

This usually occurs in adults over 20 years of age, but children can be affected. The presenting symptom is progressive pain and limitation of movement in the affected joint, which in 70% of cases is the knee. The hip and elbow can also be affected. Sometimes there are symptoms of a loose body in the joint. Some present as a persistent swelling and effusion of the joint like a monarticular inflammatory arthritis, and others as adults in the end-stage with osteoarthritis. One joint only is the rule. The synovium undergoes a metaplasia, depositing foci of cartilage in the joint and these eventually calcify.

Radiology

There is synovial thickening with a joint effusion. The ossified synovium can be seen on the plain film (*Figure 7.24*) whereas those that are purely cartilaginous can only be seen by arthrography or MRI. A large mass of intrasynovial loose bodies may cause pressure erosion on the adjacent bone. There is inevitably premature secondary degenerative change.

Management

Removal of the loose bodies can give temporary relief. There is a tendency to resolution, but if problems persist a total synovectomy is required.

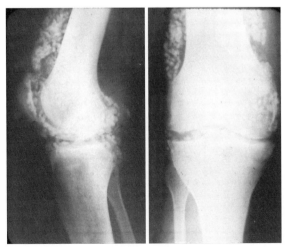

Figure 7.24 Synovial osteochondromatosis in the knee of a 19-year-old boy. There are multiple well-defined opacities within the knee extending into the suprapatellar pouch.

Sometimes only a part of the synovium of one joint is affected and the results of excision are better.

OTHER BENIGN SOFT TISSUE TUMOURS

Tumoral Calcinosis

This rare condition of unknown aetiology is characterized by the appearance of firm painless swellings adjacent to joints. It presents in the first or second decades, is often familial and affects blacks more than whites. The serum phosphate is often high. Plain films and CT show well-defined lobulated masses of calcification in periarticular soft tissue (*Figure 7.25*). As the lesions enlarge they cause disfiguration, functional impairment, and secondary ulceration and infection. Treatment consists of complete surgical resection, but recurrence is common.

Dermatomyositis

This multisystem disorder consists of non-suppurative inflammation of striated muscle. It is most common in adolescent girls and presents with skeletal muscle weakness (particularly proximal) and tenderness associated with a characteristic heliotrope facial rash. Initially plain films show muscle and subcutaneous oedema, which may be followed by extensive calcification in these sites and in the skin

(*Figure 7.26*). Spontaneous remission can occur, but in the majority tissue necrosis, muscle wasting and contractures supervene (see Chapter 10).

MALIGNANT SOFT TISSUE TUMOURS

Rhabdomyosarcoma

Rhabdomyosarcoma is a malignant tumour of muscle. It is the most common malignant soft tissue tumour in patients under 15 years of age. It may occur in the head, neck, genito-urinary tract, retroperitoneum and extremities, and also in hollow viscera. Approximately 20% occur in the pelvis, arising from the prostate, bladder, uterus and vagina. In orthopaedic practice it presents as a painless mass within the muscles, usually of the shoulder or pelvic girdle. It is highly malignant and must not be confused with a simple muscle rupture.

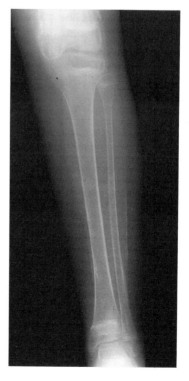
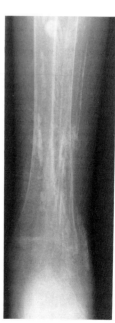

Figure 7.26 a Dermatomyositis in a ten-year-old girl. There is linear calcification in the soft tissues of the lower limb. **b** Two years later the soft tissue calcification is now florid. Note the underlying bony osteopenia.

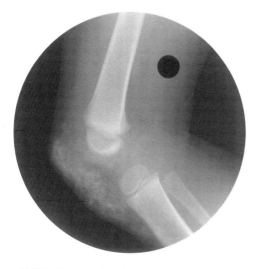

Figure 7.25 Tumoral calcinosis showing lobulated calcific densities around the knee in this four-year-old boy.

Radiology

Ultrasound, CT scan and MRI are all helpful in demonstrating the site and extent of the tumour. Both CT and MRI show an infiltrative homogeneous soft tissue mass (*Figure 7.27*).

Management

Treatment is a combination of chemotherapy and surgery. The surgery must be radical because the lesion is usually high grade and recurrence is common. If imaging shows evidence of spread across compartments, amputation may be necessary.

Liposarcoma

Liposarcoma arises from fatty tissue and is occasionally seen in children. It presents as an enlarging painful mass. Plain radiographs may show calcification and there may be erosion or scalloping of the cortex of adjacent bone. On CT there are areas of both high and low (fat) attenuation. MRI can define the extent of the tumour and shows high signal (fat) on T1- and T2-weighted images.

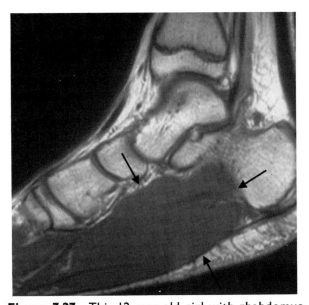

Figure 7.27 This 12-year-old girl with rhabdomyosarcoma presented with pain and a mass in the foot. A T1-weighted magnetic resonance image shows the extent of the rhabdomyosarcoma (low signal, arrows) in the soft tissues.

Table 7.7 Differential diagnosis of exquisitely tender lesions

Haemangioma
Synovial sarcoma
Neuroma
Abscess
Glomus tumour
Fibrosarcoma
Acute inflammation

Synovial Sarcoma

Synovial sarcoma is rare, but highly malignant. It often originates in the tissues surrounding the capsule of the joint rather than the synovium itself. Most are found around the hip, knee or shoulder, but it can also present in the hand and foot. Pain is the commonest presenting symptom, often occurring before the lesion becomes obvious. The lesion may present as an 'exquisitely tender' lesion. It metastasizes to lymph nodes in 25% of cases.

Radiology

There is a large soft tissue mass, usually close to a joint. Many show evidence of bone erosion, and because the lesion is painful, there is periarticular osteoporosis. Many show soft tissue calcification, which helps differentiate them from pigmented villonodular synovitis. CT is good at demonstrating the calcification; MRI shows a heterogeneous multilocular mass with internal septa.

Differential Diagnosis

The differential diagnosis of 'exquisitely tender' lesions is given in *Table 7.7*.

Management

The basic form of treatment is surgical resection, which often has to be amputation. Adjuvant chemotherapy is of equivocal efficacy, and radiotherapy is used occasionally.

FURTHER READING

Adler CP, Kozlowski K. Primary Bone Tumours and Tumorous Conditions in Children. Springer–Verlag, Berlin, 1993.

Bell SN, Campbell PE, Cole WG, Menelaus MB. Tibia vara caused by focal fibrocartilaginous dysplasia. *J Bone Joint Surg*. 1985; **67B**: 780–784.

Dahlin D. *Bone Tumours*, second edition. Charles C Thomas, Springfield, 1967.

Enneking WF. *Musculoskeletal Tumour Surgery*. Churchill Livingstone, New York, 1983.

Helms CA. *Fundamentals of Skeletal Radiology*. WB Saunders, Philadelphia, 1989.

Jaffe HL. *Tumours and Tumorous Conditions of the Bones and Joints*. Lea and Febiger, Philadelphia, 1968.

Mirra JM, Picci P, Gold R. *Bone Tumours: Clinical, Radiologic and Pathologic Correlations*. Lea and Febiger, Philadelphia, 1989.

Stoker D. *Bone Tumours in Diagnostic Radiology*, edited by RG Grainger and AJ Allison. Churchill Livingstone, Edinburgh, 1986.

Chapter 8

The Orthopaedic Management of Cerebral Palsy

H Kerr Graham

Cerebral palsy (CP) is defined as a disorder of movement and posture due to a defect or lesion in the developing brain. Cerebral palsy is not a diagnosis, rather a convenient description for a group of conditions with effects that can vary as growth takes place.

Incidence

The incidence is about two per 1000 live births and is static or even rising slightly because of the changes in neonatal intensive care and the survival of very-low-birth-weight and premature infants. About 50% of children have normal intelligence, and about 25% go on to be self-supporting as an adult.

Aetiology

Cerebral palsy may be due to many different factors, alone or in combination, and can occur before, during or after birth (*Table 8.1*). Contrary to popular and often legal opinion, the majority of children with CP are not the result of an obstetrical 'accident', which could have been avoided. Genetic factors may be implicated in about 20%. In a substantial proportion, the cause is uncertain. It is likely that the aetiology is multifactorial in some cases (e.g. a woman who smokes in pregnancy, goes into premature labour and gives birth to a low birth-weight baby in difficult circumstances). Maternal infections giving rise to CP have been given the acronym TORCH (**TO**xoplasmosis, **R**ubella, Cytomegalovirus, **H**erpes simplex).

Classification

Cerebral palsy can be described according to the types of motor disorder as:

- Spastic, pyramidal system (motor cortex).
- Athetoid, extrapyramidal system (basal ganglia).
- Ataxic (cerebellum and brain stem), often genetic.
- Rigid (basal ganglia and motor cortex).
- Mixed.

Table 8.1 Factors involved in the aetiology of cerebral palsy

Prenatal	Perinatal	Postnatal
Placental insufficiency, toxaemia Smoking, drugs and alcohol	Hypoxia due to prematurity, low birth weight, difficult delivery	Infection
Maternal infections: TORCH (toxoplasmosis, rubella, cytomegalovirus, herpes simplex)	Infections: meningitis and encephalitis	Trauma
Genetic conditions	Kernicterus, haemolytic disease of the newborn	

Spastic CP is the typical form of CP seen by the orthopaedic surgeon.

Athetoid CP is characterized by involuntary movement, variable tone and speech difficulties, which may belie the child's intelligence. Dystonic posturing is common, contractures are rare, and the role of surgery is very limited. Kernicterus used to be the main cause, but this is now uncommon because of the improved management of neonatal jaundice.

Cerebral palsy can also be classified according to the limbs involved.

- Monoplegia: one limb is involved; very rare.
- Hemiplegia: one side of the body is involved.
- Diplegia: the lower limbs are involved, often asymmetrically. The upper limbs are minimally involved.
- Triplegia: three limbs involved; very rare. The 'uninvolved limb' is usually slightly affected.
- Quadriplegia or tetraplegia: all four limbs are involved. Some of these are termed 'whole body involvement'. These children have the most severe involvement and may drool and have difficulties with sitting balance.

Clinical Features

The presentation of CP depends on three main factors: the severity and location of the neurological lesion, and the age of the child.

The children with severe CP often have absence of normal reflexes such as blinking and sucking. Some infants are ill from birth with respiratory distress, fitting, metabolic disturbance and infection. Later, persistence of abnormal reflexes such as Moro's reflex, may indicate a significant brain injury. These children are usually monitored by paediatricians as being 'at risk.' The early signs of CP are recognized and lead to early referral to orthopaedic surgeons.

Other children with less remarkable birth histories and less severe CP present at walking age with a minor gait disturbance or a delay in walking. The orthopaedic surgeon may be the first to see these children and it is important that the diagnosis is made because parents are slow to forgive a delay in diagnosis. Being sure about the diagnosis and also communicating such an emotive diagnosis to parents is daunting. Having support from paediatric colleagues in this area is essential.

After the early identification of CP many parents will ask whether their child will walk. In general terms, all hemiplegic children will walk, 75% of diplegic children walk, but less than 25% of quadriplegic children will walk. In addition, CP children who sit by two years of age are likely to walk, and those who can stand by four years of age are likely to walk. Children who have not started to walk by seven years of age are unlikely to walk.

The main problems presenting in the musculoskeletal system are spasticity, weakness, lack of voluntary control, poor coordination and sensory impairment. However, orthopaedic management can only address spasticity and the deformity it causes.

Pathology

The pathological effects of spastic cerebral palsy in the limbs can be divided into three main stages. These overlap in the same child and cannot be clearly defined from one to another. Nevertheless, the attempt to define the stage of the pathology at each joint level in each child can be useful because the management of each stage is very different (Figure 8.1).

Stage 1: Dynamic contractures
Muscle tone is increased and there are dynamic contractures. There is no fixed deformity at the joint and the dynamic contracture can be overcome during examination (e.g. the child may walk in equinus, but on the couch the foot can be corrected into dorsiflexion).

Stage 2: Muscle contractures
There is shortening of the muscle–tendon unit in relation to bone length. This produces a fixed deformity at the joint, which cannot be overcome at examination or under an anaesthetic. Throughout growth the muscles of the child with CP struggle and often fail to keep up with bone length.

Stage 3: Secondary bone changes
This is characterized by torsional abnormalities of long bones such as medial femoral torsion and lateral tibial torsion. The fixed deformities sometimes lead to joint subluxation and dislocation and even painful degenerative arthritis, especially in the hip joint.

Management

General
Cerebral palsy can involve many different parts of the developing brain and its effects are protean. Epilepsy, speech and hearing difficulties, visual defects, feeding difficulties, drooling, and learning and behavioural problems are frequent. It is therefore important that the child is looked after in a multidisciplinary setting. Usually a paediatrician with a specific interest in this area would coordinate

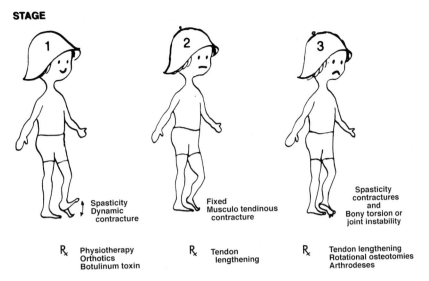

Figure 8.1   The stages of cerebral palsy and its management, modified after Rang. (Wenger DR, Rang M. *The Art and Practice of Children's Orthopaedics*. Raven Press, New York, 1993.)

such a team with the help of physiotherapists and other children's specialists where necessary. Many children with CP may not require orthopaedic involvement. More important issues for these children may include suitable education, which should be addressed by the paediatrician involved.

Orthopaedic

Orthopaedic management of CP is based on an understanding of the natural history of the condition. All forms of management are based on treating the effects of the neurological impairment rather than the lesion itself. This clearly defines the limitations of such forms of treatment.

Orthopaedic management of the child with CP can only address the problems of spasticity and the deformity caused by spasticity.

- In stage 1, where there are dynamic contractures, treatment is aimed at preventing the development of fixed contractures by stretching and casting by the physiotherapist and to a lesser extent by the use of orthoses. Other measures to reduce the spasticity can be attempted (e.g. injecting the motor nerve with phenol or the muscle belly with botulinum toxin). Selective posterior rhizotomy (SPR) has also been used to reduce the amount of spasticity.
- In stage 2, where there is fixed deformity, tendon release or lengthening is necessary to correct the deformity and to prevent recurrence. Although many different types of muscle transfer have been described their popularity has waned due to the unpredictable results. Some of these operations resulted in overcorrection with the development

of an opposite deformity, and in some the transfer did not work because the power of the transferred muscle had been overestimated. Split transfers are a major improvement because they are more likely to work in the appropriate phase and overcorrection is unlikely.
- In stage 3, where there are bone abnormalities, bone surgery such as derotation osteotomy or joint arthrodesis is necessary. This is combined with tendon lengthening to correct the underlying muscle imbalance.

The limitations of surgery

Many of the operations now used in children with CP were developed for the management of children with poliomyelitis. Poliomyelitis causes a pure lower motor neurone disorder. The resultant flaccid muscle weakness, muscle imbalance and deformities lend themselves to clear analysis then surgery with predictable and satisfying results. The upper motor neurone disorder of CP is much more complex and unpredictable. For example, dystonia can be difficult to distinguish from spasticity, but requires different management. It can be difficult to distinguish between the dynamic problems of spasticity and true musculotendinous contractures and between primary abnormalities and secondary compensations. When a child with poliomyelitis is observed walking and then examined on the couch, the findings are usually consistent. In children with CP, gait patterns and the findings on the examination couch often differ, the 'vertical examination' being much more important than the 'horizontal examination.' It can be difficult to analyse the problem scientifically and provide a basis for management. However, the increased use of gait analysis laboratories has greatly improved understanding of the problems these children encounter.

Physiotherapy

Physiotherapy is central to the management of the child with CP. The physiotherapist stimulates gross and fine motor skills and works in partnership with the family to help the child achieve his optimal motor function. As this partnership often develops over many years, the physiotherapist is in an ideal position to advise, educate and monitor the child's progress.

The physiotherapist uses exercises, stretching and positioning, together with equipment and orthoses. The aims are to achieve a good sitting posture, to help with walking, and to practice balance and coordination. The physiotherapist supervises the conservative management of the spasticity. Stretching is used to prevent the development of fixed contractures. The most important therapist in this context is the parent who performs the stretching and positioning taught by the physiotherapist at home on a regular basis. Inhibitory casting may be used in the management of dynamic equinus deformity.

The management of the child who is involved in a good physiotherapy programme is much more successful and orthopaedic intervention is much more satisfactory than for those children without physiotherapy supervision. Children who are being managed by an experienced therapist rarely present with a late problem such as hip dislocation. The experienced therapist can detect the progressive loss of hip abduction seen in hip subluxation and then refer the child on to an orthopaedic surgeon. As they can spend much longer with the child and see them in a number of different situations they are well placed to advise on goals to aim for with the child. The orthopaedic surgeon can then more easily decide on the suitable management for the child. Together with the family, the physiotherapist can also prepare the child for surgery, and following intervention, the physiotherapist supervises the postoperative rehabilitation. Clearly the surgeon and physiotherapist should work together for the good of the child; teamwork is vital.

Other therapies

Because of the incurable nature of the brain impairment and the limited ability of conventional medicine to alter the long term prognosis, many parents seek different approaches. These include conductive education, Vojta therapy, and physical techniques such as acupressure and point percussion. There is no evidence that one form of therapy is more beneficial than another. Conductive education is under evaluation in a number of centres, but the evidence so far suggests no major advantage over conventional physiotherapy.

Orthotics

The role of bracing in the management of the child with CP is limited. Fixed deformities cannot be corrected by braces, and children with dynamic deformities do not always tolerate the prescribed brace. High-level bracing is rarely indicated or helpful.

The recent development of thermoplastic materials for bracing has been a great advantage in the management of these children. They can provide effective support with a reasonable cosmetic appearance and are accepted much more readily than the old fashioned calipers made from metal and leather, which labelled the child as a 'cripple,' and were often rejected on cosmetic grounds.

The most useful and widely prescribed brace is the ankle–foot orthosis (AFO) (*Figure 8.2*). This should not be prescribed without clear goals in mind. The many variations, which can be selected intelligently to help the individual child, include the following.

- Leaf spring AFO. A child with a mild hemiplegia and a drop foot gait in the swing phase may benefit from a leaf spring AFO. The back of the AFO is ground away to allow active flexion in stance, but the foot is prevented from dropping into equinus in the swing phase of gait. This compensates for lack of phasic activity in the ankle dorsiflexors. The flexibility of the AFO also allows the ankle to dorsiflex in stance. Varus and valgus deformities of the forefoot can be controlled to some degree.

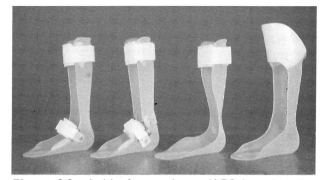

Figure 8.2 Ankle–foot orthoses (AFOs) used in the management of children with cerebral palsy. From left to right: solid AFO, hinged AFO, leaf spring AFO and ground reaction AFO.

- Hinged AFO. This provides a greater degree of adjustability in the position of the ankle and also permits dorsiflexion under the influence of weight bearing. There is also some control over varus and valgus deformities of the forefoot.
- Solid AFO. The standard solid AFO is widely prescribed because it controls forefoot deformities in stance phase. The loss of a normal heel–toe progression can be partially compensated for by accurate placement of a sole rocker.
- Floor reaction or ground reaction AFO (GRA-FO). This is used for crouch gait where there is hip and knee flexion at heel strike. This may be due to calcaneus deformity, which is sometimes seen in CP after injudicious heel cord surgery. This is in contrast to the other three types of AFO described above which are used for increasingly severe equinus gait deformities in CP. The floor reaction AFO blocks excessive dorsiflexion of the ankle in the late stance phase and knee extension can be improved, reducing the demands on the quadriceps. Active plantar flexion is possible in some designs of GRAFO.

Orthopaedic surgery

In stage 1 with dynamic contractures, tendon lengthening is unpredictable and usually not advocated. However, much recent work on CP has centred on attempts to resolve the dynamic contractures to alter the natural history of the condition.

Botulinum toxin   Injections of botulinum toxin into specific muscle groups reduce muscle tone and spasticity. Botulinum toxin blocks conduction at the neuromuscular junction by binding irreversibly with the receptors of the motor end-plate (otherwise described as a chemodenervation of muscle). The effects of the injection wear off after 3–6 months because of the sprouting of new axons from the spinal cord to reinnervate the muscle. However, in some favourable circumstances, the effects of a single injection may last longer. The most frequently injected target muscles are the calf, hamstrings and adductors.

Selective posterior rhizotomy   Selective posterior rhizotomy (SPR) is a major neurosurgical procedure in which some of the dorsal nerve rootlets in the lumbar spinal cord are sectioned, resulting in a reduction in resting muscle tone. Many children will show an improvement in their walking patterns because of the reduction in spasticity and it is possible that the incidence and severity of contractures may be reduced. There are, however, a number of complications following this type of surgery including spinal deformity, weakness of the lower limbs, hip subluxation and progression of foot deformities.

Stage 2 surgery

After progression to stage 2   Many children who have been in an optimal physiotherapy programme, including those who have been treated with botulinum toxin or SPR, eventually progress to stage 2 with fixed contractures of the muscle tendon units. These contractures may be manifested as difficulties in walking, and surgical tendon lengthening may be indicated.

The essential paradox of orthopaedic surgery in CP is that the operations are simple, but the decisions concerning timing and choice of procedure are difficult. In the past, large numbers of children who have had orthopaedic operations have had disappointing outcomes. For example, a diplegic child walking on his toes with a pattern of hip and knee flexion who has a series of tendon lengthening operations at the hip, knees and ankles can sometimes be made much better, while other apparently similar children can be made much worse. The uncertainty of outcome has led many therapists and physicians to advise against orthopaedic surgery.

Many surgeons have preferred to perform surgery in a 'piecemeal' fashion operating at one level only and studying the results before advising surgery at a second or third level. This may result in the 'birthday syndrome' identified by Mercer Rang and others. The child is admitted every year or so for orthopaedic operations, cast and mobilization and long periods of rehabilitation. He seems to spend most of his childhood birthdays in hospital having an operation or in therapy afterwards. However, an even more pressing reason to consider multiple level surgery is that the involved levels are interlinked in a way that precludes achieving the same quality of outcome from staged procedures as from surgery performed as a single event.

It is therefore important to identify all the abnormalities in the child and aim for correction at one operation to avoid the necessity of multiple admissions. It is, however, a daunting prospect to correctly identify all the musculotendinous contractures and bone torsional abnormalities by watching the child walk and static examination only.

The introduction of three-dimensional gait analysis and an understanding of the kinematics and kinetics of pathological gait have had an immense impact on improving the outcome following surgical intervention. Using three-dimensional gait analysis, a very full description of the abnormalities at the hips, knees, ankles and feet can be obtained, and a precise surgical plan can be identified and tailored to the individual child's needs. The introduction of this type of assessment has enabled a much more rapid evaluation of surgical procedures than in the past, and new procedures can be introduced and evaluated more efficiently.

HEMIPLEGIA

Children with hemiplegia are usually independent and educated in the mainstream. They have a characteristic posture, with a flexed elbow, pronated forearm, flexed wrist, internally rotated and flexed hip, flexed knee and equinus.

Hemiplegic Lower Limb

In the hemiplegic lower limb, the problems are usually most pronounced at the foot and ankle, less severe at the knee, and largely absent at the hip. Because of the 'normal' side, asymmetry is easily noted and monitored. There is usually underdevelopment of the limb, with shortening at maturity ranging from 0–5 cm with an average of 2.2 cm.

Three-dimensional gait analysis has helped to identify subgroups of hemiplegia and has therefore facilitated more logical treatment plans.

- Group 1 children have a mild 'drop foot' gait with no contracture of the Achilles tendon and no significant problem at the knee or hip level. Orthotic management by means of a leaf spring AFO is usually all that is required.
- Group 2 children have an equinus gait due to spasticity or contracture of the Achilles tendon. During the dynamic period, stretching casts, botulinum toxin injections and an AFO may be useful. When a true contracture is present many will benefit from a gastrocnemius recession or an Achilles tendon lengthening.
- Group 3 children have significant involvement of the knee as well as a contracture of the gastrosoleus. There is usually some contracture of the medial hamstrings and co-spasticity of the quadriceps. Some of these patients will require a gastrocnemius recession or Achilles tendon lengthening, combined with medial hamstring lengthening and a transfer of the distal rectus femoris tendon to the medial hamstrings.
- Group 4 children also have involvement at the hip level with some hip flexion and contracture and frequently a significant degree of medial femoral torsion (*Figure 8.3*). Exceptionally there may be

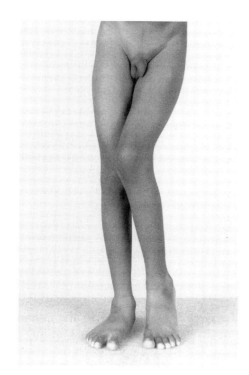

Figure 8.3 Group 4 hemiplegia with flexion, adduction and internal rotation at the hip, flexion at the knee and equinus at the ankle.

hip dysplasia. These patients may therefore require fractional lengthening of the psoas at the pelvic brim and an external rotation osteotomy of the femur, in addition to the surgery described for group 3 patients.

Management

Lengthening of the Achilles tendon
Lengthening of the Achilles tendon should only be performed when clinical examination, gait analysis data and examination under anaesthesia show that it is necessary. It is probably the most overused operation in CP surgery. Remember that 'a little equinus is better than calcaneus.' Calcaneus deformity is untreatable and the parents are not forgiving.

Clinical examination differentiates gastrocnemius contracture without involvement of the soleus from shortening of the entire calf complex. The Silverskiold test compares the range of dorsiflexion at the ankle with the knee extended (testing the length of gastrocnemius) and the knee flexed (testing the length of soleus). This test is only completely reliable under anaesthesia when spasticity is abolished by muscular relaxation. It should be performed at the time of surgery before a final decision is made about the method of lengthening.

Starting from the proximal end of the calf muscle complex, the older procedures of neurectomy

(Stoffel) and gastrocnemius origin release (Silverskiold) are of historical interest only. If the gastrocnemius is shortened, but the soleus is uninvolved a gastrocnemius recession can be performed.

The Baker procedure is carried out open at the level of the gastrocnemius aponeurosis. It is a tongue-in-groove technique and the incision in the aponeurosis is an inverted U. The aponeurosis slides apart in a controlled and stable fashion. No sutures are required. There is a high recurrence rate (up to 50%), but overlengthening is virtually impossible. This is important when it is essential to prevent overlengthening and calcaneus, especially in diplegia.

Lengthening of the Achilles tendon can also be performed closed by a percutaneous technique (the Hoke triple cut technique), semi-open by the White slide or by an open Z-lengthening with suture repair of the tendon.

- The percutaneous technique is popular because it leaves minimal scarring and can be performed as a day-case procedure. Three transverse partial tenotomies (two lateral and one medial) are made, with the tendon held under tension by an assistant. A slide lengthening is effected by forced dorsiflexion. It is mandatory to achieve controlled lengthening, and if the surgeon is not confident in his ability to avoid a complete tenotomy and overlengthening, this procedure should be avoided.
- The slide technique of White is carried out using a percutaneous or semi-open technique, through two small skin incisions. It consists of a transverse partial tenotomy proximally in the medial side of the tendon and then a second partial transverse tenotomy more distally in the anterior half of the tendon, just above the insertion on the os calcis. This relies on the spiralling nature of the tendon, and pressure on the foot will stretch the tendon up to the desired amount of dorsiflexion, but the tendon remains in continuity. DAMP is a useful acronym for remembering 'distal anterior and medial proximal'. No deep sutures are required, the scars are excellent and the risk of overlengthening is small.
- Z-lengthening is performed by open surgery and should be reserved for neglected cases with severe equinus deformity when the ability to perform a posterior release of the ankle joint may also be required. The tendon is split in the midline longitudinally and then detached by a medial transverse cut distally and a proximal lateral cut. The tendon is sutured with overlap of the two halves of the split tendon. There is a real risk of overlengthening and calcaneus deformity.

Anterior advancement of the insertion of the Achilles tendon is unnecessarily complex and offers no advantages.

Complications

Overlengthening It is very important not to overlengthen the gastrosoleus complex as this can result in a calcaneus gait and even a calcaneus deformity. This is essentially untreatable and much worse than the original equinus gait.

Recurrence of the deformity Conservative surgery such as gastrocnemius recession is associated with a high recurrence rate of up to 50% and the need for a repeat procedure. Recurrence is also likely in the younger child, and repeat surgery is often necessary if the first lengthening is carried out in a child under five years of age. However, it is preferable to have a high recurrence rate than risk calcaneus deformity.

Surgery for varus deformity of the foot

In more severe hemiplegia there may be a varus deformity of the foot. This is much more common than valgus and is usually due to overactivity of the tibialis posterior with or without some contribution from tibialis anterior. Sometimes fine-needle electromyography (EMG) is the only way to distinguish which muscle is producing the deformity. As a general rule, tibialis posterior overactivity tends to produce varus of the hind foot and forefoot throughout stance and swing. Tibialis anterior overactivity is more likely to produce supination of the forefoot in swing.

Surgery for overactivity and contracture of tibialis posterior includes simple lengthening of the tendon above the medial malleolus, the split transfer of the tendon to the lateral side of the foot, or transfer of the entire tendon anteriorly, through the interosseus membrane to the dorsum of the foot. Selection of the appropriate surgery is difficult. In the young child with a mobile deformity, the split transfer in association with a slide lengthening of the Achilles tendon gives good results. In the older hemiplegic child who has had recurrent equinus deformity and who has never developed isolated, voluntary dorsiflexion, complete transfer of the tendon to the dorsum of the foot is useful. It makes the child less dependent on orthoses and there is less risk of recurrent equinus. When the whole tendon is transferred, however, there is an increased risk of overcorrection into calcaneo valgus. This procedure should not be performed on younger children nor at the same time as Z-lengthening of the tendo Achillis (*Figure 8.4*).

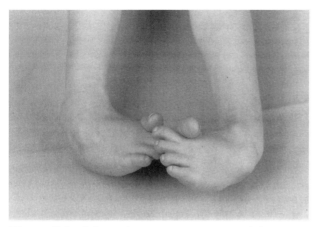

Figure 8.4 Bilateral spastic equinovarus deformities in cerebral palsy. These were managed by a combination of slide lengthening of tendo Achillis, supramalleolar lengthening of tibialis posterior and split transfer of tibialis anterior.

Surgery for valgus deformity of the foot

Valgus deformity is much less common than varus deformity, but is sometimes seen in the child with joint hypermobility and a mild contracture of the gastrosoleus. In an effort to achieve dorsiflexion of the foot, the calcaneum deviates laterally and there may be an associated 'mid-foot break.' This is also described as 'valgus ex-equino' and sometimes responds to a modest lengthening of the Achilles tendon in the growing child.

In the more severe valgus deformity, fusion of the subtalar joint is useful and there are few problems from the loss of subtalar motion. The Grice procedure is an extra-articular technique using a tibial or fibular bone graft to the sinus tarsi, but the results are unreliable. The use of internal fixation with a cannulated screw from the dorsum of the talar neck into the calcaneum and autogenous iliac cancellous bone graft have improved the results.

If the deformity is more abductus at the mid-tarsal area, correction can be achieved by lateral column lengthening. An opening wedge osteotomy of the anterior part of the calcaneum is performed and held by a wedge-shaped bone graft and internal fixation.

In hemiplegia the valgus is rarely a manifestation of peroneal muscle spasticity.

Hemiplegic Upper Limb

The upper limb posture in the hemiplegic upper limb is usually one of internal rotation and adduction at the shoulder, flexion at the elbow, pronation of the forearm, flexion of the wrist, flexion of the digits and 'thumb in palm.' The problems in the upper limbs of these children include spasticity, contracture, weakness, lack of voluntary control, and astereognosis (the inability to recognize objects put into the hand by feel). Only spasticity and its effects can be addressed by orthopaedic surgery.

Management

If there is astereognosis, correcting the posture of the hand is unlikely to produce any functional gains. However, these children are usually independent and in 'mainstream' schooling so cosmetic aspects are very important. Improving the appearance of the limb boosts the confidence of the child, but unrealistic expectations of improving function should be discussed before any surgery is attempted. Fine-wire EMG can be very useful in planning tendon transfers.

Elbow

Flexion deformity of the elbow is addressed by Z-lengthening of the biceps tendon, bicipital aponeurosis, fractional lengthening of brachialis and, occasionally, release of the anterior capsule of the elbow. Phenol block to the musculocutaneous nerve or botulinum toxin to the biceps and brachialis muscles are useful short term measures in the dynamic stage or as diagnostic procedures before surgery.

Forearm

One of the most consistent and earliest findings in the hemiplegic upper limb is loss of active supination and the insidious progression of a pronation contracture. Early release or transfer of pronator teres should be considered. In late neglected cases the pronation deformity becomes fixed due to contracture of the interosseous membrane, secondary torsional changes in the radius, and subluxation or dislocation of the radial head.

Wrist

In the younger child where the flexion deformity is not fixed, the flexed wrist can be treated by the Green transfer. The flexor carpi ulnaris is mobilized and passed around the ulna, and then sutured onto the extensor carpi radialis longus.

If there is a fixed deformity or the deformity cannot be corrected by soft tissue procedures or there is painful degenerative arthritis of the wrist, arthrodesis of the wrist is a reliable and much appreciated procedure. Internal fixation with an intramedullary (IM) rod or a well-contoured plate is required to maintain position as it may be some months before the bone fusion is sound. Tenotomy or lengthening of the long flexor tendons may also be required to protect the fusion and prevent later deformity. The indications for fusion and the position of fusion must be carefully considered for children who use crutches or wheelchairs.

Hand

In the severely involved hand, the fingers are tightly clenched, making hygiene difficult. Sensation is limited and voluntary muscle control is poor. Astereognosis is a feature of most of these hands so functional gains are unlikely and surgical goals are limited to improving the appearance and hygiene. The fingers are straightened by release of the sublimis tendons and lengthening of the profundus tendons.

The 'thumb in palm' deformity can be quite disabling, restricting grasp and the holding of objects. Functional improvements can be made where other indications are good by the Matev procedure. The contracted adductor pollicis muscle is released at its origin. Procedures to improve the position of the thumb following release include abductor pollicis longus (APL) tenodesis and extensor pollicis longus (EPL) re-routing.

Traditionally upper limb surgery is left to a later age than lower limb surgery (until the child is old enough to be assessed more precisely and to participate in a rehabilitation programme). However, some muscles form fixed contractures at an early stage with secondary effects that can be difficult to overcome. In particular, pronation of the forearm becomes fixed much earlier than elbow, wrist or finger flexion. It can then be difficult, even after pronator teres lengthening or transfer, to regain a good range of supination. Release of pronator teres should therefore be considered at an early age.

Botulinum toxin can be useful in the upper limb for dystonic posturing and also for assessing the need for more definitive surgery. It can be used to demonstrate the degree of control and strength in the extensors when considering tendon transfers in the forearm.

SPASTIC DIPLEGIA

The typical child with diplegia only slowly becomes an independent walker, but will eventually achieve a good standard of independence. Many of the lower limb muscle groups are 'spring loaded' and prone to contracture. The most affected muscles include the hip flexors, the hamstrings and the calf muscles. There may also, however, be contractures in the adductors, the medial rotators of the hip and the quadriceps. Secondary bone torsional problems are common, including medial femoral torsion, lateral tibial torsion, and valgus of the foot and ankle.

Management

Surgery is directed at releasing the overactive muscles and correcting the contracture, starting at the hip and working downwards. Many of the previously described tendon transfers that worked well in polio have now been abandoned. The transferred muscle power was unpredictable and sometimes ineffective, and sometimes led to overcorrection.

An analysis of the problems and an appropriate surgical prescription is daunting without three-dimensional gait analysis. There is growing evidence that 'single event' bilateral multilevel soft tissue and bone surgery is preferable to piecemeal surgery. The information gained from three-dimensional gait analysis would suggest the following principles at the hip, the knee and the ankle.

At the hip

Psoas power should be preserved at all costs by fractional lengthening at the pelvic brim. Tenotomy at the lesser trochanter should be avoided in ambulators. Adductor surgery should be modest and usually restricted to a simple percutaneous tenotomy of adductor longus. Three-dimensional gait analysis reveals that most of what appears to be adduction and scissoring is often medial femoral torsion and should not be addressed by adductor release.

At the knee

Hamstring surgery should be approached with great care. In the past, the flexed or crouched gait has been treated with distal hamstring lengthening. However, hamstring contracture is frequently overestimated by ignoring the effects of hip flexion contracture on the measurement of the popliteal angle. Distal hamstring lengthening consists of Z-lengthening the round tendons (semitendinosus, gracilis) and 'ringbarking' or fractional lengthening the flat tendons (semimembranosus, biceps). If at all possible, only the medial hamstrings should be lengthened. Lengthening of the medial and lateral hamstrings together is associated with prolonged weakness of knee flexion and increased anterior pelvic tilt due to the reduction in hip extensor power proximally. This is more of a problem if the psoas muscle is spastic or contracted. Transfer of the hamstrings to the distal femur (Egger procedure) is of historical interest only. At best, the result was a totally stiff-knee gait and at worst, a gross recurvatum deformity.

Distal hamstring lengthening alone frequently results in a stiff-knee gait. This is because the effects of quadriceps–hamstring co-spasticity have been ignored. Weakening of the hamstrings reveals the overactivity in the quadriceps, giving rise to the stiff-knee gait. This problem can be addressed by transfer of the distal rectus femoris tendon to the semitendinosus. In late cases in which a distal rectus transfer has not been carried out, proximal rectus femoris lengthening may be more appropriate.

At the ankle

Equinus can be much more apparent than real. The flexion at the hip and knee may dictate that the child walks on his toes with no effective contact between the heels and the ground. However, gait analysis may show that in this position there is already an adequate range of dorsiflexion at the ankle and sometimes a relative calcaneus. Overlengthening of the

tendo Achillis in this situation can lead to disastrous 'crouch gait' and calcaneus deformity and is to be completely avoided (*Figure 8.5*).

Bone surgery

As a result of muscle imbalance, children with diplegia develop torsional abnormalities of the long bones, typically medial femoral torsion, lateral tibial torsion and planovalgus feet. The muscle–tendon units work most efficiently by producing moments around stable joints in the line of progression of gait. Where there are torsional abnormalities the muscle–tendon unit cannot work effectively and this can be described as 'lever arm disease.' In these children the knees may face 50° inwards (medial femoral torsion) and the ankles 50° outwards (lateral tibial torsion). This results in a dissipation of much of the effort of walking and an awkward and ungainly gait.

Correction of bone torsion should be considered as part of 'single event' surgery in diplegia. The torsional problems can be identified by clinical examination and confirmed by CT measurements. Correction can be achieved by rotational osteotomies which require precise planning and stable fixation (*Figure 8.6*).

The effects of bone rotation on soft tissue tension must be considered. If the hamstrings have a

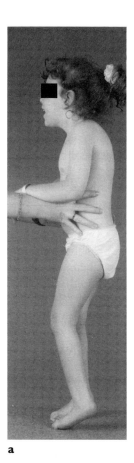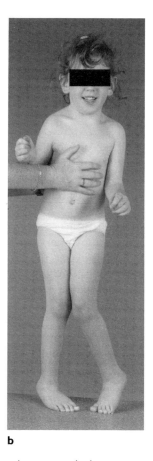

a   b

Figure 8.5a,b Asymmetrical spastic diplegia in a four-year-old girl. Note the posture of flexion, adduction and internal rotation at the hips, flexed knees and equinus feet. The equinus is apparent and not real; the crouch posture is dictated by psoas and hamstring spasticity and contracture.

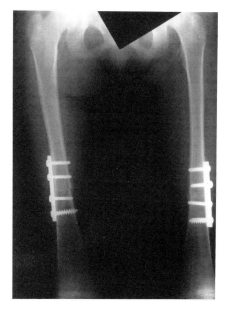

Figure 8.6 Bilateral femoral external rotation osteotomies with compression plate fixation for severe intoeing gait in spastic diplegia. This boy had multiple soft tissue procedures as part of his single-event multilevel surgery including distal hamstring lengthening and transfer of the rectus femoris tendon to semitendinosus.

borderline contracture before femoral osteotomy they may be tightened by femoral derotation to the point that lengthening is necessary. Rotation at one level may dictate surgery at another level. Most parents clearly see the inwardly-facing knees as a problem, but are less aware that if external rotation osteotomy of the femur is performed in isolation then lateral tibial torsion may be exposed resulting in a very out-toed gait. Osteotomy at both levels may be required.

Femoral osteotomy may be proximal or distal. Proximal intertrochanteric osteotomy with AO blade plate fixation is performed when there is hip subluxation. Distal femoral osteotomies are easier to perform and can be more precisely controlled, so are preferred if hip subluxation is not a problem. Supra-condylar femoral osteotomy is best performed after the age of 12 years because before this age the deformity may recur during the remainder of the growth period.

The amount of derotation is important. Children with CP often walk at the limit of their range of internal rotation at the hip. If they have 90° of internal rotation at the hip preoperatively and an external rotation osteotomy of only 45° is performed, there may be significant residual intoeing. Much more derotation is required in comparison to that required for children without CP who are intoeing because of persistent femoral anteversion.

Similar considerations apply to the tibia. Proximal osteotomies carry a risk of compartment syndrome and neurological complications. In the absence of genu varum or valgum a supramalleolar osteotomy is to be preferred.

In the foot valgus deformities are corrected by the Grice subtalar fusion using screw fixation and a cancellous iliac graft from the hip. In the older child with forefoot deformities the lateral inlay triple arthrodesis is ideal.

SPASTIC QUADRIPLEGIA

Less than 25% of children with whole body involvement will be able to walk. A few will become household ambulators, but will be reliant on orthoses and aids. Many are dependent on carers and have very limited ability to communicate. For those who show the ability to develop useful walking, the principles of lower limb surgery are similar to those with severe spastic diplegia. In the much larger group of non-ambulators surgical intervention is designed for the comfort of the child and to help the burden of carers. The priorities are a straight spine, level pelvis and mobile enlocated hips. Contractures of the knees and feet are much less important. If possible, major foot deformities should be avoided so that the child can wear 'normal' shoes.

Many of these children have asymmetries in their lower limbs and there can be a causal relationship between unilateral hip dislocation, pelvic obliquity and scoliosis. However, the relationship is not always uniform.

The majority of children with spasticity of the hip adductors and flexors will demonstrate a progressive reduction of passive abduction at the hips as the contracture of these muscles develop. Secondary bone abnormalities will then develop on both the femoral and pelvic sides of the hip joint. These may include medial femoral torsion, coxa valga, and acetabular dysplasia. Instability of the hip may develop and then progress to subluxation and then dislocation.

The hip abnormality should not be allowed to progress because the adduction deformity leads to seating, toileting and perineal care difficulties. It can also cause problems with transfer ability and lead to a painful degenerative arthritis.

Management

Preventive hip surgery: soft tissue release
The majority of these hips can be protected against subluxation and dislocation by a well-timed adductor release procedure. Hips at risk are identified by progressive loss of abduction and by serial radiography. Helpful radiological indices are the acetabular index and Reimer migration percentage. In an extensive study from this hospital, guidelines have been established in which the acetabular index measured at the age of two and then four years can be used to predict which hips are likely to dislocate without treatment, those hips that are likely to dislocate only in the presence of scoliosis, and those hips that are likely to remain stable without treatment.

Soft tissue surgery for the prevention of hip dislocation consists of an open release of adductor longus, adductor brevis, and gracilis, and recession of the psoas tendon from the lesser trochanter. The anterior branch of the obturator nerve is divided.

This operation requires good perioperative management. Although the surgical incision is small and the extent of the soft tissue surgery limited, it is frequently associated with a stormy course for the child. Good postoperative analgesia using local anaesthetic techniques (caudal, epidural or local wound infiltration) as well as opiate infusions and muscle relaxants are required. Many of these children develop a cycle of muscle spasm that produces increased pain followed by increased muscle spasm, exhausting child and parents within 24 hours of surgery. The administration of rectal diazepam can usually break this difficult cycle.

Abduction splintage after the surgery is most important, either in an adjustable brace or in cylinder plasters held apart with an adjustable 'broomstick.' If the adduction deformity is asymmetrical before surgery an effort should be made to perform graduated surgery on both sides in an attempt to balance the deformities. If there is asymmetry of adduction spasm postoperatively, 'broomstick' plasters may allow the tighter hip to be in adduction and the other hip to be hyperabducted. There may be little improvement following the operation and this will

lead to the tendons healing with minimal lengthening on the hip at-risk side and an early 'recurrence' of the deformity.

Reconstructive hip surgery

Many cases present late with severe subluxation or established dislocation. Management is then much more difficult and should be tailored to the individual needs of the patient, taking into account awareness, ability to communicate, and the presence or absence of pain. About 50% of subluxed and dislocated hips in children with CP seem to cause pain and there is therefore a role for secondary bone reconstructive operations. Frequently there are abnormalities on both the femoral and pelvic sides, and in the majority

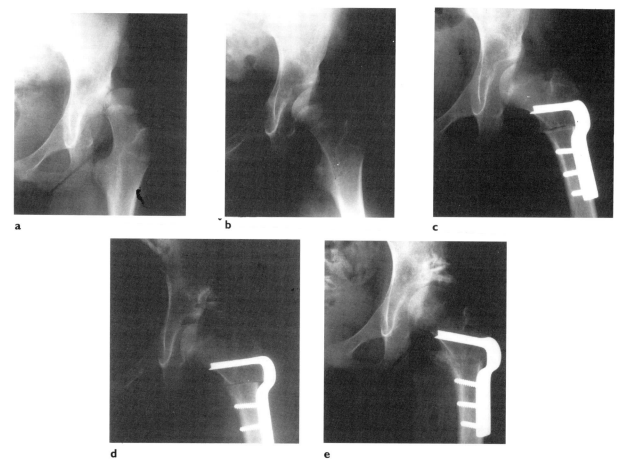

Figure 8.7 **a** Dislocation of the left hip in a 12-year-old girl with mild spastic quadriplegia who was a household ambulator. **b** Following adductor and psoas lengthening, the hip was reducible. **c** The amount of abduction and internal rotation required to reduce the hip dictated the amount of rotation (50°) and varus (20°) of the femoral osteotomy to achieve best congruence. **d** The hip was still uncovered after femoral osteotomy, so at the same surgery a slotted acetabular augmentation (Staheli shelf) was performed. **e** At three-year follow-up the osteotomies have united and the hip is mobile and pain-free. The acetabular augmentation has matured and hypertrophied as a result of loading and weight-bearing.

of cases both have to be addressed. If soft tissue releases have not previously been performed, these are usually necessary before bone surgery (*Figure 8.7*).

On the femoral side, a femoral derotation osteotomy is performed at the intertrochanteric level using blade plate fixation. Correction of the femoral medial torsion is achieved with derotation of 40–80°. A small varus component can be added to the procedure, but the neck–shaft angle should not be overcorrected into varus, but only to a normal value. Overcorrection may aid hip stability, but abolishes the abduction gained at earlier soft tissue release and leaves carers questioning the value of the surgery.

On the pelvic side, a number of procedures may be helpful. The acetabulum may be globally deficient or the deficiency may be mainly anterolateral. If there is significant doubt regarding the precise bone architecture, then CT scanning sometimes with three-dimensional reconstruction can be helpful. Primary reconstructive pelvic osteotomies of the Salter, Steele and Sutherland types have a limited indication in this situation because they sacrifice posterior cover to achieve more anterior cover and can result in posterior subluxation in these circumstances. Capsular arthroplasty of the Chiari or shelf types are usually more appropriate. The Staheli shelf procedure has much to commend it because anterior, lateral and posterior deficiencies can be addressed without the need for internal fixation or prolonged immobilization.

The complication rate from this type of surgery can be high and the results are not uniformly good. Bone surgery in these children with severe CP should be avoided if at all possible by early radical soft tissue releases.

Salvage hip surgery

If bone reconstruction of the hip fails in these children, there are four remaining salvage procedures to be considered; each being a major undertaking and having major associated complications and problems.

- Femoral valgus osteotomy under a dislocated hip is a reasonable procedure for deformity, but not for pain.
- Excision of the proximal femur is associated with a stormy and prolonged postoperative course. The long term results can be good in selected cases.
- Arthrodesis is accepted by very few children because of the constraints of deformities and stiffness at other joints.

- Total joint replacement is useful in carefully-selected patients with pain but not much deformity. The low demands on the arthroplasty may ensure longevity if the early risks of dislocation are avoided.

REFERENCES AND FURTHER READING

Bleck EE. Locomotor prognosis in cerebral palsy. *Devel Med Child Neurol* 1975; **17**: 18–25.

Bleck EE. *Orthopaedic Management in Cerebral Palsy*. JB Lippincott Co, Philadelphia, 1987.

Bleck EE. Current concepts review. Management of the lower extremities in children who have cerebral palsy. *J Bone Joint Surg* 1990; **72A**: 140–144.

Cosgrove AP, Corry IS, Graham HK. Botulinum toxin in the management of the lower limb in cerebral palsy. *Develop Med Child Neurol* 1994; **36**: 379–385.

Cooke PH, Carey RPL, Williams PF. Lower femoral osteotomy in cerebral palsy: brief report. *J Bone Joint Surg* 1989; **71B**: 146–147.

Cooke PH, Cole WG, Carey RPL. Dislocation of the hip in cerebral palsy. Natural history and predictability. *J Bone Joint Surg* 1989; **71B**: 441–6.

Ferguson RL, Allen BL. Considerations in the treatment of cerebral palsy patients with spinal deformities. *Orthop Clin North Am* 1987; **19**: 419–426.

Gage J. Gait analysis. An essential tool in the treatment of cerebral palsy. *Clin Orthop* 1993; **288**: 126–134.

Graham HK, Fixsen JA. Lengthening of the calcaneal tendon in spastic hemiplegia by the White slide technique. A long-term review. *J Bone Joint Surg* 1988; **70B**: 472–475.

Koman LA, Gelberman RH, Toby EB, Poehling GG. Cerebral palsy. Management of the upper extremity. *Clin Orthop* 1990; **253**: 62–74.

Mubarak SJ, Valencia FG, Wenger DR. One-stage correction of the spastic dislocated hip. Use of pericapsular acetabuloplasty to improve coverage. *J Bone Joint Surg* 1992; **74A**: 1347–1357.

Olney BW, Williams PF, Menelaus MB. Treatment of spastic equinus by aponeurosis lengthening. *J Pediatr Orthop* 1988; **8**: 422–425.

Oppenheim WD. Selective posterior rhizotomy for spastic cerebral palsy. A review. *Clin Orthop* 1990; **253**: 20–29.

Root L, Laplaza FJ, Brourman SN, Angel DH. The severely unstable hip in cerebral palsy, treatment with open reduction, pelvic osteotomy, and femoral osteotomy with shortening. *J Bone Joint Surg* 1995; **77A**: 703–712.

Sutherland DH. Gait analysis in neuromuscular diseases. In: *American Academy of Orthopaedic Surgeons Instructional Course Lectures, XXXIX*, edited by WB Greene. pp. 333–341. American Academy of Orthopaedic Surgeons, Park Ridge, Illinois, 1990.

Chapter 9
Spina Bifida

Malcolm B Menelaus

Neural tube defects are congenital anomalies characterized by abnormal closure of the neural tube. Anencephaly represents the abnormality at the cranial end of the tube. Spina bifida describes a group of disorders including failure of full development of the vertebral arches and abnormalities in the development of structures derived from the neural tube and the meninges. This results in abnormal innervation of those organs supplied by the affected part of the spinal cord. There is multiple organ involvement with effects on the bladder and bowel as well as denervation of muscles and sensory organs. Spinal dysraphism refers to hidden abnormalities affecting the spinal cord or cauda equina and these may produce subtle neurological disturbances.

Aetiology

Neural tube defects follow a multifactorial pattern of inheritance. There is an increased familial incidence of all types of neural tube defects, but the inheritance would seem to be polygenic.

Environmental factors that have been implicated include folate deficiency, other vitamin deficiencies, absence of selenium from the regional soil, poor maternal nutrition, a high maternal alcohol intake, maternal diabetes mellitus, fever at a critical stage of pregnancy and other factors (Shurtleff, 1986).

Incidence

The incidence of spina bifida varies in different areas. In addition, there are racial differences and seasonal variations. Over the past 20 years the incidence has fallen in regions where the incidence has been high, but no such fall has been observed in other areas. The fall in incidence might be partly explained by pre-natal diagnosis and selective abortion and the administration of folate to women who are likely to become pregnant, and partly by emigration from high-risk areas.

The highest incidence has been in Ireland, Wales and the north of England (about five per 1000 live births). In North America and Australia the incidence is less than one per 1000 live births.

Pathology

Spina bifida may be subdivided into:

- Spina bifida cystica, where there is a visible cyst present.
- Spina bifida occulta (*Figure 9.1a*), where the defect is hidden, but may be suspected because of the presence of a dimple (which may connect with the dura by a fibrous cord), a patch of hair, pigmentation or a lipoma (which can be continuous with an intradural lipoma).

These conditions represent abnormalities of separation of the skin from neural tissue during the closure of the neural tube.

Types of spina bifida cystica
Myeloschisis or myelocoele (*Figure 9.1b*) is the most severe form of defect. The vertebral arches are deficient with neural plate material spread out on the surface, sometimes in a shallow depression, but more commonly over a cystic swelling of the meninges.

Myelomeningocoele (*Figure 9.1c*) is a cystic swelling lined by dura and arachnoid, protruding through a defect in the vertebral arches. The spinal cord and nerve roots are carried out into the fundus of the sac. This is the commonest form. In the clinical setting, as in this chapter, the terms spina bifida and myelomeningocoele are used interchangeably. Both refer to children with neuromuscular deficiencies due to failure of the neural tube to close.

Meningocoele (*Figure 9.1d*) is a cystic swelling of dura and arachnoid, protruding through a defect in the vertebral arches under the skin. The spinal cord is entirely confined within the vertebral arches, but may show abnormalities.

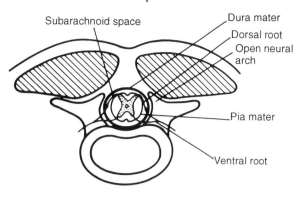

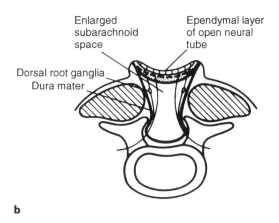

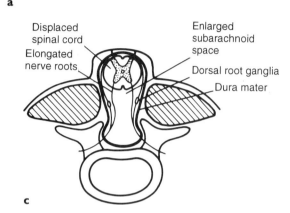

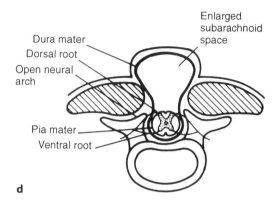

Figure 9.1   **a** Spina bifida occulta.   **b** Myelocoele.   **c** Myelomeningocoele.   **d** Meningocoele

Multisystem Involvement

In addition to the gross spinal abnormality, other pathology is usually present. In the central nervous system (CNS) there may be the Arnold–Chiari malformation leading to hydrocephalus. Approximately 72% of patients develop significant hydrocephalus and require ventriculoperitoneal shunts. In addition there may also be cerebellar hypoplasia, hydromyelia, syringomyelia and diastematomyelia. The majority of patients have upper limb disabilities due to a variety of subtle neurological lesions, but 50–65% of patients have normal intelligence. Children with myelomeningocoele generally have paralysis of the bladder and bowel incontinence and a tendency to trophic ulceration in areas of skin anaesthesia over the sacrum, buttocks and feet.

Multidisciplinary Management

An appropriate management programme for children with myelomeningocoele can only be carried out at a large paediatric institution where there is a coordinated team of specialists and allied health personnel made up of the following:

- A coordinator, who is usually a paediatrician with expertise in the management of children with multiple disabilities.
- A neurosurgeon, who is concerned with the early surgical repair of the spinal lesion and supervises serial evaluation of head circumference and ventricular size by ultrasound or computerized tomography (CT) to determine whether hydrocephalus is developing.
- An orthopaedic surgeon, who in the neonatal period treats conditions such as talipes equinovarus and at a later stage is concerned with managing deformity.
- A urologist, who is concerned with the management of bladder paralysis. The aim of such management is to minimize urinary infections and prevent chronic renal disease. His aim is to enable the child to be dry by nursery school or school age. Clean intermittent catheterization (CIC) is now the first line of management and most children have substantially improved continence with this technique. Bladder augmentation and artificial sphincter operations are appropriate for some children.
- A paediatric surgeon, who is involved in the management of the neurogenic bowel. His aim is

to enable the child to defecate at a time and place of his choosing and to be clean in between. Chronic constipation, faecal impaction and overflow incontinence are common.

- A psychiatrist and psychologist, who are necessary to a greater or lesser extent to help with the management of psychological problems experienced by the child and family.
- A medical social worker, who is necessary to advise the family on social services available for the child with severe disabilities.
- A physiotherapist and occupational therapist, who play a large part in improving upper and lower limb function.
- An appliance specialist, who advises on the many types of urinary and bowel aids.
- An orthotist, who plays a major part in the conservative management of limb disability.

The coordinator advises the family of appropriate skin care to avoid pressure sores and burns. Thorough education in this area is needed and the aid of a plastic surgeon is necessary if there is established skin loss. The coordinator will also advise children and adolescents at an appropriate age about sexual function.

Most children with spina bifida need assistance at school because of difficulties with access, mobility and continence. Children with shunted hydrocephalus have specific learning problems. There may be difficulty in concentration span and fine motor and perceptual functioning. Nevertheless, the majority of children can attend 'normal' schools.

Genetic counselling

Genetic counselling should provide the family with information that allows them to make a decision about having further children. Counselling should involve careful discussion of the recurrence risk for further pregnancies, the availability of antenatal diagnosis, and an explanation of the variability of the condition.

Recurrence risk Recurrence risk varies in different areas, so counselling should be based on local experience. In general, it is approximately 1 in 25 following the birth of an affected baby; of which 50% is for anencephaly and 50% for other neural tube defects. If the parents have had two affected children, the risk rises to approximately 1 in 10 and after three affected children to approximately 1 in 4. The birth of a child with anencephaly, multiple congenital vertebral anomalies or spinal dysraphism indicates the same predisposition to the recurrence of neural tube defects. Adult survivors with spina bifida who

are contemplating having a family face the same risk as the parents of a single child with spina bifida.

Antenatal diagnosis Maternal serum alpha-fetoprotein is usually tested routinely as a screening test between the 16th and 20th week of pregnancy. If the serum level is high, then ultrasound and amniocentesis are performed.

Ultrasound can detect most anencephalics and a few spina bifidas at 10–12 weeks of pregnancy using vaginal ultrasound. Standard ultrasound at 16–18 weeks identifies virtually all anencephalics and over 80% of spina bifidas. Although neural tube defects can usually be identified they cannot be excluded with certainty and therefore the technique is often used with amniocentesis.

Amniocentesis is always carried out with ultrasound control to localize the placenta, confirm gestational age, exclude multiple pregnancy and visible malformations. In experienced hands, the risk of producing a miscarriage is about 1 in 200.

The fluid is submitted for alpha-fetoprotein estimation and in some laboratories acetylcholine esterase levels. The values obtained are compared with the ranges of normal established in that laboratory for each particular week of gestation. By a combination of ultrasonography and maternal alpha-fetoprotein levels almost all fetuses with anencephaly and at least 90% of those with spina bifida can be recognized. Small skin-covered lesions may be missed. In addition the amniotic fluid cells are examined for chromosome disorders such as Down's syndrome.

Prevention

Multivitamins, and especially folate, may have a role in preventing neural tube defects. These vitamins are recommended for the mother during the period in which she may become pregnant.

Intrauterine diagnosis allows the abortion of babies with neural tube defects when this is acceptable to the parents. Screening of all pregnancies has the potential to reduce the incidence of this disorder. However, prediction of the severity of the neural tube defect is often difficult *in utero*. Ultrasound can be used to look at the muscles affected to see if there are strong quadriceps.

It has also been shown that there is a lower incidence of severe neurological deficit in those spina bifida babies who are delivered by caesarean section at the 36th week of pregnancy compared with those delivered vaginally at term. Presumably this is due to less trauma to the exposed neural plate during delivery. The parents who wish to continue the pregnancy should be offered this option.

Goals of management and expectations of outcome

The main goal of orthopaedic management is to allow the child to be mobile in the community. This does not necessarily imply walking as many are more mobile in a wheelchair. However, Mazur *et al.* (1989) established that children who have walked for a period in childhood, even if they later cease walking, are better at many functions of daily living than those who have never walked.

These children should be given the best chance of walking by establishing a stable posture (*Figure 9.2*). This means that they must have their centre of gravity directly over their feet with minimal flexion deformities at hips and knees. Approximately 60% of spina bifida children have neurological deficiencies in their upper limbs and often need to use both hands for activities that normally can be carried out single-handed. For this reason as well we aim, wherever possible, to enable them to stand for long periods without using their hands for support.

Orthopaedic surgery has different goals according to the level of neurosegmental lesion. Most children with thoracic lesions will not continue useful walking in adult life. Children with lumbar lesions may continue useful walking in adult life if they have

strong quadriceps muscles and do not develop significant deformity at their hips. Those with strong quadriceps muscles require only below-knee orthoses, but may need sticks or crutches for hip stability if the abductors are weak. Children with sacral lesions can be expected to be useful walkers without orthoses into adult life.

Those children who will not continue walking into adult life require simple surgery to provide them with a stable posture in childhood. Those who will continue walking require more sophisticated surgery to meet the demands of their way of life. The development of a reciprocating gait orthosis has enabled children who are completely paraplegic or merely have some hip flexor power to walk effectively and with minimal energy expenditure. Some of these children will continue to walk well into adolescence whereas those requiring knee–ankle–foot orthoses (KAFOs) and who walk with a swing-through gait expend much more energy and generally cease walking at an earlier age.

Because the surgery necessary in children with high lesions is relatively minor, it can and should be performed at several levels and in both limbs under one anaesthetic. Muscle imbalance must be corrected in all circumstances so that recurrent deformity does not occur. Radical surgery is necessary to correct rigid, arthrogrypotic-type deformities and care must be taken to avoid pressure on anaesthetic skin. For this and other reasons, operative correction of deformities is preferable to conservative methods. In all management in spina bifida, immobilization of the child and of the uninvolved limbs must be for as short a time as possible so that the incidence of pathological fractures is minimized.

There are some children who are severely retarded or have gross spasticity and multiple congenital anomalies who are clearly not going to walk and these children should be provided with a powered wheelchair early, such as at two years of age.

Assessment of neurosegmental level

The assessment of the neurosegmental level allows some predictions to be made about the child's likely walking abilities. It can generally be carried out fairly accurately in the neonatal period. If the child is not moving the lower limbs at all the lesion is at a high level. Those children who can move their ankles and extend their knees have a low-level lesion with a high probability of walking. Nevertheless, there are difficulties in such assessment. Some muscle activities seen in the neonatal period are due to purely reflex activity and not to voluntary activity. This may be obvious if there is a continuous and uninterrupted activity of a muscle or continuous 'flickering activity'

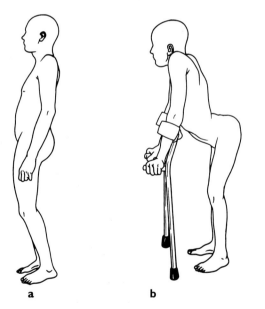

a   b

Figure 9.2 **a** Extension posture: the centre of gravity of the body lies directly above the feet. The hips will extend beyond neutral, which allows the hips to remain extended in the absence of any gluteal activity. **b** Flexion posture at the hips, secondary to fixed flexion deformity and reduced hip extensor power imposes a lumbar lordosis, which becomes fixed. The centre of gravity lies in front of the feet and crutches are needed for stability.

Table 9.1   Assessment of neurosegmental level

Thoracic	No active movement at the hip
L1	Iliopsoas grade 2 or better
L2	Iliopsoas, sartorius and adductors grade 3 or better
L3	Quadriceps grade 3 or better and meet criteria for L2
L4	Medial hamstring or tibialis anterior grade 3 or better and meet criteria for L3
L5	Lateral hamstrings grade 3 or better and meet criteria for L4 plus one of the following: gluteus medius grade 2 or better; peroneus tertius grade 4 or better; tibialis posterior grade 3 or better
Sacral	Two of the following and meet criteria for L5: gastrocnemius/soleus grade 2 or better; gluteus medius grade 3 or better; gluteus maximus grade 3 or better
No loss	All leg muscles normal strength

of a muscle. As the child gets older it becomes easier for the clinician to define the level of lesion based on muscle power as indicated in *Table 9.1.*

There will be a corresponding sensory defect, but this is difficult to determine clinically until the child is old enough to cooperate and by that time the level of the neurosegmental defect has become clear using muscle testing.

Problems in Children with Myelomeningocoele

Skin anaesthesia

Pressure sores and chilblains are common. If serial plasters are necessary to correct deformity they should be carefully padded because there is no pain to warn the surgeon of pressure on the skin. In most instances, plaster casts should only be used to maintain the correction of deformity that has been achieved by soft tissue surgery. The routine use of lambs' wool-lined boots reduces the risk of chilblains and pressure sores. Hip spicas should include paralysed feet. Varus feet are always unacceptable and pressure sores are inevitable. Parents should be warned to inspect their children's feet daily and to protect them from extremes of temperature.

Bone fragility

Pathological fractures occur in approximately 20% of patients with paralysis in the lower limbs. Epiphyseal displacements and hyperplastic callus formation are common (*Figure 9.3*). Occasionally pathological fractures occur in spina bifida due to renal rickets.

Pathological fractures in patients with spina bifida are commonly mistaken for bone or joint infection. The patient may present with a red, hot and swollen limb without a history of trauma, and radiographs often reveal a fracture or an epiphyseal displacement that has occurred days or weeks previously. There may be hyperplastic callus formation.

Immobilization of the child and the fractured limb should be the minimum compatible with union in a satisfactory position. Epiphyseal displacements will unite in four weeks. Patients who are unable to walk require less perfect reduction of such fractures. Supracondylar fracture of the femur is the most common pathological fracture and is frequently seen 7–10 days following the injury. It should be immobilized in a rigid splint that can be removed for appropriate skin care.

Heterotopic ossification

This is likely to occur in patients with thoracic and upper lumbar level lesions who undergo surgery about the hip. The ossification may lead to restricted hip movement and is an additional reason for avoiding hip surgery in patients with high level lesions.

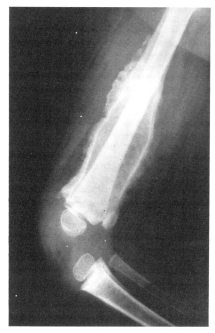

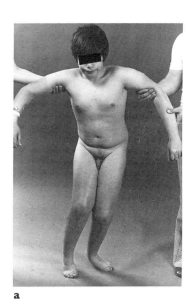

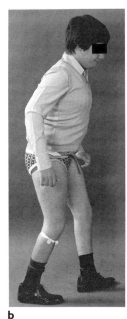

a   b

Figure 9.3 Hypertrophic callous formation following a minimal lower femoral epiphyseal displacement. This girl, with a high lumbar lesion, had no history of trauma and presented with a tense red thigh, which was initially diagnosed as infection. (Reproduced with permission from Menelaus MB (1980). *The Orthopaedic Management of Spina Bifida Cystica*. Churchill Livingstone, Edinburgh.)

Figure 9.4 a A 12-year-old boy with an L5 lesion plus spasticity in the hamstring and calves. He could not walk unless supported. **b** Following hamstring and calf releases he became a community ambulator. (Reproduced with permission from Menelaus MB (1980). *The Orthopaedic Management of Spina Bifida Cystica*. Churchill Livingstone, Edinburgh.)

Deformity

Mobile and rigid deformities are seen. They vary from minor and mobile deformity to severe and rigid deformity similar to that seen in arthrogryposis multiplex congenita. The causes of deformity are:

- Muscle imbalance due to lower motor neurone lesions.
- Muscle imbalance due to upper motor neurone lesions.
- Intrauterine posture.
- Habitually-assumed posture after birth.
- Coexistent congenital malformation.
- Arthrogryposis.

Muscle imbalance due to lower motor neurone lesions is largely due to the developmental defect with paralysed agonists and normally-functioning antagonists. Various patterns of deformity are seen. Some are due to muscle imbalance as described by Sharrard (1964). However, recent studies raise doubt about the influence of muscle imbalance as the major cause of deformity. Hip flexion deformity is most common in children with a thoracic level

lesion where there is no muscle activity and hip dislocation is more common in these children than in children with an L4 lesion where the muscle imbalance is at its greatest (Shurtleff, 1986; Broughton *et al.*, 1993).

Nevertheless, there is some correlation between the lowest functioning neurosegmental level, the muscles acting and the limb posture. This correlation is certainly constant in those patients in whom L5 is spared and who have a calcaneus deformity of the foot due to activity in the tibialis anterior yet no activity in the gastrocnemius–soleus complex. Such muscle imbalance leads to fixed deformity.

Approximately 65% of infants with myelomeningocoele have some degree of spasticity as a result of muscle imbalance due to an upper motor neurone lesion (*Figure 9.4*). There is an interruption of the long spinal tracts with preservation of purely reflex activity in isolated distal segments.

The muscle imbalance producing deformity in spina bifida may therefore be due to:

- Normal muscle versus flaccid antagonist.
- Spastic muscle versus normal antagonist.
- Spastic muscle versus flaccid antagonist.

Deformities due to spasticity may not be present at birth, but develop in the early months of life.

Sometimes deformity is present at birth in totally-paralysed lower limbs and seems to result from the child's position *in utero*. In some of these cases the deformity may be fixed, which suggests that muscle imbalance has been present in fetal life.

Habitually-assumed posture after birth can lead to deformities in flaccid legs that are allowed to lie in one particular position. The hips may therefore develop a fixed external rotation, flexion, and abduction deformity. The knees may develop flexion and the feet an equinus deformity.

Coexistent congenital malformations may include some of the club feet encountered. Syndactyly of the second and third toes and renal anomalies are also associated with spina bifida.

Some of the limb deformities resemble those seen in arthrogryposis multiplex congenita with rigidity and a lack of normal flexion creases. Such deformities are very resistant to treatment.

Tethering of the cord

Some children, who have had a myelomeningocoele closed at birth present later with a progressive foot deformity, which is usually cavus. If tethering is confirmed on a magnetic resonance imaging (MRI) scan it should be treated by surgical release. Some present as teenagers with a rapid deterioration in quadriceps power and again require urgent surgical release of the tethering.

Orthopaedic Management

Orthoses

Bracing is arranged when the child shows some interest in pulling himself into a vertical position on feet or knees. Ankle–foot orthoses (AFOs) are ordered to control mobile ankle or foot deformities. Some recommend AFOs for most of these patients to protect the insensate foot and to transmit forces higher up the leg to areas with sensation.

Floor reaction orthoses may be sufficient if there is some quadriceps weakness, but more commonly quadriceps weakness demands the use of KAFOs. Children will not tolerate these above-knee orthoses for long periods until they have reached an age when they no longer prefer to crawl.

For children with extensive paralysis the parapodium or Shrewsbury swivel walker is appropriate. For children who have no muscle power or just some hip flexor power, have good upper limb function and enjoy walking, a reciprocating-gait orthosis is appropriate. This is useful between the ages of about 20 months and ten years. For larger and heavier children the parawalker (or hip guidance orthosis) is helpful.

Wheelchairs

Children with severe disability will commonly walk during early childhood and then find that they are more mobile using a wheelchair between the ages of 10 and 16 years, and seldom stand or walk subsequently. The parents of children with high-level lesions should be informed at an early stage that a wheelchair is likely to be preferred to walking in the long term. It is important that this is not interpreted as a failure and there should not be overenthusiastic insistence on walking despite many difficulties throughout the child's development. These children have other important areas of learning and socializing on which to spend time.

THE FOOT

The foot may deform in various ways at the heel, ankle and forefoot. In the non-walker, deformity is worth correcting so that the child can look normal and wear normal shoes. This is important to the child's self-esteem. In the walker, deformity should be avoided so that the child has a stable base on which to walk and because deformity leads to neuropathic ulceration.

Fixed varus deformity invariably causes complications due to weight-bearing on a small area of the sole. It should be corrected by surgery. Undercorrection should not be accepted because further surgery is usually necessary.

Valgus feet that remain mobile can usually be controlled with appropriate footwear and orthoses until adolescence. Mobile valgus deformity of the subtalar joint is commonly complicated by external torsion and valgus deformity of the ankle mortice; the deformity is difficult to control by bracing and it is often necessary to correct this complex deformity by surgery.

Whenever possible, operations on the foot and leg should be performed under the same anaesthetic as other limb surgery, urological surgery or neurosurgery.

Although mobile feet are preferable to stiff feet, we have found triple arthrodesis at maturity useful in the management of both varus and valgus deformity (Olney and Menelaus, 1988).

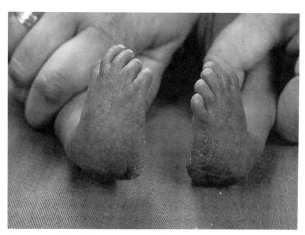

Figure 9.5 One-month-old baby with a thoracic-level lesion and rigid talipes equinovarus. This is best treated by immediate tenotomy of the tendo Achillis (the skin is insensitive), and cautious serial casting, avoiding pressure.

Equinovarus Deformity

The rigidity of this deformity varies from that seen in the usual form of talipes equinovarus to the extreme rigidity of arthrogryposis (*Figure 9.5*). This is the most troublesome foot deformity because of its tendency to recur despite apparently adequate initial correction.

Management

Unless survival is unlikely, the deformity should be treated from birth. The feet are placed in well-padded plaster casts, which are changed frequently while the baby is in hospital and then at intervals of 4–6 weeks. Before treatment, the feet may appear to be purely varus or even calcaneovarus, but as the varus is corrected, it is usually apparent that there is tightness of the Achilles tendon. In these circumstances closed tenotomy is indicated. Despite this early management, a posteromedial soft-tissue release will generally be necessary between the ages of four months and one year. Portions of the tendons of the Achilles tendon, tibialis posterior and the long toe flexors are excised rather than just divided. Only occasionally will the degree of deformity be so mild that conservative treatment will correct the varus and adductus, leaving only equinus to be corrected by posterior release. Tendon transfers have no place in the management of this condition.

Should the deformity recur, a repeat soft-tissue release is performed. However, if recurrent deformity occurs between 5–14 years of age, it is generally wise to accept the deformity, provide surgical footwear

and perform triple arthrodesis at skeletal maturity. If the child has considerable paralysis, the demands on the feet may be such that pressure effects do not present a problem. Should trophic ulcers appear, then soft-tissue releases are preferable to talectomy.

Equinus Deformity

This deformity usually responds to closed or open tenotomy of the Achilles tendon, depending on the severity of the deformity and the age of the child.

Cavus Deformity

The management of this condition will depend on the degree of rigidity of the deformity and the age of the child. Minor deformity in a young child may be corrected by open division of the tight plantar structures. If there is heel varus and the child is over four years of age, then osteotomy of the os calcis is appropriate. If the deformity then recurs and the child is too young for triple arthrodesis, it may be necessary to osteotomize all the metatarsals at their bases. The surgical management of severe cavovalgus deformity in the immature foot is demonstrated in *Figure 9.6*. Triple arthrodesis is carried out if there is a combination of cavus and varus deformity in a patient close to skeletal maturity.

Calcaneus Deformity

Generally this deformity is left untreated until muscle power can be properly assessed at 3–5 years of age. Stiffening the tongue of the boot may control minor degrees of deformity in the young child.

If the strength of the tibialis anterior is normal then this tendon is transferred through the interosseous membrane to the heel. Any other active ankle dorsiflexors are divided and if there is fixed calcaneus deformity an anterior ankle release is combined with this tendon transfer. If the anterior muscles are spastic or if they are weak, they are divided and the Achilles tendon is tenodesed to the fibular metaphysis. The drill hole through the fibula stimulates growth at the lower end of the fibula and this may correct valgus deformity at the ankle mortice (a deformity that commonly occurs in combination with calcaneus deformity). The late-developing calcaneus deformity with a 'pistol grip' heel is best treated by osteotomy of the os calcis, removing a wedge based posteriorly so that the tuberosity lies less vertically. At the same time, restoration of

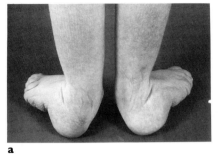
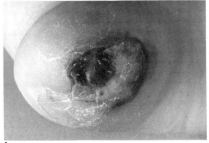
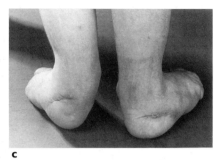

a   b   c

Figure 9.6 a Calcaneocavovalgus deformity of both feet in four-year-old child with an L4 lesion plus spasticity of tibialis anterior and peroneus tertius. **b** Trophic ulcer on the left heel. Note the thick surrounding skin resulting from weight-bearing in calcaneus. **c** Posture of the feet two years after bilateral excision of 1 cm of tibialis anterior and peroneus tertius plus os calcis osteotomy displaced to correct valgus and to horizontalize the formerly vertical tuberosity of the os calcis. (Reproduced with permission from Menelaus MB (1980). *The Orthopaedic Management of Spina Bifida Cystica*. Churchill Livingstone, Edinburgh.)

muscle balance is achieved by tenodesis or tendon transfer.

Valgus Deformity

This deformity may occur at the ankle mortice, the subtalar joint or at both these sites. Clinical examination and weight-bearing radiographs or CT scans will identify the site of the deformity.

Valgus at the Ankle

Clinically this can be detected because the distal end of the fibula lies more proximal than normal when compared with the level of the medial malleolus. Radiographs demonstrate that the lower fibular growth plate, which should be at the same level as the ankle joint, lies proximal to this. The lower tibial epiphysis is wedge-shaped; the medial portion of the epiphysis is wider than the lateral (*Figure 9.7*).

Under six years of age this deformity may be reversed by arresting the medial portion of the lower tibial growth plate. This arrest can be performed either with staples, by the Phemister technique, or by closed drilling.

Deformity at a later age and of a degree sufficient to present a problem should be corrected by supra-malleolar osteotomy of the tibia. This is performed with excision of a medially-based wedge of lower tibia and an oblique osteotomy of the fibula. The tibial osteotomy should be approximately 1 cm proximal to the lower tibial growth plate. Any external tibial torsion can be corrected at the same

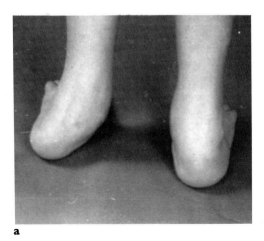
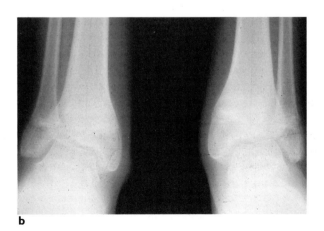

a   b

Figure 9.7 a There is valgus of the ankle mortice on either side, more severe on the left, in a 14-year-old girl with an L5 lesion. **b** Note the proximal situation of the tip of the lateral malleolus and of the growth plate of the lower fibula and the wedge-shaped lower tibial epiphysis characteristic of this condition.

time. The osteotomy may be secured with a single staple or with two crossed K wires. There is a risk of wound breakdown and delayed union following this procedure.

Valgus at the Subtalar Joint

If this is so gross that it cannot be controlled by an AFO under the age of ten years then an os calcis osteotomy is performed. A wedge of os calcis based medially is excised and the tuberosity of the os calcis displaced medially. The position is held by a heavy K wire. Some prefer an extraarticular subtalar fusion as described by Grice. Care should be taken to avoid overcorrection.

If the patient is approaching maturity then there is commonly a plano-abductus deformity of the forefoot in association with the subtalar valgus. This is best corrected by triple arthrodesis. The most satisfactory form of triple arthrodesis for the valgus foot (which generally lacks any fixed deformity, but sweeps into valgus on weight-bearing) is the lateral inlay arthrodesis (Williams and Menelaus, 1977).

Valgus at the Ankle and Subtalar Joint

This requires surgery at two sites. Supramalleolar osteotomy of the tibia and fibula may be combined with either os calcis osteotomy or lateral inlay triple fusion (Nicol and Menelaus, 1983) depending on the nature of the foot deformity.

Paralytic Convex Pes Valgus (Vertical Talus)

This occurs in less than 2% of children with spina bifida. It can be present at birth and is then similar to the congenital vertical talus not associated with spina bifida. It can also occur in a less rigid form, which develops slowly over the first years of life.

Surgical correction is necessary and involves reduction of the talonavicular and sometimes the calcaneocuboid joint and correction of the ankle equinus and of the heel valgus. These objectives can be achieved through a Cincinnati approach. The operation is best performed in the first year of life. The tibialis anterior, extensor digitorum longus and the peroneal muscles are sectioned and the tendo Achillis lengthened. A lateral release of the subtalar joint is performed and if the valgus deformity is great, an extraarticular subtalar fusion is performed using a lateral bone block. The correction is maintained with longitudinal vertical K wires for 4–6

weeks and plaster immobilization maintained for three months postoperatively. A carefully moulded AFO is then used to control planus, heel valgus and a flail ankle.

TORSIONAL DEFORMITIES OF THE TIBIA

External Rotation of the Tibia

This is commonly associated with valgus at the ankle. It should be treated after eight years of age by supramalleolar rotational osteotomy of the tibia, which can be combined with correction of the valgus ankle at the supramalleolar level (see above) (*Figure 9.8*).

Internal Rotation of the Tibia

Gross degrees of the deformity in the first three years of life are corrected by osteoclasis of the tibia and fibula or at a later stage by supramalleolar external rotation osteotomy.

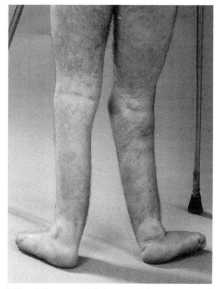

Figure 9.8   14-year-old boy with no muscle power below the knee level. The right leg has gross external tibial torsion and there is valgus deformity of the ankle mortice. The left leg has undergone supramalleolar osteotomy of the tibia to correct these deformities.

THE KNEE

The Flail Undeformed Knee

This is found in approximately 30% of those children who survive to an age at which walking may occur. Bracing is necessary to support the knees if the child is to be ambulatory.

The Undeformed Knee with Quadriceps Weakness

This situation is common. Early in life bracing annoys these children because they want to crawl on the floor. Later a floor reaction orthosis may be useful. For some children a long brace on one leg and a short one on the other with alternate bracing on alternate days may provide an answer.

Fixed Flexion Deformity

Fixed flexion deformity is most common in children with thoracic level spina bifida. A deformity of less than 20° can generally be ignored. More than 20° fixed flexion deformity in walkers is usually best treated surgically. A posterior release of all the hamstring tendons is performed together with a posterior capsular release when necessary. Postoperatively the knee is immobilized in a well-padded cast.

Rarely, a supracondylar osteotomy of the femur is necessary to obtain a full correction.

Limited Flexion with Recurvatum

The knee may be rigid in extension and may have the featureless appearance seen in arthrogryposis multiplex congenita. They become troublesome at the age of about six years when they become awkward in cars and classrooms. Such knees may be treated by subcutaneous tenotomy of the ligamentum patellae. At the age of six years the child is able to manage knee locks on KAFOs without assistance.

THE HIP

Children with spina bifida have three problems with their hips: deformity, dislocation and a lack of power for extension and abduction.

Hip Deformity

The commonest deformity is fixed flexion. It is seen in its most severe form and tends to be most progressive in patients with flail hips (Shurtleff, 1986). It is also seen in patients with low-level lesions. Should the patient have good walking potential and the deformity be more than 20° and progressive, a soft-tissue release of all the tight structures in front of and lateral to the hip is performed.

An anterior hip release is performed through the incision described by Salter (1961) for innominate osteotomy. The muscles are swept off both the inner and outer surfaces of the ilium, the psoas tendon is divided, sartorius and rectus femoris are released, and if necessary, the anterior capsule of the hip joint is divided transversely. At the conclusion of the procedure the anterior superior iliac spine and adjacent portions of the iliac crest protrude forward and are excised. Commonly both hips require this procedure and both can be corrected under one anaesthetic. Postoperatively the patient is nursed on a Bradford frame and may lie prone or supine.

Rarely, extension osteotomy of the upper femur is necessary to correct gross hip flexion deformity in children over ten years of age.

Hip Dislocation

It is now generally agreed that reduction of the dislocated hip in spina bifida does not improve walking ability. Nevertheless some patients, particularly if the dislocation is unilateral, have a troublesome leg length discrepancy if the hip remains dislocated (*Figure 9.9*). The indications for reduction of the dislocated hip are summarized in *Table 9.2*.

If the hip is to be reduced it is important to minimize the duration of plaster immobilization. Hip reduction should be stabilized by pelvic osteotomy using either Pemberton (1965) or Chiari procedures. Plaster immobilization is required for 6–8 weeks postoperatively.

Provision of Abductor and Extensor Power

Sharrard (1964) stressed the importance of providing abductor and extensor power and weakening the strong flexors by performing iliopsoas transfer. It is now clear that dislocation of the hip is most common in patients with flail hips and there is doubt about the need to correct muscle balance at the hip in the

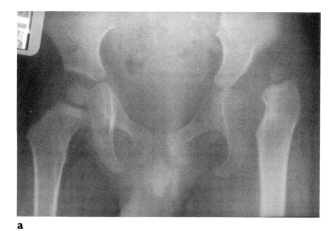

a

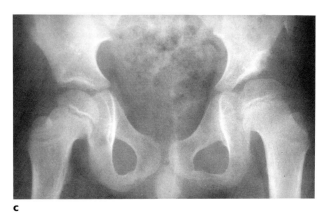

c

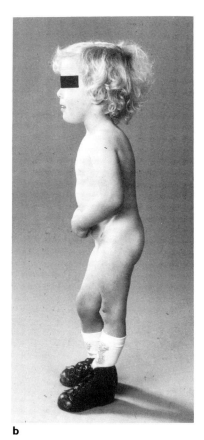

b

Figure 9.9 a Unilateral left hip dislocation in an 18-month-old child with a lesion at L4 neurosegmental level. Note the gross acetabular dysplasia. **b** The child standing at the age of two years: note the short left leg and the good standing ability. **c** Radiograph of the same child at eight years of age. At three years of age she had undergone open reduction, adductor and psoas release plus Pemberton osteotomy followed by ten weeks of plaster immobilization. She is a community ambulator and has no limb length inequality. (Reproduced with permission from Williams PF, Cole WG. *Orthopaedic Management in Childhood*. Chapman & Hall, London.)

prevention of hip dislocation. On the other hand stance and gait may be improved by providing a strong abductor and extensor. This can be obtained by posterior iliopsoas transfer or by one or more of the following procedures (Yngve and Lindseth, 1982):

- External oblique transfer to the greater trochanter.
- Transfer of the adductor origin posteriorly.
- Posterior transfer of the origin of tensor fascia lata.

THE SPINE

Spinal deformity prevents effective walking, and can make sitting difficult. It is a drastic impairment of function if the child has to use one hand to keep him upright because of spinal deformity. Because of subtle neurological disturbances in the upper limbs, spina bifida patients commonly need to use both hands for functions that people without spina bifida can carry out with one hand.

In treating the deforming spine surgically, every effort must be made to avoid prolonged immobilization. Osteoporosis, fractures, genitourinary complications and psychological disturbance may develop, and a child with spina bifida off his feet for as little as three months may never walk again.

Classification of Spinal Deformity

Spinal deformities in spina bifida may take one or more of the following forms:

Table 9.2   The indications for reducing hip dislocation in spina bifida

	Bilateral	Unilateral

High lesions
Weak quadriceps, require
   above-knee bracing.
Short-term walkers.
	Never reduce dislocation	**Seldom reduce**
		May do so if:
		Dislocation is not gross.
		The other leg has a low lesion.
		Surgery is necessary for hip flexion
		   deformity.

Low lesions
Strong quadriceps, may require
   below-knee bracing.
Lifetime walkers.
	Seldom reduce
	May do so if:
	Dislocation is not gross.
	Surgery is necessary for hip
	   flexion deformity.
		Always reduce

- Kyphosis, paralytic and congenital forms.
- Scoliosis, the most common form occurring in myelomeningocoele patients being paralytic in type, but congenital and mixed congenital and paralytic curves also occur. The curve may be a lordoscoliosis or a kyphoscoliosis.
- Lordosis, which is commonly secondary to fixed flexion deformity of the hip.
- Spondylolisthesis.
- Absence of the sacrum (partial or complete).
- Defects of the neural arch and wide separation of the pedicles at the level of the neurological and meningeal lesion.
- Diastematomyelia.
- The full range of vertebral body anomalies seen in congenital scoliosis and occurring either at the level of the spina bifida or any other level of the spine. These anomalies include defects of segmentation, defects of formation and mixed defects.

Kyphosis

Children who are born with kyphosis generally have hydrocephalus and are among the most severely affected children. Some of these children do not survive. The kyphosis is generally in the lumbar spine. It can measure as much as 80° at birth, and increases by an average of 8° per annum. Portions of the erector spinae muscles lie anterior to the axis of flexion and therefore become flexors of the spine and aggravate the tendency to kyphosis.

Management

The indication for correction is recurrent skin ulceration. A variety of surgical techniques are available and the choice will depend on the age of the child and the severity of the kyphosis. Procedures available include correction and anterior strut graft fusion, or one-stage excision followed by posterior fixation.

Scoliosis

Although the curve is most commonly paralytic in origin it may be congenital or mixed. Furthermore patients who have hydrosyringomyelia may develop scoliosis secondary to this cause and drainage of the syrinx may prevent progression or lead to some reversal of the scoliosis. Severe and progressive scoliosis is most common in patients with thoracic-level lesions. The incidence progressively diminishes with lesser degrees of neurological deficit.

Management

There is a small place for bracing in children with rapidly progressive scoliosis who are considered too young for surgery.

Indications for operative management
The main aims of surgery are:

- To provide a stable posture for standing and sitting. The pelvis should be level and the trunk should sit vertical on this level pelvis without the need for hand support. This aim is frequently not achieved.
- To produce a stable fusion and prevent recurrence.
- To remove the convexities that may be the site of pressure, maintain maximum length of the trunk, preserve good respiratory function and achieve satisfactory cosmesis.

Usually this means operating on a deformity over 35° between 8–14 years of age.

The principles of surgery

Stable fusion by both anterior and posterior approaches should be achieved. Anterior instrumentation enables correction of the tight curve at the apex of the primary curve (which is usually at the thoracolumbar junction) and this procedure has a high fusion rate. Posterior instrumentation increases the length of spine that can be fused and allows better correction of pelvic obliquity.

SUMMARY OF ORTHOPAEDIC MANAGEMENT OF SPINA BIFIDA

Orthopaedic management of spina bifida patients must be tailored to meet the future demands of the child. In general, those with high-level lesions and weak quadriceps muscles will place minimal demands on their feet and legs during the period when they are walking and are best served by simple surgery. This simple surgery will generally take the form of soft-tissue release to rid the patient of fixed deformity. However, those with high-level lesions more frequently require radical surgery for scoliosis and this surgery will take the form of anterior and posterior fusion.

Children with low-level lesions and strong quadriceps muscles are likely to walk throughout life. They put greater demands on their feet and legs and benefit more from a good range of movement at the hip and knee. They need plantigrade feet.

SPINAL DYSRAPHISM

Spinal dysraphism refers to the abnormalities of formation of dorsal midline structures. Approximately 10–30% of the population have a degree of this abnormality, but in most it is a coincidental radiological finding of spina bifida occulta affecting one vertebral arch. Clinically significant spinal dysraphism is rare.

The condition may affect all or some of the primary embryonic layers. The type of dysplasia and the resultant conditions are described in *Table 9.3*.

The commonest forms of pathology are as follows:

- Diastematomyelia, where the spinal cord or filum terminale, or both, are split sagittally by a bony or fibrocartilaginous septum (*Figure 9.10*).
- Lumbosacral lipoma.
- Meningocoele manqué, in which a loop of nerve root or trunk emerges from the spinal cord, cauda equina or filum terminale, becomes adherent to the dura, and then returns to the cauda equina or filum near its point of origin.
- Dermoid cyst.
- Tight filum terminale resulting in a tethered cord and the conus lying at a lower level than expected. Normally the conus is at the level of the coccyx in the fetus, at the upper border of the third lumbar vertebra at birth, and at the upper border of the second lumbar vertebra at the age of five years.
- Hydromyelia.
- Atrophy meningocoele.
- Arachnoid cyst.
- Various forms of myelodysplasia.

Frequently more than one of these abnormalities is present in combination.

Diagnosis

Patients may present to the orthopaedic surgeon at any age from birth to maturity with one of the following features:

- A short, often wasted, leg.
- A small foot.
- Cavovarus foot deformity.
- Paralytic valgus foot deformity.
- Trophic ulceration.

In addition to the above features there may be a cutaneous lesion such as a patch of hair, a naevus, a lipoma, a scarred area, or a sinus or dimple in the midline over the lumbar spine. In James and Lassman's classic series of 200 cases (1981), about 25% had no external cutaneous manifestation. It is therefore imperative that the clinician has a high level of suspicion of this condition in association with the deformities listed above and investigations undertaken as outlined below.

Differential Diagnosis

This depends to some extent on the presenting features. If the patient presents with a short leg or small foot then the common differential diagnosis is hemihypertrophy or hemiatrophy. If neurological features are present then the differential diagnosis includes the hereditary motor and sensory neuropathies and cerebral palsy (see Chapter 10).

Table 9.3 Spina bifida, spinal dysraphism or the spinal dysraphic state

Embryonal origin	Type of dysplasia	Resultant condition
Somatic ectodermal	Cutaneous	Cutaneous defect (e.g. hypertrichosis, naevus, dermal sinus)
Mesodermal	Vertebral	Split in spinous process Laminal defects Rachischisis
	Dural	Non-fusion of dura mater
Neurectodermal	Neural tube	Myelodysplasia Intramedullary and extramedullary growths associated with dysraphia
	Neural crest	Ectopia of spinal ganglia and of posterior nerve roots

Adapted from Lichtenstein (1940). Details of all aspects of the condition have been described by James and Lassman (1972, 1981).

Radiology

Ultrasound is the investigation of choice in children under six months of age presenting with midline lumbar dermal abnormalities.

After six months, a plain radiograph should be taken of the full length of the spine. It may show a widened interpeduncular distance, varying degrees of spina bifida, anomalies of formation of the vertebrae or a bony spur if diastematomyelia is present. CT scanning, with or without myelography, and MRI are useful in defining the precise nature of the abnormality when planning surgery.

Management

Management consists of recognizing the condition, arresting any further neurological deterioration and then correcting any foot deformity that has arisen.

Having diagnosed the condition it is then necessary to decide whether it is worthwhile excising any

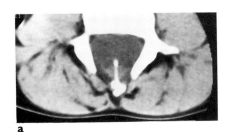
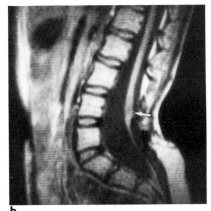
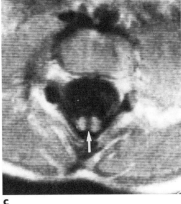

a   b   c

Figure 9.10 a Investigations of a 10-year-old girl with diastematomyelia. There is an incomplete spur at the level of the fourth lumbar vertebra. Axial computerized tomography section showing the incomplete bony spur between hemicords. **b** Midsagittal magnetic resonance imaging section. Note a focal abnormality where the cord is less well defined at the site of the lesion (arrow). Note also that the cord extends abnormally distally to L5 level and a thickened filum terminale extends below it. **c** Axial magnetic resonance imaging section at L4 showing the bifid spinal cord (arrowed) lying posteriorly suggesting tethering. (Reproduced with permission from Benson M *et al.* (1994). *Children's Orthopaedics and Fractures.* Churchill Livingstone, Edinburgh.)

bony spur or releasing cord tethering to prevent the progression of the neurological abnormality. These decisions can only be made in a centre of expertise with neurosurgical involvement.

The foot deformity should be addressed when the neurological abnormality has stabilized. Surgery involves correction of the deformity and correction of any muscle imbalance causing the deformity. If there is doubt as to the most appropriate action or as to the precise nature of any muscle imbalance, then cast correction of the deformity is of value. A later deterioration will occur, but by then the appropriate course of action may be clearer.

Surgical correction of the deformity follows the usual rules for foot deformity surgery. Soft-tissue releases are used in the under five-year-olds, limited bony procedures such as metatarsal osteotomies or osteotomies of the os calcis for children aged 5–10 years, and bony fusions such as a triple or wedge tarsectomy are used in the over 12-year-olds.

REFERENCES AND FURTHER READING

Broughton NS, Menelaus MB, Cole WG, Shurtleff DB. The natural history of hip deformity in myelomeningocoele. *J Bone Joint Surg* 1993; **75B**: 760–763.

James CCM, Lassman LP. *Spinal Dysraphism. Spina Bifida Occulta.* Butterworths, London, 1972.

James CCM, Lassman LP. *Spina Bifida Occulta. Orthopaedic, Radiological and Neurosurgical Aspects.* Academic Press, London/Grune & Stratton, New York, 1981.

Lichtenstein BW. Spinal dysraphism. Spina bifida and myelodysplasia. *Arch Neurol Psych* 1940; **44**: 792–810.

Mazur J, Shurtleff D, Menelaus MB. Orthopaedic management of high-level spina bifida. *J Bone Joint Surg* 1989; **71A**: 56–61.

Menelaus MB. *The Orthopaedic Management of Spina Bifida Cystica.* Churchill Livingstone, Edinburgh, 1980.

Nicol RO, Menelaus MB. Correction of combined tibial torsion and valgus deformity of the foot. *J Bone Joint Surg* 1983; **65B**: 641–645.

Olney BW, Menelaus MB. Triple arthrodesis of the foot in spina bifida patients. *J Bone Joint Surg* 1988; **70B**: 234–235.

Salter RB. Innominate osteotomy in the treatment of congenital dislocation and subluxation of the hip. *J Bone Joint Surg* 1961; **43B**: 44–61.

Schafer MF, Dias LS. *Myelomeningocoele; Orthopaedic Treatment.* Williams & Wilkins, Baltimore, London, 1983.

Sharrard WJW. Posterior iliopsoas transplantation in the treatment of paralytic dislocation of the hip. *J Bone Joint Surg* 1964; **46B**: 426–444.

Shurtleff DB. *Myelodysplasias and Exstrophies: Significance, Prevention and Treatment.* Grune & Stratton, Orlando, Florida, 1986.

Torode IP, Godette G. Surgical correction of congenital kyphosis in myelomeningocoele. *J Pediatr Orthop* 1995; **15**: 202–205.

Williams PF, Menelaus MB. Triple arthrodesis by inlay grafting: a method suitable for the undeformed or valgus foot. *J Bone Joint Surg* 1977; **59B**: 333–336.

Wright JG, Menelaus MB, Broughton NS, Shurtleff D. Natural history of knee contractures in myelocoele. *J Pediatr Orthop* 1991; **11**: 725–730.

Yngve DA, Lindseth RE. Effectiveness of muscle tansfer in myelomeningocoele hips measured by radiographic indices. *J Pediatr Orthop* 1982; **2**: 121–125.

Chapter 10
Neuromuscular Disorders of Childhood

Gary R Nattrass

The neuromuscular disorders of childhood are a spectrum of conditions that have a wide range of aetiologies and variability in manifestation yet share many common clinical traits. The challenge to the clinician is first to detect if there is a neuromuscular problem and then, by diagnosing the specific condition, provide guidance about the natural history of the disorder. Consideration can then be given to whether orthopaedic intervention is appropriate. Since many of these conditions are hereditary it is essential to be able to tell the family what the implications are for the patient, siblings, the extended family and further pregnancies.

History

The presentation may take many forms and it is vital to understand exactly what the parents consider to be abnormal. They may be concerned about a delay in walking or that the child was walking and has now stopped. They may be describing an abnormal gait pattern. The timing of the development of abnormalities is important as is the rate of progression.

Developmental history is discussed. Specifically one should note any problem in the pre- or perinatal period as well as the achievement of development milestones (*Table 10.1*). Parents are often concerned that their child is not walking 'soon enough'. While it is 'normal' to be walking by oneself by 14 months of age, concern is not indicated until 18 months of age.

The family history will often provide the diagnosis as many of these conditions are hereditary.

A review of systems should be directed at gaining information about the general health of the child. The feeding pattern should be noted, together with any weight change or fever.

Table 10.1 Motor milestones

Age	Skill
3 months	Lifts head when prone
6 months	Rolls over
9 months	Sits without support
12 months	Walks with one-hand support
15 months	Walks on own
2 years	Ascends stairs; runs forward
3 years	Pedals tricycle
4 years	Balances on one foot
5 years	Hops on one foot

Physical Examination

Examination of the child begins with a general assessment of the child's well-being, including their reaction to the environment. Their stage of sitting or walking is noted.

A full neurological examination is performed with assessment of the power of muscles, any spasticity and increased tendon jerks. Sensation, coordination and proprioception are all tested.

In paediatric orthopaedic practice one soon starts to recognize various patterns of weakness and there are common patterns of presentation.

The floppy baby
The hypotonic baby without weakness usually has a central nervous system (CNS) aetiology (e.g. cerebral palsy). Hypotonia accompanied by weakness usually signifies a peripheral neuromuscular cause (e.g. spinal muscle atrophy or congenital myopathy).

Proximal muscle weakness
Gowers sign is evident when the patient is placed supine on the floor and then asked to rise from the

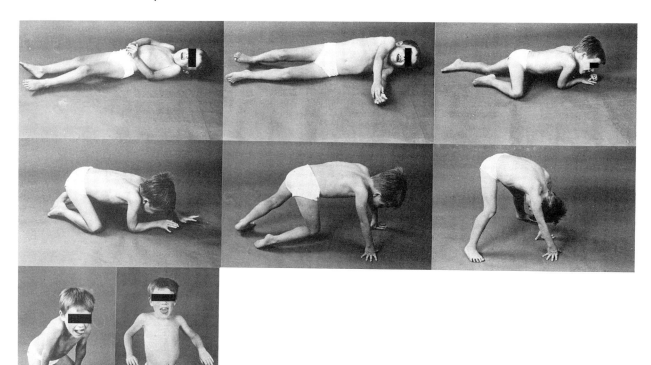

Figure 10.1 Gowers sign: this child with marked proximal muscle weakness (quadriceps and gluteus maximus) stands from the supine position by using his arms to 'climb' up his legs. (Reproduced with permission from Williams PF, Cole WG. *Orthopaedic Management in Childhood*. Chapman & Hall, London.)

floor (*Figure 10.1*). Because of the marked proximal muscle wasting (quadriceps and gluteus maximus) the child will only be able to rise after 'climbing up his legs' by pushing his hands against his knees to extend them and then pushing his trunk upward by working his hands up his thigh. This fully developed picture is a sign of severe weakness. Children with lesser degrees of weakness may only put the legs apart and push the bottom upwards and then extend the trunk using the hands.

The Meryon ('fall through') sign is evident when the patient is lifted up under the axillae and slides through due to weakness of the shoulder girdle.

Differential diagnosis includes muscular dystrophies, spinal motor atrophy, and congenital myopathies.

Differentiation of upper motor neurone lesion from lower motor neurone lesion

Upper motor neurone lesions occur above the level of the anterior horn cell. The lower motor neurone includes the anterior horn cell and distal to it (*Table 10.2*).

Table 10.2 Clinical features of upper and lower motor neurone lesions

	Upper motor neurone	Lower motor neurone
Tone	Increased (spasticity)	Decreased (flaccid)
Wasting	Late	Early
Plantar reflex	Upgoing	Downgoing
Clonus	Yes	No
Fasciculation (rare)	No	Yes

Table 10.3   Differential diagnosis of the cavovarus foot

Neuromuscular

Brain	Cerebral palsy
Spinal cord	Spinal dysraphism
	Diastematomyelia
	Tethered cord
	Friedreich's ataxia
	Spinal cord tumour
	Polio
Peripheral	Hereditary motor and sensory neuropathy
	Nerve trauma

Structural

Sequelae of talipes equinovarus
Soft tissue injury (trauma, burns, irradiation)

Idiopathic

Cavovarus feet

Cavovarus feet (pes cavus) has many different causes of muscle imbalance and may be the only sign to alert the physician to underlying disease (*Table 10.3*). Weakness in the intrinsic muscles of the foot result in a 'claw toe' deformity with extension at the metatarsophalangeal joint and flexion at the inter-phalangeal joints (*Figure 10.2*). There is then a relative plantar flexion of the first metatarsal and subsequently contracture and thickening of the plantar fascia. With time, the deformity becomes worse and eventually becomes fixed.

Toe walking

A diagnosis of 'idiopathic toe walker' can only be given after other causes have been eliminated (*Table 10.4*). The important point to help confirm the diagnosis in the toe walker is whether this is a new pattern or whether the child has always walked in this manner. A late onset of toe walking must raise the immediate suspicion of a neurological condition such as muscular dystrophy, peripheral neuropathy or cord tethering from spinal dysraphism.

Laboratory Tests

Creatinine phosphokinase (CPK)

This is an intracellular enzyme released from muscle cells with degeneration (or trauma). The level is greatly increased in muscular dystrophy (Duchenne or Becker), but only mildly increased in the other dystrophic disorders (facioscapulohumeral, Emery–Dreifuss). It is only slightly elevated or normal in the congenital myopathies. CPK is normal in diseases that primarily affect nerve (peripheral neuropathy, spinal muscle atrophy or Friedreich ataxia).

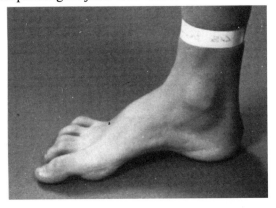
a

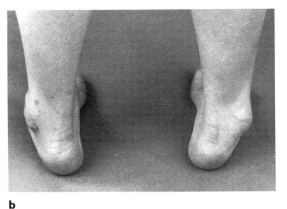
b

Figure 10.2a,b   Cavovarus feet: the metatarsophalangeal joints are hyperextended and there is flexion at the interphalangeal joints and subsequent plantar flexion of the first metatarsal. The hindfoot is in varus.

Table 10.4   Differential diagnosis of toe walking

'Always walked that way'	'Late onset'
Cerebral palsy	Muscular dystrophy
Leg length discrepancy	Peripheral neuropathy
Congenital short tendo Achillis	Spinal dysraphism (tethered cord)
Idiopathic (habitual)	Spinal cord tumour

Aldolase

This is an enzyme that catalyses the breakdown of glucose and is found in most tissues. It is markedly elevated in Duchenne muscular dystrophy, moderately elevated in other myopathies, and essentially normal in neural atrophies.

DNA diagnosis

This is now possible for a number of neuromuscular disorders and may be performed on either a small quantity of blood or amniotic fluid. Detection of a deletion in the dystrophin gene on the X chromosome confirms a diagnosis of Duchenne or Becker muscular dystrophy and may be used for antenatal diagnosis.

Electrophysiology

Electromyography (EMG)

This is used to differentiate myopathic from neurogenic disorders (*Figure 10.3*). Denervation results in fibrillation potentials (i.e. the muscle fires sponta-

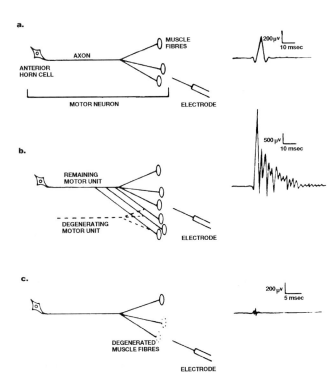

Figure 10.3 Electromyography studies the motor unit potentials to aid in the differentiation of a neuropathic process from a myopathic process. **a** Normal motor unit; **b**, neuropathic motor unit; **c**, myopathic motor unit. (Reproduced with permission from Kaplan J *et al*. Modern electrodiagnostic studies in infants and children. *Pediatric Annals*, **13**: 2, 150–164, 1984.)

neously without the organizational effect of the nerve) whereas a myopathy results in a low-amplitude polyphasic pattern.

Nerve conduction studies

These are used to determine if the process is localized to a single nerve or is generalized. Nerve conduction studies are typically carried out over the median, ulnar, peroneal and posterior tibial nerves. Conduction velocity will be normal in anterior horn disease, root disease and myopathies, but will be markedly decreased in demyelinating neuropathies. The normal value in a child over five years of age is 45–65 m s^{-1} although this does vary with age and from nerve to nerve. The velocity is slower in younger children because myelination is incomplete.

Biopsy

Muscle biopsy (*Figure 10.4*) is important in the diagnostic process and is usually indicated unless a definitive diagnosis has been made by other means. The biopsy should be performed on the least affected muscle when dealing with a chronic disease, while the most affected muscles should be biopsied in an acute disease. If the muscle weakness is mainly proximal, vastus lateralis is used. If the weakness is mainly distal, gastrocnemius is used.

Histological findings in myopathic disorders typically include:

- A variation in size of the fibres.
- A central location of nuclei.
- Degenerating and regenerating fibres.

Neuropathic disorders will tend to show atrophy of the fibre group with all the fibres in an abnormal group having a uniformly small diameter. An inflammatory cellular reaction will be seen in an inflammatory myopathy.

Dystrophin testing can now be carried out through dystrophin immunoblotting of a small amount of frozen muscle. It is absent in Duchenne muscular dystrophy and reduced in Becker muscular dystrophy.

Nerve biopsy is carried out much less frequently than muscle biopsy. It is used to determine the type of peripheral neuropathy because they are defined by their pattern of demyelination. The sural nerve is used.

MUSCULAR DYSTROPHY

The muscular dystrophies are a group of non-inflammatory inherited primary disorders of muscle that

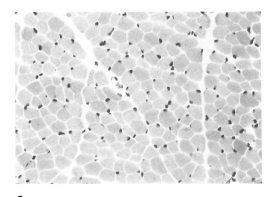

a

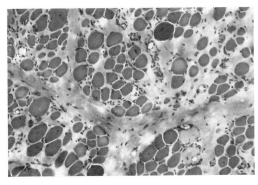

b

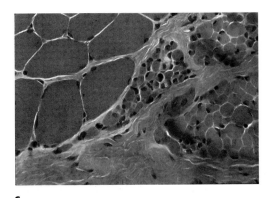

c

Figure 10.4 a The pattern of a normal muscle biopsy. **b** The pattern of Duchenne muscular dystrophy in a muscle biopsy, which is characterized by degeneration, fibrosis, and fatty replacement of the muscle fibres. **c** Muscle biopsy from a patient with spinal muscular atrophy (SMA). Neuropathic processes such as SMA result in atrophy of the muscle fibre.

result in progressive degeneration and weakness of skeletal muscle. They can be classified on the basis of their genetic transmission (*Table 10.5*).

Duchenne and Becker muscular dystrophy are myopathic disorders caused by an abnormality of the muscle protein dystrophin, which is a component

Table 10.5   Genetic basis of the muscular dystrophies

Sex-linked
Duchenne, Becker, Emery–Dreifuss

Autosomal recessive
Limb-girdle

Autosomal dominant
Facioscapulohumeral

of the cell membrane cytoskeleton. Duchenne muscular dystrophy is characterized by a complete absence of dystrophin. In Becker muscular dystrophy dystrophin is present, but is either altered in size or decreased in amount or both. The gene responsible for both disorders is located on the xp21 region of the X chromosome.

Duchenne Muscular Dystrophy

Duchenne muscular dystrophy occurs almost exclusively in males because it is X-linked. The incidence is around 20 per 100,000 male births. Approximately 30% of affected children are thought to have new mutations.

Clinical Features

Children are usually brought for consultation either because they are slow to walk or because their other motor milestones are delayed. They may have an awkward gait or a known family history. Sometimes they present with flat feet, or knock knees, but with parental concern that there is something not quite right about their progress (*Figure 10.5*).

The natural progression of the disease is to present at 3–5 years of age, and then to develop increasing weakness and contractures over the next five years, becoming wheelchair bound by 10–12 years of age. This is followed by severe scoliosis. Death usually occurs at 18–25 years of age due to pulmonary failure and cardiomyopathy.

Management

Orthopaedic management in these children should be tailored to the stage of the disease and the goals should be realistic in view of its natural history. The goal in the ambulating child is therefore to prolong his ambulation, and in the non-ambulator to

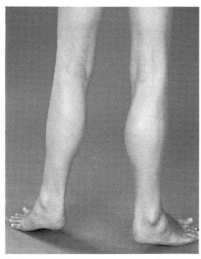

Figure 10.5   Pseudohypertrophy of the calf muscle is a classic sign of Duchenne or Becker muscle dystrophy. Note that this patient with Becker muscle dystrophy has also developed an equinus deformity at the ankle.

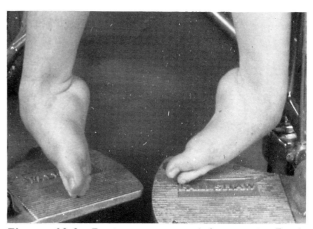

Figure 10.6   Equinocavovarus deformity in Duchenne muscular dystrophy may require surgical correction to overcome difficulties using a wheelchair.

produce a stable posture for sitting by correction of the scoliosis.

The lower limb

The management of lower limb contractures depends on the expectations of the family and on the philosophy of the treating surgeon. With aggressive intervention, ambulation can be prolonged from 1–3 years through bracing and surgery.

Usually the tibialis posterior is the last muscle to be affected in the lower limb. The resultant equinovarus deformity is treated by tendo Achillis lengthening, and transfer of the tibialis posterior through the interosseous membrane to the dorsum of the foot. Timing of the surgery is controversial. It has been tried early before there is deformity, but this does not seem to change the natural history. It is usually carried out when the patient's walking ability is markedly worsening, and if performed within six months of losing the ability to walk, the results can be successful for up to three years. Surgery is also useful for the wheelchair-bound patient who develops a rigid equinovarus deformity so that normal shoes can be worn and the foot does not rest abnormally on the foot plate of the wheelchair (*Figure 10.6*).

Posterior releases around the knee are sometimes performed to aid the weakened quadriceps in extending the knee and to correct flexion deformity of the knee.

Bracing can be used with or without surgery, but because of the added weight the brace might actually hinder the patient's efforts at walking.

Flexion–abduction contractures about the hip have been released by some, but there does not appear to be good evidence that this changes the natural history.

Scoliosis

Scoliosis develops in 95% of patients with Duchenne's muscular dystrophy. About 25% of patients develop some scoliosis while still walking, but after the patient becomes wheelchair-bound the curve often progresses rapidly. Bracing and specialized wheelchair modifications can slow but not prevent the development of the curve. Severe scoliosis in these children causes difficulty in sitting due to pain and pressure sores. In some this is so severe that it prevents sitting. The goal of spinal stabilization is to aid the child in wheelchair sitting.

Children with Duchenne's muscular dystrophy develop a restrictive pulmonary pattern due to muscle weakness and contractures rather than the scoliosis. Pulmonary function, as measured by the forced expiratory volume (FEV), declines most rapidly during the adolescent growth spurt. Once the FEV is less than 35% there are concerns about the patients becoming ventilator-dependent after surgery. Lung function tests can be unreliable in these children so it is difficult to define a specific figure below which surgery should not be attempted. However, spinal stabilization is best undertaken in the time between the curve developing and before the FEV decreases to less than 35% of normal. In those who will obviously require surgery, this should not be delayed. Instrumentation is usually to the pelvis using the Luque or Unit Rod and sublaminar wiring. This is a major undertaking producing more blood loss than with scoliosis surgery in normal children as well as increased respiratory problems postoperatively.

Becker Muscular Dystrophy

Becker muscular dystrophy presents with similar problems to those seen in Duchenne muscular dystrophy but the age of onset of symptoms is about twice that for Duchenne. Lower limb contractures develop at a slower rate, but surgical correction is worthwhile, as outlined above. Scoliosis occurs in those children with a severe form of the disease, but the incidence is much less than that with Duchenne muscular dystrophy. Life expectancy is greater than that with Duchenne with the majority living into their forties or beyond.

Emery–Dreifuss Muscular Dystrophy

Emery–Dreifuss muscular dystrophy is rare and primarily affects the humoroperoneal muscles producing elbow flexion contractures and ankle equinus contractures. Dystrophin production is normal. Presentation is usually before the age of five years, with toe walking and an awkward gait. Elbow contractures and extensor muscle contractures of the neck develop later. Cardiac consultation is mandatory because of the high incidence of cardiac abnormalities and premature sudden death. Cardiac pacemakers are often implanted even if the patient is asymptomatic. If cardiac complications are avoided life expectancy is normal.

Limb-Girdle Muscular Dystrophy

Limb-girdle muscular dystrophy is an autosomal recessive disorder with a variable presentation. It is usually diagnosed in the late teens and primarily affects the shoulders and hips with weakness of the distal muscles of the limbs in more severely affected individuals. Since CPK is elevated, and EMG and biopsy are that of a myopathy, a normal dystrophin assay is necessary to exclude Becker muscular dystrophy. Orthopaedic treatment is again directed at treating the contractures.

Facioscapulohumeral Muscular Dystrophy

Facioscapulohumeral muscular dystrophy is an autosomal dominant disorder that is characterized by a slowly progressive weakness of the face, shoulder girdle and arm muscles. This disorder also has a very wide range of clinical presentations. It is slowly progressive and patients have a normal life expectancy. The usual onset is in late childhood or early adulthood, though there is a more severe autosomal recessive infantile form.

The most common findings are facial weakness and scapular winging. This may weaken the shoulder girdle considerably and require treatment by scapulothoracic fusion. Other patterns of weakness are variably present including foot drop due to involvement of the peroneal muscles and dorsiflexors of the foot, which may require bracing or tibialis posterior transfer. There may be weakness of the forearm, pelvis and thigh, and rarely scoliosis.

Congenital Muscular Dystrophy

Congenital muscular dystrophy usually presents as hypotonia and weakness at birth. There is marked variation in its clinical course. Diagnosis is made by muscle biopsy, which reveals variation in the diameter of the fibres within each fascicle and increased perimysial and endomysial fibrosis. The CPK is usually elevated and EMG changes are myopathic. Some forms of congenital muscular dystrophy are due to a deficiency of merosin, a membrane protein. Some patients die early in life, but many stabilize and live well into adult life. Orthopaedic management involves attention to contractures and secondary deformity.

CONGENITAL MYOPATHY

The congenital myopathies are a group of diseases that have a primary defect in a specific component of the muscle fibre. They cause muscle weakness and tend to involve the proximal muscles of the limbs. They differ from the muscular dystrophies because they present earlier, usually as 'the floppy baby' and the progression of the weakness is often slow. Inheritance varies with autosomal recessive, autosomal dominant, and X-linked patterns being seen. Serum enzymes are normal or slightly elevated. Muscle biopsy reveals that the abnormality is in the myofibril, which is distinct from the pathology of the muscular dystrophies where there is replacement of muscle fibres by adipose tissue. The individual diseases are named by the abnormality seen on histochemical and electromicroscopic evaluation of the muscle biopsy:

- Central core disease is characterized by a local absence of mitochondria and sarcoplasmic reticulum, giving the appearance of a 'core' within the muscle fibre. These children also have an increased incidence of malignant hyperthermia.
- Nemaline (rod–body) myopathy is characterized by the presence of 'rod–bodies' within the muscle fibre.
- Other types of congenital myopathy include myotubular (centronuclear) myopathy, congenital fibre-type disproportion myopathy and various metabolic myopathies.

Clinical Features

Cases may present to orthopaedic surgeons with joint contractures and scoliosis. The underlying myopathy may go unrecognized and be the cause of a failure of treatment for congenital dislocation of the hip.

MYOTONIC SYNDROMES

These syndromes are characterized by an inability of skeletal muscle to relax after a strong contraction on voluntary movement or mechanical stimulation. This is noticeable in the 'lingering handshake' – patients are unable to relax their grip after a handshake.

Myotonic Dystrophy (Steinert Disease)

This is an autosomal dominant condition involving chromosome 19. It usually presents in late adolescence or early adulthood as a steadily progressive condition that affects distal muscles first. As the disease progresses, there is a gradual proximal spread with increasing difficulty in walking. Patients tend to have an associated facial weakness resulting in an expressionless facies and ptosis. In the congenital form, the child has a 'fish-mouth', which is difficult to close. Enzyme studies are often normal and the EMG shows a characteristic loud 'dive bomber' pattern. Orthopaedic intervention is rarely required in childhood.

Congenital Myotonic Dystrophy

This is a more severe form of myotonic dystrophy. It is passed on from a mother with myotonic dystrophy. These children are affected more than their mother and present with expressionless facies, hypotonia, difficulty in feeding and respiratory failure. Orthopaedic problems are severe talipes equinovarus (similar to arthrogryposis), dislocated hips, joint contractures and difficulty in walking.

Mytonia Congenita (Thomsen Disease)

This presents as a generalized muscle hypertrophy and myotonia. Specific orthopaedic problems are rare in childhood.

INFLAMMATORY MYOPATHIES

Acute muscle pain with inflammation may be the presentation of dermatomyositis or polymyositis. This febrile illness, which affects females more than males, results in very tender, brawny and indurated muscles. Its aetiology is unknown, but it is believed that both genetics and exposure to a virus may be important. The muscle weakness tends to be proximal and symmetrical and there may be muscle calcinosis. In dermatomyositis the patient develops an erythematous rash over the malar area of the face as a butterfly rash and this may spread to the upper chest. There may also be dark lilac discoloration of the eyelids, known as heliotrope eyelids, which is said to be pathognomonic.

Management

Management of these conditions consists of attempting to arrest the acute inflammatory picture with prednisone or other immunosuppressive agents along with splinting any painful extremities. If joint contractures develop the orthopaedic surgeon may be involved in soft-tissue releases, but surgery may be extensive yet unrewarding.

HEREDITARY MOTOR AND SENSORY NEUROPATHIES

The hereditary motor and sensory neuropathies (HMSN) include a range of inherited neuropathies that have variable inheritance patterns, clinical expression and pathological findings. In the past, they have been given many different names, which have added to the confusion (*Table 10.6*). There are seven types of HMSN, with types I–III being most commonly seen by orthopaedic surgeons.

Pathology

Types I and II HMSN are usually autosomal dominant conditions, but may show autosomal recessive or X-linked patterns. Type III is an autosomal recessive disorder that begins in infancy and is more severe at presentation than types I or II.

Types I and III differ from type II in that they are due to demyelination of the peripheral nerve whereas type II is due to an abnormality in the axon of the spinal cord neurone with peripheral nerve myelination being normal.

Clinical Features

Types I and III produce muscle weakness of the hands and feet and absent reflexes. There is reduced distal sensory capability, particularly involving light touch and position and vibration sense. The EMG indicates a neuropathic disorder and nerve conduction study (NCS) show a marked slowing of the rate of impulse conduction. Muscle biopsy demonstrates a neuropathic pattern and nerve biopsy shows demyelination. Type I presents in the first or second decade of life. Progression is slow and only rarely is a wheelchair required in middle to late adult life.

Since type II is an abnormality of the neurone there are persistently normal reflexes and minimal if any sensory involvement. The sensory and motor nerve conduction times are only slightly abnormal. The EMG findings are similar to those of a neuropathy of the anterior horn cell, and nerve biopsy shows the persistence of myelin. Type II tends to present in the second or third decade with more severe involvement of the lower extremities (stork-leg appearance), but less upper limb involvement than type I or III.

Management

Orthopaedic management in these conditions is directed primarily at the foot deformity, hip dysplasia and scoliosis.

Foot deformity

The peripheral neuropathies affect the intrinsic muscles of the foot first, and the initial deformities are claw toes. Progression takes place proximally with adduction of the metatarsals and plantar flexion of the first metatarsal. A cavus deformity of the foot then occurs followed by varus of the hindfoot, to give the typical appearance of the cavovarus foot.

The block test of Coleman helps to determine whether varus of the hindfoot seen on walking is due to a fixed varus deformity of the hindfoot or whether it is secondary to a fixed pronation deformity of the forefoot. The block is placed obliquely under the heel and lateral aspect of the forefoot and the head of the first metatarsal is allowed to fall into its natural position. If the hindfoot corrects with this manoeuvre the standing varus is not fixed and is a

Table 10.6 Hereditary and motor sensory neuropathies

Type	Other names	Nerve conduction velocity
I	Charcot–Marie–Tooth (hypertrophic form) Peroneal muscle atrophy Roussey–Lévy syndrome (hereditary areflexic dystaxia)	Delayed
II	Charcot–Marie–Tooth (axonal form) Peroneal muscle atrophy	Normal
III	Dejerine–Sottas disease Hypertrophic neuropathy of infancy	Delayed
IV	Refsum disease (phytanic acid storage neuropathy)	Very delayed
V	Neuropathy with spastic paraplegia Familial spastic paraplegia	Delayed
VI	Optic atrophy with peroneal muscle atrophy	Delayed
VII	Retinitis pigmentosa with distal motor weakness	Delayed

secondary phenomenon due to fixed pronation of the forefoot. If the varus does not correct with this manoeuvre, the varus is fixed.

Management is based on the location and degree of deformity and whether it is correctable. A deformity that is not passively correctable cannot be cured by soft-tissue procedures. A deformity that has not yet become fixed will usually respond to soft-tissue surgery.

Clawing of the toes is treated by open flexor tenotomy if the deformity is correctable. Transfer of the flexor tendons to the extensor hood (Girdlestone transfer) is now rarely employed. When the deformity is fixed a fusion of the proximal interphalangeal joint with K-wire fixation is combined with extensor tenotomy and dorsal capsulotomy of the metatarso-phalangeal joints.

Clawing of the big toe is treated by fusion of the interphalangeal joint and transfer of the extensor hallucis longus to the neck of the first metatarsal (as described by Robert Jones).

In the younger child with a mobile cavus deformity an open release of the plantar fascia (Steindler operation) may prevent progression. Once the deformity is fixed it can only be improved by bony correction. This may be by a triple arthrodesis if there is varus at the hindfoot. If there is no varus then it can be corrected by a closing dorsal wedge tarsectomy, but this shortens the foot considerably and the correction is best carried out using a cresentic or V-shaped osteotomy through the midfoot as described by Japas.

If the Coleman block test has identified a significant amount of fixed pronation of the forefoot this can be addressed by a dorsiflexion osteotomy at the base of the first and second metatarsals.

Fixed varus of the hindfoot in the young child is best treated by a calcaneal osteotomy. This can be carried out as a closing lateral wedge in the manner of Dwyer or as a sliding displacement osteotomy or as a combination of the two. Triple arthrodesis is the treatment of choice if the deformity is combined with midtarsal deformity and in the older child.

Often there is associated equinus, which should be treated by lengthening of the tendo Achillis. Any muscle imbalance should be addressed, even if the deformity is fixed. This usually implies lengthening or division of the tibialis posterior, although sometimes the tendon can be usefully transferred to the dorsum or lateral aspect of the dorsum of the foot through the interosseous membrane.

Treatment is based on the physical findings and whether the deformity is fixed. But in general terms for the child less than ten years of age soft-tissue

release with or without a transfer of the tibialis posterior and a calcaneal osteotomy for heel varus is appropriate. For the child over 14 years of age with a fixed deformity, triple arthrodesis is usually the best surgical option.

Hip dysplasia

This is not uncommon in these children. There is acetabular dysplasia and the femoral head subluxes superiorly. This is best treated by innominate osteotomy or a shelf augmentation. During this procedure great care is taken to avoid damaging the sciatic nerve as it seems to be more susceptible to minor stretching than in the normal child.

Scoliosis

Scoliosis is seen in about 50% of these children in a mild form. Treatment is similar to that for idiopathic scoliosis.

SPINAL MUSCULAR ATROPHY

Spinal muscular atrophy (SMA) is an autosomal recessive disorder resulting in degeneration of the anterior horn cells of the spinal cord with associated muscle weakness and atrophy (*Figure 10.7*). It occurs in one in 20,000 live births. Since it is the anterior horn cells that are involved, sensation remains normal. The present classification is based on clinical severity, but confusion may exist because of the old eponymous nomenclature (*Table 10.7*). All three types have different mutations at the same locus on chromosome 5q.

Type I presents with severe involvement in the first six months of life. The child remains markedly weak

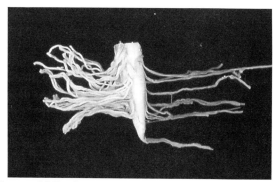

Figure 10.7 Spinal muscular atrophy: section of the spinal cord demonstrating atrophy of the ventral roots resulting from degeneration of the anterior horn cell. In contrast, the dorsal roots are normal.

Table 10.7 Classification of spinal muscular atrophy

Spinal muscular atrophy	Old nomenclature
Type I	Acute Werdnig–Hoffman
Type II	Chronic Werdnig–Hoffman
Type III	Kugelberg–Welander

and generally dies as a result of respiratory failure by 18 months of age.

Type II presents between six months and two years of age. These children may or may not walk. Those that do walk often lose this ability later in life. They are strong enough to survive for many years and although some do die in their teenage years, many live into their thirties and forties.

Type III is diagnosed later, usually after two years of age. The children are initially able to walk, although with difficulty. Walking ability may be lost late in the first decade or in the teenage years.

The natural history of SMA correlates with the maximum function attained rather than with the age of the original presentation. These children have normal intelligence and benefit greatly from orthopaedic procedures that can improve their function, for example sitting upright to use a computer and interact socially.

Management

Scoliosis

Scoliosis occurs in all children with type II SMA and all those with type III who lose the ability to walk. The scoliosis affects the ability of the child to sit. Bracing and wheelchair modifications can be used to aid in sitting, but progression of the curve is inevitable. Timing of spinal stabilization, as with Duchenne muscular dystrophy, must be balanced between the age of the patient, worsening pulmonary function, increasing curve and increasing rigidity. In general, children over ten years of age with a flexible curve greater than 40° and an FEV greater than 40% should be considered for posterior instrumentation and fusion to the pelvis.

Scoliosis in the type III SMA patients who can walk should be managed expectantly. Bracing can be tried, but may be found to limit walking ability. Spinal surgery can result in a loss of lordosis, which is necessary for them to walk, but should be considered when the child stops walking.

Hip dysplasia

Hip dysplasia may occur as a result of muscle imbalance. Dislocation of the hip results in pelvic obliquity and affects sitting balance. Coxa valga can be treated with varus osteotomy of the proximal femur, with acetabular procedures if necessary. The type III SMA patient who is walking may develop dysplasia. It is then difficult to determine whether poor walking ability relates to progression of the disease or the hip subluxation or both. A varus femoral osteotomy can weaken the already compromised abductors of the hip, so it is usually better to address the acetabular side first with an innominate osteotomy.

FRIEDREICH ATAXIA

Friedreich ataxia (hereditary spinal cerebellar ataxia) is an autosomal recessive disorder characterized by spinocerebellar degeneration. Atrophy occurs in the dorsal and ventral cerebellar tracts, the corticospinal tracts and the posterior column. The incidence is approximately one in 50,000. The abnormal gene responsible for this disorder is on chromosome 9.

Nerve conduction studies show a markedly decreased sensory action potential and only a slight decrease in motor nerve conduction velocity. This differs from the findings in motor and sensory neuropathies where the motor nerve conduction velocity is significantly decreased.

Clinical Features

The usual presentation is with an ataxic gait or a cavus foot between 7–15 years of age. The diagnosis is suggested by the triad of ataxia, areflexia and an extensor plantar response.

The natural history of this disorder is a gradual progression, resulting in wheelchair dependency during the second or third decade of life. Death usually occurs in the fourth or fifth decade due to a progressive hypertrophic cardiomyopathy, pneumonia or aspiration.

Management

The major orthopaedic manifestations are scoliosis and cavovarus foot deformities.

Scoliosis

The structural scoliosis is more like an idiopathic scoliosis than a neuromuscular scoliosis. In the non-walker, single-stage posterior instrumentation and fusion should be carried out when the curve is over

40°. In the walker, loss of walking ability has been reported following spinal surgery, so if the curve is less than 25°, a brace may be useful in those patients who can tolerate it.

Cavovarus foot deformity

The cavovarus foot deformity contributes to the difficulties that these patients develop in walking. The goal is to give the patient a stable plantigrade foot. Early management of the mobile cavovarus foot consists of bracing and soft-tissue procedures, such as plantar release and tibialis posterior lengthening or transfer. These may be combined with calcaneal osteotomy performed as a displacement or a closing wedge. Later a triple arthrodesis may be required to stabilize a rigid deformity.

ARTHROGRYPOSIS

Arthrogryposis is a general term referring to a congenital non-progressive limitation of joint movement due to soft-tissue contractures affecting two or more joints. Included under this term is a heterogeneous group of over 150 syndromes. The most common of these is arthrogryposis multiplex congenita ('amyoplasia'), which is a condition of multiple congenital contractures with typical and symmetrical positioning of the limbs and decreased girth in the muscular areas of the limbs. It occurs sporadically with no known hereditary pattern. Distal arthrogryposis is an autosomal dominant condition producing clenched fist and foot deformities, while multiple pterygium syndrome results in a vertical talus in 80% of patients.

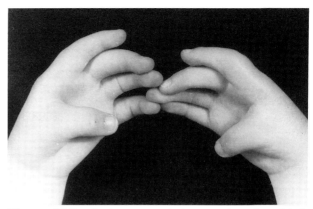

Figure 10.8 Arthrogryposis has produced multiple joint contractures in these hands. The skin is shiny and there are few skin creases.

Aetiology

The aetiology most commonly relates to a defect in the anterior horn cell, which is believed to be an intrauterine event occurring at weeks 8–12. The exact causative agent is unknown, but the possibilities include a virus, a teratogen, local environment, or a metabolic cause. Other causes of intrauterine immobility such as neuropathies and myopathies can also result in a failure of normal intrauterine joint movement with subsequent contracture. A similar condition reported in sheep, cows and horses is due to maternal exposure to the Akabane virus in early pregnancy. No such virus has ever been identified in human cases of arthrogryposis.

Clinical Features

Typically skin creases are absent and the skin is tense and glossy (*Figure 10.8*). Muscle volume is decreased and sensation is intact. However, the clinical presentation of this group of disorders is extremely varied

Table 10.8 Patterns of involvement in arthrogryposis

Upper limb
Shoulder: adduction and internal rotation contracture
Elbow: extension contracture (occasionally flexion)
Wrist: flexion, ulnar deviation, pronation
Hand: variable flexion at the metacarpophalangeal and interphalangeal joints

Lower limb
Hips: flexion, abduction, external rotation contracture, dislocation (uni- or bilateral) in 35%
Knees: flexion (occasionally hyperextension)
Foot and ankle: equinovarus, vertical talus

Spine
Scoliosis: 35% in infancy, childhood or adolescence

in both site and degree of involvement. All four limbs are affected in 92%, lower limbs only in 7%, and upper limbs only in 1%. The patterns of involvement are described in *Table 10.8*.

Differential Diagnosis

Differential diagnoses include primary neuromuscular disorders, lumbosacral agenesis and multiple congenital anomalies.

Management

It is important that an orthopaedic surgeon familiar with the condition is involved at an early stage. The prognosis and overall plan of management can be discussed. These children are generally of normal intelligence and well motivated and tend to do well if left alone. Early management consists of improving the range of movement with the help of a physiotherapist and the parents at home and splinting.

The underlying surgical principle in arthrogryposis is to 'do no harm'. It is essential that any surgical intervention is carefully considered for the individual to improve the child's function rather than merely make them 'different' (*Figure 10.9*).

The lower limb

Management of dislocated hips in children with arthrogryposis is controversial. If the hip is stiff and dislocated, closed reduction is unlikely to be beneficial. Open reduction of a unilateral hip dislocation may be justified. Bilateral dislocations are generally left unreduced because of the risks of further stiffening and development of asymmetry if one side is unsuccessful. Open reduction if attempted should be carried out at about one year and after the knee and feet have been treated.

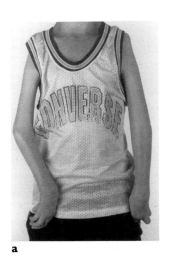

a

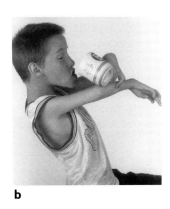

b

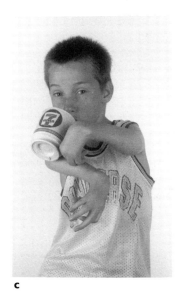

c

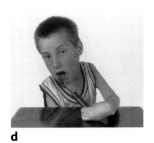

d

Figure 10.9   Although the deformity caused by arthrogryposis can be severe, patients usually develop unique ways of coping with day to day activity. Care must therefore be taken to ensure that any surgery that is carried out will at least maintain the patient's level of function and independence.

Knee flexion contracture may be treated early by posterior capsulotomy and hamstring division, generally at about six months, after the feet have been treated. Later, supracondylar osteotomy of the femur may be necessary for recurrent deformity. The advantage of osteotomy is that when combined with shortening, the neurovascular bundle is not stretched, and since the correction is internally fixed above the knee, the knee can be flexed postoperatively. With an osteotomy, correction of up to 90° can be performed in one sitting (*Figure 10.10*). Regardless of the method used, the natural history is for recurrence of the flexion deformity with growth, and multiple operations are usually necessary.

Extension deformity of the knee is less common. Soft-tissue procedures such as quadriceps lengthening and anterior capsulotomy are usually tried first, but flexion osteotomy of the femur may be required.

Talipes equinovarus is very common. It is often rigid and has a high recurrence rate despite extensive soft-tissue release. The goal of reconstruction is to produce a plantigrade foot. Subtalar release and a posteromedial release are required at about the age of three months, and in the more severe cases talectomy may be necessary. Adequate soft tissue cover is important with these procedures. Significant deformity in children over ten years of age should be treated by triple arthrodesis.

The upper limb

In assessing the upper extremity, the elbow and shoulder should be examined together. In bilateral

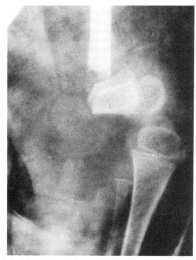

Figure 10.10 The flexion deformity at the knee in arthrogryposis may be resistant to soft-tissue releases and require an extensive extension osteotomy.

disease, only one side would be operated upon to give the patient two ranges of movement in which to function. For example, surgery should preserve one limb for perineal care and the other for strength activities. Surgical options include humeral derotation osteotomy, flexion or extension osteotomies of the humerus in the supracondylar region and elbow capsulotomy. If there is an acceptable range of movement, muscle transfers may be of help.

The approach to the involved wrists depends on whether the hand is functional. If the hand is functional, anterior wrist capsulotomy and fusion may be considered. If the hand is not functional, the wrist should be left alone.

Hand deformities are varied and difficult to deal with. A thumb-in-palm deformity may be treated by Z-plasty and release of adductors. Metacarpophalangeal joint fusion of the thumb is sometimes appropriate.

The spine

Scoliosis may be managed in a similar manner to that of idiopathic curves, using bracing for mild curves, and instrumentation and fusion for those that progress. However, less correction with instrumentation can be expected in the child with arthrogryposis because of the severe contractures.

POLIOMYELITIS

Poliomyelitis is a viral infection that affects the anterior horn cells in the spinal cord with subsequent impairment or paralysis of the supplied muscle. While prophylactic vaccination has eliminated new cases in the developed world, the orthopaedic surgeon will regularly see patients with the musculoskeletal sequelae of the disease. About ten million people worldwide have residual muscle weakness due to poliomyelitis.

Diagnosis of poliomyelitis can usually be made clinically on the basis of neurological loss, which is strictly motor (lower motor neurone pattern) without any associated sensory loss. It differs from the symmetrical paralysis of Guillain–Barré syndrome in the progression and distribution of the paralysis and in the analysis of the cerebral spinal fluid.

Clinical Features

Poliomyelitis results in a broad range of presentation, depending on the position and extent of cord involvement (*Figure 10.11*). Certain patterns are common as muscles innervated by a short column of

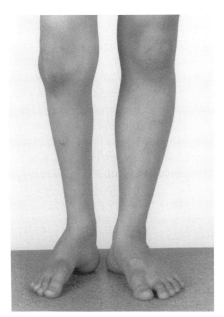

Figure 10.11 This child with poliomyelitis has been left with a hypoplastic right leg resulting in a marked leg length discrepancy. She also has a calcaneocavus foot as a result of residual muscle imbalance.

anterior horn cells tend to be more severely affected than those innervated by a long column covering multiple levels of the spinal cord. Paralysis of tibialis anterior, which has a discrete supply at one level in the cord is very common and results in foot drop. Total paralysis of the hamstrings is unusual because they have a motor supply from anterior horn cells at multiple levels.

Management

Treatment should be directed towards improving function and can be guided by the following principles.

Get the child walking

One must first assess whether the child has the potential to walk. If so, correction of contractures is the main concern. The most common contractures are flexion and abduction at the hip. These are treated by proximal surgical release of the abductors and flexors and distal release of the iliotibial band and intramuscular septum. Knee flexion contractures may be corrected by serial casting, but posterior and lateral soft-tissue releases may be necessary, or even an extension femoral osteotomy in the supracondylar area. Equinus is common and treated by open tendo Achillis lengthening. Walking can then be started using simple bracing – knee–ankle–

foot orthosis (KAFO) with a pelvic band and hip hinges if necessary – and a walker.

Prevent deformity

Equinus deformity increases with growth. However, if a tendo Achillis lengthening is combined with a transfer to replace the non-functioning tibialis anterior, recurrent equinus is less likely. In these circumstances the first choice for transfer, tibialis posterior, is often also paralysed so the weaker peroneals or extensor hallucis longus to the first metatarsal (the Jones transfer) can be used. It should, however, be noted that the child often uses the equinus deformity to make up for a weak quadriceps. After placing the foot on the ground in walking the hip extensors are used to pull the leg back and produce knee extension. This may go to the point of recurvatum and be known as back-kneeing. Lengthening the tendo Achillis in these circumstances decreases the ability to extend the knee and makes walking more difficult.

Leg length discrepancy (LLD) should be evaluated in terms of the child's long-term bracing requirements. If it is likely that the child will always require a brace, that side should be allowed to remain short to help in clearance during swing phase of gait (e.g. 2 cm shorter for a long leg brace). Similarly, if a hip is dysplastic, leaving that leg short will tend to increase its coverage as the hip automatically assumes a valgus posture because of the pelvic obliquity. LLD in polio does not behave in the predictable manner that it does in many conditions and limb lengthening should be left until maturity. During limb lengthening it is important to work closely with the orthotist so that bracing can be continued during the process.

Decrease bracing

Lower limb stability depends on the ability to extend the knee. If this can be achieved surgically, it may be possible to free the patient of a brace or reduce the requirement from a KAFO to an ankle–foot orthosis (AFO). If the quadriceps is weak or absent, the flexion contractures of the knee should be corrected by either serial casting or surgical release. Knee stability can then be restored by bracing with a floor reaction AFO or by surgery. Surgery consists of increasing the push-off by transferring the peroneals into the os calcis and fusing the subtalar joint or by an extension osteotomy of the distal femur.

Correct upper extremity problems

A flail shoulder is common in polio. If the patient has a functioning serratus anterior a shoulder fusion can be extremely beneficial so that the arm is moved by scapular–thoracic movement. At the elbow, flexion may be restored by transferring the origin of the wrist flexors or extensors more proximally on the humerus (known as the Steindler flexorplasty).

Treat scoliosis

Curves in the early stages are more flexible than in idiopathic scoliosis, but subsequently become very stiff. Management depends not only on the extent of the curve, but also on the degree of rigidity. Bracing can be used in the early stages for flexible moderate curves. When the curve has progressed to over 40°, instrumentation and fusion are carried out. In a walker, great care must be taken to preserve as many movement segments as possible in the lumbo-sacral region so as not to convert the patient into a non-walker.

GUILLIAN–BARRÉ SYNDROME

Guillian–Barré paralysis (acute polyradiculoneuritis) presents as an ascending symmetrical motor paresis. Its effects range from a mild gait abnormality to acute flaccid paralysis with respiratory failure requiring ventilator support.

The disease classically follows a viral prodrome. Diagnosis is made on clinical examination, which shows a diffuse lower motor neurone pattern of flaccid paresis with relative preservation of sensation. The weakness progresses from the lower limbs and gradually ascends to a variable degree over a few hours or days. Cerebrospinal fluid shows a normal cell count with an increased protein level. Nerve conduction studies show delay in both motor and sensory conduction. Nerve biopsy confirms an inflammatory pattern, but is usually not necessary for diagnosis.

The greatest concern with this disease is paralysis of the muscles of respiration and bulbar muscles. These patients should be admitted to hospital as 30–40% may require respiratory support with a ventilator. Death is now uncommon with modern intensive care management.

Acute orthopaedic management consists of splinting the involved extremities to avoid contractures. While the usual course of the disease is a full recovery in strength, approximately 20% of patients may be left with some motor deficit. This is almost always a weakness of ankle dorsiflexion and foot eversion that may require a foot drop splint, muscle transfer or corrective bony procedures. Rarely, muscle transfer procedures may be helpful in the upper limbs.

CONGENITAL SENSORY NEUROPATHIES

Congenital sensory neuropathy is an inherited condition that may have an autosomal dominant or recessive pattern or may present as a new mutation.

The most common orthopaedic conditions that occur as a result of the indifference to pain are neuropathic joints, recurrent fractures, osteomyelitis and skin ulcerations (*Figure 10.12*). A Charcot joint of the ankle or knee is common.

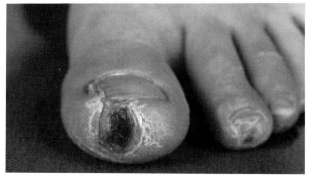

Figure 10.12 Indolent toe ulcers are common in congenital sensory neuropathy and can result in a chronic infection.

Management

These patients are often very difficult to deal with because they suffer a great deal of psychological distress including self-mutilation. Although treatment of the orthopaedic conditions relating to the disorder are managed according to standard principles, the orthopaedic surgeon should ensure that a paediatrician is involved in the overall care of these patients.

REFERENCES AND FURTHER READING

Bowen JR, MacEwen GD. Muscle and nerve disorders in children. In: *Operative Orthopaedics*, second edition, edited by M W Chapman. pp. 3277–3313. JB Lippincott, Philadelphia, 1993.

DelBello DA, Watts H.G. Distal femoral extension osteotomy of knee flexion contracture in patients with arthrogryposis. *J Pediatr Orthop* 1996; **16**: 122–126.

Drennan JC. Neuromuscular disorders. In: *Lovell and Winter Pediatric Orthopaedics*, third edition, edited by RT Morrissy. pp. 381–463. JB Lippincott, Philadelphia, 1990.

Galasko CS, Delaney C, Morris P. Spinal stabilisation in Duchenne muscular dystrophy. *J Bone Joint Surg* 1992; **74B**: 210–214.

James JIP. *Poliomyelitis: Essentials of Surgical Management.* Edward Arnold, London, 1987.

Sarwark JF, MacEwen GD, Scott CI, Jr. Current concepts review. Amyoplasia (a common form of arthrogryposis). *J Bone Joint Surg* 1990; **72A**: 465–469.

Shapiro F, Bresnan MJ. Current concepts review. Orthopaedic management of childhood neuromuscular disease. Part I: spinal muscular atrophy. *J Bone Joint Surg* 1982; **64A**: 785–789.

Shapiro F, Bresnan MJ. Current concepts review. Orthopaedic management of childhood neuromuscular disease. Part II: peripheral neuropathies, Friedreich's ataxia, and arthrogryposis multiplex congenita. *J Bone Joint Surg* 1982; **64A**: 949–953.

Shapiro F, Bresnan M. Current concepts review. Orthopaedic management of childhood neuromuscular disease. Part III diseases of muscle. *J Bone Joint Surg* 1982; **64A**: 1102–1107.

Shapiro F, Specht L. Current concepts review. The diagnosis and orthopaedic treatment of childhood spinal muscular atrophy, peripheral neuropathy, Friedreich's ataxia, and arthrogryposis. *J Bone Joint Surg* 1993; **75A**: 1699–1713.

Shapiro F, Specht I. Current concepts review. The diagnosis and orthopaedic treatment of inherited muscular diseases of childhood. *J Bone Joint Surg* 1993; **64A**: 439–454.

Shapiro F, Specht I. Orthopaedic deformities in Emery–Dreifuss muscular dystrophy. *J Pediatr Orthop* 1991; **11**: 336–339.

Smith AD, Koreska J, Moseley CF. Progression of scoliosis in Duchenne muscular dystrophy. *J Bone Joint Surg* 1989; **71A**: 1066–1074.

Torode IP, Lee PYC. Luque instrumentation for spinal deformity in Duchenne muscular dystrophy. *J Orthop Surg* 1994; **2**: 55–60.

Watts HG. Management of common third world orthopaedic problems: paralytic poliomyelitis, tuberculosis of bones and joints, Hansen's disease (leprosy), and chronic osteomyelitis. In: *Instructional Course Lectures*, edited by RE Eilert. pp. 471–478. American Academy of Orthopaedic Surgeons, Park Ridge, Illinois, 1992.

Williams P. The management of arthrogryposis. *Orthop Clin North Am* 1978; **9**: 67–88.

Chapter 11
Bone and Joint Infection

Virginia J Saxton and Mark D O'Sullivan

ACUTE OSTEOMYELITIS

Acute osteomyelitis is a bacterial infection of bone associated with a pyrexial illness. It is predominantly a disease of childhood, affecting males twice as often as females. It is usually caused by the spread of organisms in the blood (haematogenous), but can be secondary to direct spread from adjacent tissues or through an open wound (surgical or traumatic). There is an increased incidence in lower socio-economic groups and it is more common in the immunocompromised. There is a seasonal variation, with the incidence peaking in autumn.

Subacute osteomyelitis produces less severe constitutional changes and the history is longer than two weeks. There is minimal loss of limb function and there are established radiological changes at presentation.

Aetiology

In the course of a bacteraemia, organisms occasionally settle in the metaphysis of a long bone. The reasons for this metaphyseal site include:

- Increased blood flow at the growing ends of long bones.
- Possible trauma with haematoma formation.
- Hairpin arrangement of the terminal branches of blood vessels in the metaphysis.
- Endothelial gaps in these vessels.
- Large cavernous sinuses with sluggish flow at the arteriovenous junction.

Clinical Features

The child with acute osteomyelitis presents with a rapid onset of pain and reluctance to use the affected limb. There is a history of recent infection such as a skin or respiratory infection in about 25% of cases. The child is febrile, appears unwell and may be septicaemic. The affected limb is held still and there may be warmth and redness over the area. The site is exquisitely tender and adjacent joint movement is reduced, but not absent.

In infants, the picture may be completely different because the typical constitutional changes of the older child are usually absent. Failure to thrive and irritability may be the only early indications of sepsis. At all ages, the most common bones affected are the long bones, particularly of the lower limbs. Other sites include the pelvis and long bones of the upper limbs.

Pathology

Bacterial invasion of the bone sets up local inflammation with associated hyperaemia and a cellular response. Pus forms within the medullary cavity of the bone, resulting in bone necrosis and resorption. The pus may then track through the cortex to form a subperiosteal collection, lifting the periosteum, which lays down new bone (*Table 11.1*). If the metaphysis is intraarticular, as in the hip, pus may spread into the joint. The epiphysis may be directly involved in children less than one year of age because they have transphyseal vessels, which communicate between the metaphysis and the epiphysis (*Figure 11.1*).

Sequestrum is necrotic bone, formed when cortical bone is deprived of its blood supply after periosteal stripping. It remains dense and does not become demineralized unlike vital hyperaemic bone.

Involucrum is the periosteal new bone, which forms over the cortex surrounding the infected area.

Cloacae are the channels that form in the cortex between the medulla and the surrounding soft tissue in chronic osteomyelitis. They allow free flow of pus and may communicate with the surface via a sinus.

Organisms

The organism most commonly involved is *Staphylococcus aureus*, which causes 60–90% of all such

Table 11.1   General and focal causes of periosteal reaction seen on plain radiographs.

Traumatic	Stress fractures
	Non-accidental injuries
Infective	Osteomyelitis (acute, chronic, multifocal)
	Syphilis
Metabolic	Scurvy
	Healing rickets
Tumour	Osteosarcoma
	Ewing sarcoma
	Neuroblastoma
Miscellaneous	Caffey disease (infantile cortical hyperostosis)
	Hypertrophic pulmonary osteoarthropathy

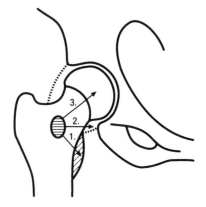

Figure 11.1   The spread of acute osteomyelitis. **1.** To form a subperiosteal abscess. **2.** Acute septic arthritis may develop if the metaphysis is intra-articular (e.g. hip and shoulder). **3.** In infants, infection may spread to the physis and epiphysis.

infections in childhood. Other organisms include streptococcal species including *Pneumococcus, Haemophilus influenzae* type b (Hib), *Escherichia coli, Pseudomonas* and other gram-negative organisms.

In children under four years of age about 20% of infections were due to Hib, but following the introduction of the Hib vaccine the incidence is much reduced. In infants, gram-negative organisms (e.g. *E. coli*) and group B β-haemolytic streptococci may be involved, particularly in infants who have had an infection or catheterization of the umbilical vessels. *Salmonella* is not uncommon in sickle cell disease. In the immunocompromised patient, due to for example acquired immunodeficiency syndrome (AIDS), tuberculosis and *Candida* may be seen. In pre-existing soft tissue infection osteomyelitis may be caused by anaerobes. Puncture wounds in the feet through trainers may lead to *Pseudomonas* osteomyelitis of the calcaneum (*Figure 11.2*).

Laboratory Investigations

Investigations are an aid to diagnosis in uncertain cases and important in the determination of the organism. The white cell count (WCC) and erythrocyte sedimentation rate (ESR) are generally raised, although the WCC may be normal initially. The ESR tends to be raised early and is often around 40–80 mm h^{-1}. It remains high after the infection subsides. It must be remembered that this test may be normal in neonates with osteomyelitis. C-reactive protein

(CRP) is usually raised and can be useful for monitoring response to treatment.

Blood cultures must be taken before any antibiotics are given and grow the infecting organism in about 50% of cases.

In the presence of a subperiosteal abscess, aspiration of pus is a good method for identifying the organism. This can be carried out using a needle under local or general anaesthesia or as an open incision with drainage. Bone aspiration is occasionally warranted. The yield of organisms by local aspiration is about 60–70%.

Cases of Hib infection can be identified by examining the urine with a latex agglutination test for Hib antigen.

Radiology

Plain films

The first visible changes are loss of the normal fascial planes and fat shadows due to soft tissue and muscle oedema. Bony changes are not normally visible before 7–10 days and are typically in the metaphysis, although diaphyseal involvement can occur (*Figures 11.3, 11.4*). There is metaphyseal rarefaction due to hyperaemia and bone destruction. These changes are initially poorly circumscribed, but may subsequently become better defined. Periosteal reaction does not normally occur until about 14 days after the onset of the illness.

Bone scan

The three-phase technetium-99m bone scan is very sensitive in detecting infection at all ages. It is

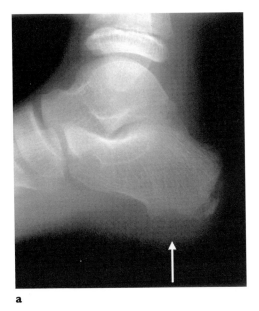
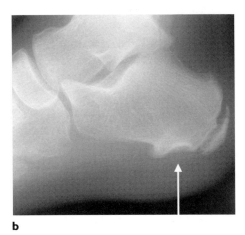

a

b

Figure 11.2 a Acute osteomyelitis of the calcaneum (due to *Pseudomonas*) in a ten-year-old boy secondary to a puncture wound through his trainers. This lateral view shows cortical destruction inferiorly (arrow) in the calcaneum with associated soft tissue swelling. **b** Two months later following treatment with antibiotics there has been considerable healing of the osteomyelitis with residual sclerosis and deformity (arrow).

generally positive 24–72 hours after the start of infection. There is increased uptake in the affected area in all three phases of the scan. There may, however, be a cold spot if the underlying bone has infarcted. The scan is particularly useful in detecting the site of the infection and showing if multiple sites are affected. If the scan is negative and the clinical suspicion is high then other nuclear studies such as technetium-99m-labelled white cells or a gallium-67

citrate scan is helpful. Both concentrate in acutely-infected tissues.

Ultrasound
This is very useful in detecting a joint effusion (see septic arthritis). In acute osteomyelitis it may show fluid under the periosteum. Ultrasound is helpful in defining soft tissue abscesses and in guiding aspiration.

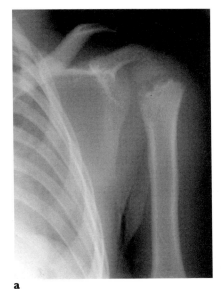
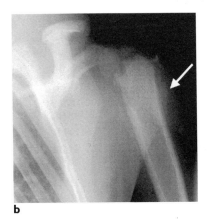
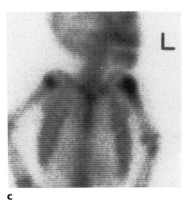

a

b

c

Figure 11.3 a Soft tissue swelling with metaphyseal irregularity and destruction due to acute osteomyelitis of the left humerus in a three-year-old boy. **b** Two weeks later (without treatment) there is now further bony destruction and a periosteal reaction (arrow) extending down the shaft of the humerus. **c** Technetium-99 bone scan shows increased uptake in the left humeral metaphysis and proximal shaft consistent with osteomyelitis.

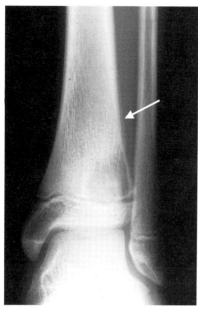

Figure 11.4 Acute osteomyelitis in the distal tibial metaphysis of an 11-year-old girl. The area of bone destruction is fairly well defined and there is an associated periosteal reaction (arrow) extending up the shaft laterally.

Computerized tomography

This is most useful in subacute and chronic osteomyelitis because computerized tomography (CT) is good at showing cortical bone. Soft tissue swelling, abscess formation, gas in the marrow, sacroiliac involvement, foreign bodies and bony sequestra may be seen with CT when they are not visible on the plain films as a result of overlying soft tissue change.

Magnetic resonance imaging

Magnetic resonance imaging (MRI) is probably the most sensitive test for detecting infection. Marrow oedema is well seen and is the earliest MRI finding in acute osteomyelitis. There is a decreased signal intensity on T1- and increased signal on T2-weighted scans. MRI is very sensitive to marrow and soft tissue changes, but cortical changes are best seen with CT. MRI can also show joint fluid, cartilage damage and soft tissue sinus tracks. It is as accurate as a bone scan in detecting osteomyelitis, but is much more sensitive in detecting soft tissue involvement.

Differential Diagnosis

The differential diagnosis of osteomyelitis includes the following:

- Septic arthritis which may be difficult to differentiate, particularly if it affects the hip and spine. In septic arthritis there is usually virtually no movement in the joint. Both septic arthritis and osteomyelitis may coexist in the proximal femur.
- Tumours such as Ewing's sarcoma, which may have a clinical course and produce radiological appearances very similar to those of acute or subacute osteomyelitis. If there is doubt about the diagnosis, a biopsy must be performed.
- Sickle cell crisis, which may be difficult to differentiate initially from bone infection. The course of the disease, blood parameters and blood cultures are all useful in this situation.

Management

The child is admitted to hospital and management should start as soon as possible. Pain relief is given and the investigations are completed so that antibiotic treatment can be started.

Antibiotics

Intravenous flucloxacillin is started as soon as the diagnosis is suspected and blood cultures have been taken. This is continued until the child has been afebrile for 24 hours. Oral antibiotics are then continued for 3–6 weeks. Early acute osteomyelitis that settles quickly can be treated for three weeks. Subacute osteomyelitis should be treated for the full six weeks.

In the child under four years of age who has not been given Hib vaccination, antibiotics should cover *Haemophilus*. Ampicillin, chloramphenicol or a third-generation cephalosporin may be administered with the flucloxacillin. However 20% of *Haemophilus* are resistant to ampicillin and there are concerns about the grey-baby complication of chloramphenicol. Third-generation cephalosporins are expensive and can only be given parenterally. Amoxycillin with clavulinic acid (trade name Augmentin) is another option.

Immobilization

A plaster backslab is used until the initial pain and swelling settles. For more central lesions, bed rest or traction is used.

Surgery

Drainage is occasionally required if an abscess forms or when the osteomyelitis fails to settle after 48 hours of antibiotics. Ultrasound is useful in detecting a soft tissue collection, but usually the site of most tenderness is the best guide as to where the incision should be made. At the time of surgery, the periosteum is opened and the pus is released. If there is a periosteal collection there is no indication to drill the cortex because there must have been cortical penetration.

Occasionally a bone biopsy is taken for culture if there is no subperiosteal collection and the patient is failing to settle.

Complications

The complications of osteomyelitis include:

- Septic arthritis if the metaphysis is intraarticular (e.g. hip and shoulder), which demands surgical exploration.
- Septicaemia.
- Premature growth plate arrest causing lower limb discrepancy and progressive deformity (Chapter 24)
- Chronic osteomyelitis.

Neonatal Osteomyelitis

The infant presents with swelling of the limb or septicaemia. Complete refusal to move the limb is the most obvious sign and may be described as a 'pseudoparalysis.' Multiple sites are typical of neonatal osteomyelitis due to the poor immune response. Extension into the adjacent joint is common (70%) via transphyseal vessels or because the metaphysis is intraarticular. The source of the infecting organism may be the umbilicus. Infecting bacteria include group B β-haemolytic *Streptococcus*, *S. aureus* and *E. coli*.

Detecting the involved area may be difficult and a bone scan is helpful in determining all the sites of involvement. It may show a cold spot if there is infarction. The bone scan may be relatively less sensitive in neonatal osteomyelitis. A negative study when there is a high clinical suspicion of disease should be followed by a gallium study, which is highly sensitive in this age group. Late complications include growth plate arrest, joint surface deformity with subsequent degenerative change, and avascular necrosis in the hip.

Epiphyseal Osteomyelitis

This is unusual, but may occur in infants due to spread from the metaphysis across the growth plate. In the older child it may occur as a primary site. It is particularly seen in the knee, most commonly the distal femoral epiphysis. Plain films show a well-defined epiphyseal lucency that is hot on a bone scan (*Figure 11.5*). MRI is very sensitive in this condition. Associated septic arthritis is common, so arthrotomy is usually required. Biopsy may be required if the diagnosis or organism is in doubt.

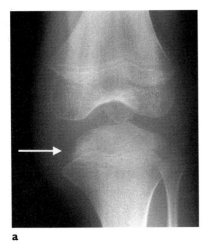 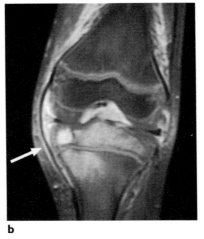 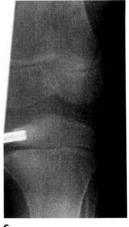

a   b   c

Figure 11.5 a Epiphyseal osteomyelitis in a seven-year-old boy in the proximal tibial epiphysis. There is soft tissue swelling medially around the joint and cortical destruction of the medial aspect of the tibial epiphysis (arrow). **b** A T1-weighted magnetic resonance scan with fat suppression and gadolinium (contrast agent) shows intense enhancement of a focal area of osteomyelitis (arrow) in the medial epiphysis. **c** The patient failed to settle with 12 weeks of antibiotic treatment and therefore underwent biopsy and curettage of the lesion. Appropriate antibiotics were then continued.

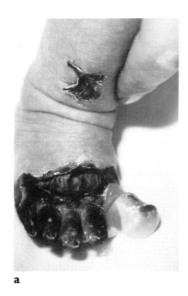 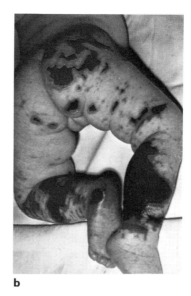

a   b

Figure 11.6 a Meningococcal septicaemia may result in distal gangrene.   **b** Patches of gangrene are another feature of meningococcal septicaemia.

Meningococcal Septicaemia

This potentially fatal disease may have musculoskeletal manifestations. Patches of gangrene on the skin and gangrene of the digits or limbs may be features. There may also be partial growth plate arrest (*Figure 11.6*).

SEPTIC ARTHRITIS

The causes of acute septic arthritis are similar to those of acute osteomyelitis. The most common cause is haematogenous. It may also result from surgery, trauma with penetration of the joint, or spread from adjacent tissues (e.g. from adjacent osteomyelitis when the metaphysis is intraarticular). Septic arthritis is less common than osteomyelitis. The joints most commonly involved are the hip, knee and shoulder.

Pathology

Infection within the joint creates a synovitis. Articular cartilage is gradually destroyed by the release of enzymes, increased intraarticular pressure and lack of movement and later by the spread of granulation tissue over the articular cartilage.

Complete healing may occur if treatment is started early. However, if there is a delay in presentation or diagnosis, healing may result in fibrous or bony ankylosis. Avascular necrosis and dislocation can occur as a result of compression of the blood vessels by pus.

Organisms

The organisms involved are similar to those seen in acute osteomyelitis. Culture of the synovial fluid reveals the organism in only 50% of patients. *S. aureus* accounts for 60–80% of the cases where an organism is identified. Other common organisms are *Streptococcus* and *Haemophilus*.

Clinical Features

Septic arthritis presents in a similar way to osteomyelitis. The child is unwell, has a high fever and does not move the affected limb. In peripheral joints there is swelling, redness, and tenderness, with very restricted movements.

In infants, a delay in diagnosis is common because the usual signs of inflammation are lacking. Careful examination may be required to determine the site of infection. The umbilicus should be examined when looking for an infective focus.

Laboratory Investigations

Diagnosis relies on the demonstration of bacteria in the synovial fluid or bacterial growth on culture. As in osteomyelitis, the WCC and ESR may be raised. Blood cultures are taken and the joint aspirated before starting antibiotics.

Radiology

Plain radiographs

These may not be helpful. In the hip, intraarticular pus and fluid may displace the femoral head laterally and cause dislocation (Tom Smith arthritis) (*Figure 11.7*). However, a normal plain film does not exclude an effusion. An untreated septic arthritis will show osteopenia and subarticular bone destruction on the plain films .

Ultrasound

This is a sensitive method of detecting a joint effusion, especially in the hip. It can pick up as little as 1 ml of fluid, but it cannot reliably distinguish pus from serous fluid.

Bone scan

This will show increased activity around the joint in the first two phases of the scan. The static phase will show increased uptake if there is osteomyelitis. There may be a 'cold' region suggesting an avascular or hypovascular zone if the sepsis has compromised the blood supply to the epiphysis.

Differential Diagnosis

The differential diagnosis of septic arthritis includes:

- Irritable hip.
- Acute osteomyelitis of the adjacent bone.

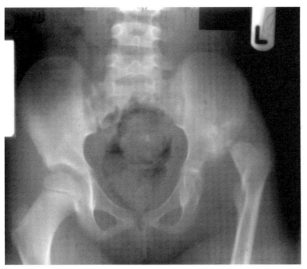

Figure 11.7 Dislocation of the left hip secondary to previous septic arthritis. There has been destruction on both sides of the joint resulting in a shallow acetabulum, almost complete destruction of the epiphysis, and subsequent dislocation.

- Monarticular arthritis as seen in juvenile chronic arthritis.
- Rheumatic fever (rare).

Management

If septic arthritis is suspected, the child should be fasted and appropriate investigations performed as soon as possible. Septic joints should be washed out to obtain fluid for culture and to prevent any long term sequelae. Parenteral antibiotics are started after specimens have been taken. We advocate that all infected joints are opened and washed out, either by arthrotomy or arthroscopy. However, there are units where septic arthritis is treated by aspiration and then parenteral antibiotics, but even in these units, septic arthritis of the hip in a child over two years of age is treated by arthrotomy and washout.

Aspiration and washout

The first stage is to obtain a specimen of joint fluid, which is then sent for microbiological examination. The second stage is to release the pus and irrigate the joint to prevent articular cartilage degeneration. This can be carried out by arthrotomy, arthroscopy or by aspiration. In general it will depend on the joint involved, the consistency of the pus and the experience of the surgeon. The hip is usually released by arthrotomy whereas the knee is initially washed out with the arthroscope. If the pus is thick an arthrotomy may be required.

Hip arthrotomy is performed as follows. A small incision is made in the groin crease and continued down in the interval between sartorius and tensor fascia lata. The hip capsule is identified with the reflected head of rectus femoris overlying it. The capsule is incised to release the pus and a square section of capsule excised to allow continued drainage of the hip. The joint is irrigated with saline through an infant feeding tube until the fluid is clear. The tube is then removed and the wound is closed and dressed. A drain tube is not usually inserted.

Antibiotics

Antibiotics are started after joint fluid has been taken for examination. Flucloxacillin is used until the culture results are available. In children less than four years of age, ampicillin is added to cover *Haemophilus*. Intravenous antibiotics are continued until the child is symptomatically well and has been apyrexial for 24 hours. The appropriate oral antibiotic is continued for at least three weeks.

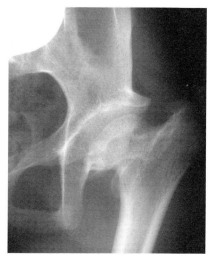

Figure 11.8 Late sequelae of septic arthritis. There has been destruction in the proximal femoral epiphysis and growth plate resulting in coxa breva and coxa vara. This will lead to a leg length discrepancy, loss of joint movement and premature secondary osteoarthritis.

Immobilization

The limb is rested in either a plaster backslab or traction until it has improved symptomatically. The use of continuous passive motion (CPM) is controversial in septic arthritis and is not used in our institution.

Complications

The complications of septic arthritis include:

- Avascular necrosis (particularly hip and shoulder).
- Dislocation (particularly hip).
- Joint destruction with secondary osteoarthritis or ankylosis.
- Growth plate arrest causing leg length discrepancy and progressive deformity (*Figure 11.8*).

CHRONIC OSTEOMYELITIS

Sequel to Acute Osteomyelitis

This is an uncommon condition in children in developed countries because acute osteomyelitis is now so well treated by antibiotics. However, bacteria may remain quiescent for long periods in bone following an acute infection. Chronic osteomyelitis is characterized by recurrent episodes of infection with pain, fevers and discharge from sinuses.

Secondary to an Open Fracture or Surgery

This is the most common cause today, particularly chronic osteomyelitis secondary to an open fracture in patients from developing countries.

Clinical Features

Patients usually present with a recurrence of their chronic osteomyelitis. Pain, fevers, redness, tenderness and discharge are the most common symptoms and there is often a history of an open fracture or surgery. There may be a discharging sinus.

Radiology

With continuing osteomyelitis, part of the bony cortex may infarct producing a sequestrum. This is surrounded by an extensive envelope of new periosteal bone, which is called the involucrum. Running through the involucrum are tracks (cloacae) which decompress the medullary abscess into the soft tissues (*Figures 11.9, 11.10*). In older children the periosteum is more firmly attached and there is a greater tendency for the infection to spread along the marrow cavity producing extensive patchy bone destruction with the formation of a cortical sinus.

Pathology

The area of involved bone contains cavities surrounded by sclerotic bone. Retained sequestra are common and increase the frequency of acute episodes. They are occasionally discharged through sinuses. The sclerotic new bone is reactive due to endosteal and periosteal new bone formation (involucrum). The bone has a poor blood supply and resistant organisms eventually infect the involved area.

Organisms

Although *S. aureus* is still the most common causative organism it only accounts for 30–50% of cases of chronic osteomyelitis. Mixed organisms are grown in 25%. Other organisms involved include gram-negative organisms, anaerobes, *S. epidermidis* and *Streptococcus*. It is important to remember that the organisms involved may change from time to time and may be multiple. Skin commensals may grow from superficial swabs and tend to overestimate the number of polymicrobial infections. Deep swabs must be taken with bone biopsies if possible.

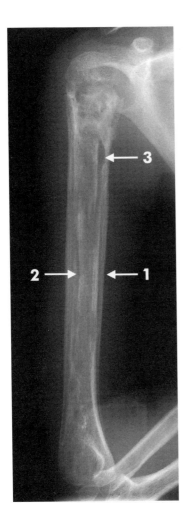

Figure 11.9   Chronic osteomyelitis in a four-year-old girl. This shows classical appearances of chronic osteomyelitis. There is an envelope of new periosteal bone (involucrum) (1) involving most of the humerus and an extensive sequestrum has formed throughout the length of the shaft (2). There is a cloaca proximally and medially (3), which discharged into the soft tissues and eventually out through a sinus.

Management

The treatment in childhood is generally conservative.

Non-operative

The child is admitted to hospital and bed rest is started. Swabs are taken (both deep and superficial) and the affected limb is placed in a plaster backslab. Antibiotics are useful for controlling acute flares and in preventing the spread of infection to healthy bone. There is doubt about the ability of antibiotics to eradicate chronic osteomyelitis as it has been shown that the identified and treated organisms persist in 30% of cases. Sinuses are dressed on a regular basis.

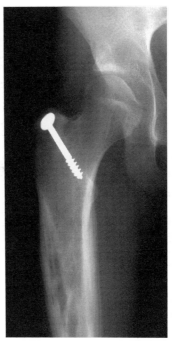

Figure 11.10   Chronic osteomyelitis. In this case the infection is centred in the diaphysis with a more focal area of bony destruction and marked surrounding sclerosis. There is a periosteal reaction, some of which has consolidated.

Operative

Surgical treatment of chronic osteomyelitis is controversial, but there are several definite indications. Abscesses require drainage and in the presence of recurrent flares of infection with a sequestrum, sequestrectomy should be undertaken.

Options to try to eradicate the infection include:

- Saucerization.
- Debridement with or without muscle or skin flaps.
- Bone grafting (either cancellous or vascularized).
- Antibiotic-impregnated polymethylmethacrylate beads.
- Excision of infected bone and bone transport, using ring fixators.
- Amputation.

Brodie's Abscess

Clinical Features

The patients present with pain and local tenderness and there may be swelling. The child is usually over eight years of age. The pain may fluctuate with exacerbations superimposed on constant aching discomfort. Fever is mild or absent and constitutional symptoms are rare.

Radiology

Plain films show a circumscribed area of bone destruction between 0.5–5 cm in diameter. There is a variable degree of surrounding sclerosis, but this is well demarcated and is often extensive (*Figure 11.11*). Approximately 40% show periosteal new bone and 20% have a sequestrum, which is best seen on CT. MRI demonstrates any fistulous tracks running through the bone into soft tissues. The lesion may resemble an osteoid osteoma.

Management

Episodes are usually treated conservatively with immobilization and antibiotics. Recurrent episodes are treated surgically with removal of the abscess roof, curettage and removal of the abscess wall. Antibiotics are continued for six weeks. *En bloc* resection is an alternative to curettage for easily resectable bones.

Sclerosing Osteomyelitis of Garré

Garré described a diffuse inflammatory lesion affecting the shafts of the long bones or the jaw. There is thickening of the corticocancellous bone and partial obliteration of the marrow space. Suppuration does not occur and sequestra and sinuses do not form. It is uncertain whether the lesion is of bacterial origin. Plain films show marked sclerosis with periosteal and endosteal cortical thickening with no evidence of bone destruction. It may be confused with an osteoid osteoma or a sclerosing bone tumour as seen in a Ewing sarcoma. It is rarely seen today.

Treatment follows the guidelines given above.

Chronic Recurrent Multifocal Osteomyelitis

This disorder is most common in the 7–14 years age group and has no known cause. It presents with a gradual onset of malaise and a low-grade fever. There is local pain and tenderness at the affected site. Bone lesions may occur sequentially and are located predominantly in the metaphyses of long bones of the lower limb, but may involve the medial end of the clavicle, a vertebral body or the sacroiliac

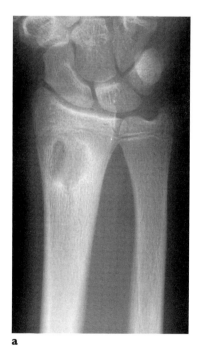
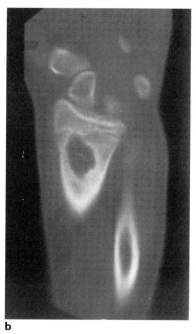

a   b

Figure 11.11   a Brodie's abscess in a 13-year-old girl. There is a well-defined area of focal destruction in the distal radial metaphysis with some surrounding sclerosis and no periosteal reaction. The patient had been symptomatic for a year.   **b** Computerized tomographic scan shows the well-demarcated abscess with surrounding sclerosis.

joint. The bone lesions are frequently relapsing and may be symmetrical. Associations have been reported with arthritis (20–30%) and with palmoplantar pustulosis. The disease tends to have a prolonged duration with exacerbations and remissions, and residual bony swelling is common. There is no response to antibiotics.

Laboratory Investigations

The ESR is usually raised. Biopsy shows a nonspecific inflammatory reaction. Organisms are rarely grown.

Radiology

The lesions appear as a destructive lucency in the metaphysis with a variable degree of surrounding sclerosis (*Figure 11.12*). They are occasionally symmetrical and may extend into the epiphysis. When involved, the clavicle is affected at the medial end with both lucent and sclerotic areas with periosteal reaction and expansion. The vertebrae may show changes similar to discitis or there may be vertebra plana. The bone scan is hot at the site of lesions and may show clinically-silent lesions.

Management

Non-steroidal anti-inflammatory drugs are the mainstay of treatment and corticosteroids may be useful. In general antibiotics are not used.

TUBERCULOSIS

Tuberculosis is a chronic infection caused by *Mycobacterium tuberculosis* and can present as either a septic arthritis or osteomyelitis. Although uncommon the incidence is higher in the Asian population. It is also more common in the homeless and the immunocompromised such as children with AIDS. Musculoskeletal disease is usually secondary to an established focus elsewhere in the body. The primary infection occurs in the lungs, tonsils or the alimentary tract. Infection is more likely to affect a synovial joint than the shaft of a bone in contrast to haematogenous osteomyelitis. Of those with active tuberculosis only 5–10% have bone and joint involvement. Approximately 50% of those with bone and joint involvement have spinal tuberculosis while 15% have tuberculosis in the hip, 15% in the knee, 10% in other joints and 10% in bone without joint involvement.

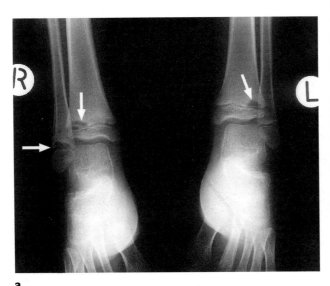
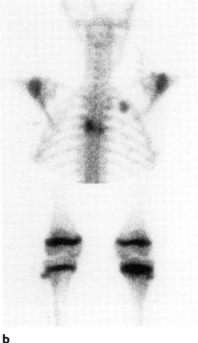

a   b

Figure 11.12 **a** Chronic recurrent multifocal osteomyelitis in a nine-year-old girl. There are symmetrical changes of chronic recurrent osteomyelitis in both distal tibias and the right fibula (arrows). **b** The bone scan of the girl shown in Figure 11.12a shows increased uptake in the left proximal tibial metaphysis and also in T5.

Clinical Features

Tuberculosis usually presents insidiously. There may be a history of previous infection or of contact with tuberculosis. The patient may present with pain, swelling, fever, weight loss and muscle wasting. The pain of spinal disease may not be severe and patients may not present until the appearance of an abscess in the groin (cold abscess) or until a kyphus develops (Pott disease). Cord compression can occur resulting in paraplegia.

Radiology

The natural history is of a subacute or chronic infection so radiological changes are usually present by the time of presentation. The initial lesion is at a bone end or tuberosity. Plain films show rarefaction around the affected area (*Figure 11.13a*). Later bone destruction may occur. There is a marked absence of bone sclerosis and periosteal reaction even though the disease is active. The growth plate is not a barrier to infection so the epiphysis is often involved.

In the spine the focus of infection may be in the disc or at the anterior aspect of the vertebral body and causes early loss of the disc space. The infection tracks up and down beneath the anterior longitudinal ligament involving adjacent vertebrae. The cervicothoracic, thoracolumbar and lumbosacral areas are particularly affected. An angular kyphosis develops as the bone and disc destruction continue (*Figure 11.13b*). The caseous material eventually calcifies and this is a characteristic but late feature of previous tuberculous infection.

Diagnosis

The only absolute evidence that a lesion is of tuberculous origin is the identification of the mycobacterium from the affected bone or joint. The diagnosis is often delayed because the condition is not suspected. Tuberculosis should be considered if:

- The patient is from a high risk group.
- There is a long history.
- There is marked muscle wasting or joint swelling.
- There is periarticular osteoporosis.
- The patient has a positive Mantoux test.

The ESR may be normal.

Management

Rest
In the pre-antibiotic era, the mainstay of treatment was rest. Following the introduction of chemotherapy, rest is no longer mandatory. In the initial management of the disease, the patient is usually admitted to hospital and drug therapy is started. Most patients are kept in bed with or without traction until the pain subsides and then kept on restricted activities until the joint changes resolve.

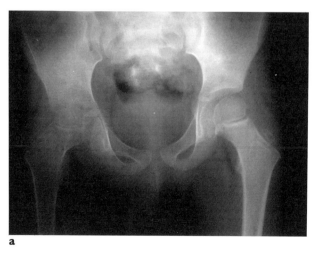
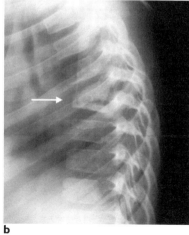

a   b

Figure 11.13 a Tuberculosis of the right hip. There is extensive rarefaction around the right hip joint and there is loss of the cortical outline of the acetabulum and of the femoral epiphysis. Note the lack of both periosteal reaction and osteoblastic response. **b** Spinal tuberculosis. There is almost total collapse of T5 and T6 with loss of the disc space (arrowed). Ankylosis is beginning to occur between the vertebrae. This has resulted in a severe kyphosis.

Chemotherapy

Isoniazid and rifampicin are the first-line drugs and are continued for nine months. Pyrazinamide is also used during the first two months. If drug resistance is suspected, ethambutol can be added, but may cause retrobulbar neuritis. Streptomycin is now rarely used because of its nephrotoxicity and ototoxicity.

Surgery

This may be required to drain pus, remove necrotic bone or soft tissues or correct deformity. Occasionally arthrodesis is necessary for a destroyed joint. There is debate about the use of surgical debridement for spinal tuberculosis versus the use of chemotherapy alone.

SYPHILIS OF BONE

Syphilis is usually congenital in infants and children. It is now rare in developed countries. Syphilis causes a laminated periosteal reaction, which consolidates to new bone as may be seen in the sabre tibia. It also causes a metaphysitis, typically in the upper medial tibia and seen as local destruction.

VIRAL OSTEOPATHY

This can occur following an intrauterine infection with a virus such as rubella or cytomegalovirus. The bone changes mainly affect the metaphyses and show alternating longitudinal streaks of increased and decreased density giving a 'celery stalk' appearance (*Figure 11.14*). A transverse metaphyseal band of reduced density behind the zone of provisional calcification may also be seen.

PERIOSTEAL REACTION

The periosteum can be elevated by a variety of causes (blood, pus, oedema, tumour or trauma). The elevated periosteum is only visible once new bone is laid down on its deep surface and this is not visible for 10–14 days. Initially it is separate from the underlying cortex and is seen as a fine line of calcific density parallel to the underlying bone. This new bone may become incorporated into the cortex or there may be further elevation depending on the pathological process. If there are successive episodes in the pathological process this can produce several layers of new bone giving an 'onion-peel' appearance. This can be seen in infection and other non-malignant processes as well as in Ewing sarcoma.

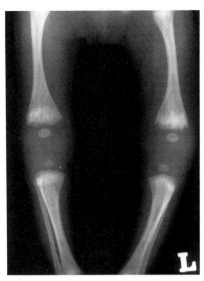

Figure 11.14 Viral osteopathy. This shows the classical changes of rubella osteopathy with irregularity of the metaphysis and longitudinal sclerosis and lucency in the distal femora. These appearances have been likened to a 'celery stalk'.

Infantile Cortical Hyperostosis (Caffey Disease)

This rare disorder consists of irritability, fever and constitutional upset in the first six months of life. The aetiology is unknown. There is irregular periosteal elevation of affected bone, which results in extensive irregular cortical thickening. The mandible, scapulae, clavicles, ribs and long bones are most commonly affected. Ultimately most of the bones remodel to a normal shape.

DISCITIS

Discitis is a painful condition of the back in children associated with a radiological loss of disc space. In severe cases it behaves as a bacterial condition, with osteomyelitis of the adjacent vertebral bodies, and responds to antibiotics. In others the changes are less severe, with no evidence of involvement of the adjacent vertebral bodies on plain radiography, and no bacteria can be grown: antibiotics are ineffective and the condition may be an autoimmune phenomenon.

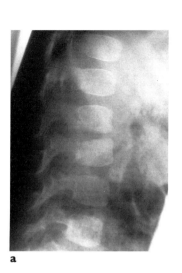 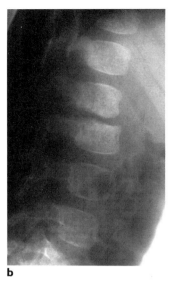 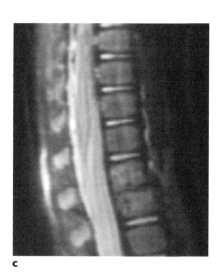

a   b   c

Figure 11.15 **a** Discitis in an 18-month-old child. There is loss of L1/L2 disc height with destruction of the adjacent end-plates. **b** Two months later there has been further loss of disc height and some sclerosis in the adjacent end-plates. **c** T2-weighted sagittal magnetic resonance image scan shows the disc destruction and also shows the full extent of the adjacent vertebral body involvement.

Clinical Features

Discitis usually affects children aged 1–12 years. The lumbar spine is most commonly affected and the child presents with back pain, stiffness and refusal to walk. Examination may show that the child is febrile, has decreased straight-leg raising and is tender in the affected area.

Laboratory Investigations

The ESR is usually raised, and the WCC is variable.

Radiology

In the initial phase the plain films are normal. The bone scan, however, is sensitive very early in the disease, showing a hot spot at the affected disc. Single photon emission computed tomography (SPECT) helps with detection and localization of the lesion. As the condition progresses, the plain films show loss of disc height with some end-plate irregularity (*Figure 11.15*). Later endplate sclerosis develops. CT shows any bone destruction, paravertebral or psoas abscess and intraspinal extension. MRI also shows intravertebral and paravertebral changes. Intravertebral involvement is seen as a low signal on T1- and high signal on T2-weighted scans. The posterior elements are not affected. The disc may eventually regain height although the sclerosis and end-plate irregularity may persist.

Management

The child is treated with bed rest until the symptoms improve. A plaster jacket is then applied for 3–6 weeks. The role of antibiotics is controversial. They are used if there are features suggestive of osteomyelitis, but the majority of children do not require them. A biopsy is performed if the discitis fails to resolve despite adequate treatment. This can be carried out using a CT-guided needle aspirate.

TRANSIENT SYNOVITIS OF THE HIP

Transient synovitis of the hip is very common but poorly understood. It is by far the commonest cause of a limp in children aged 2–10 years. Because the precise aetiology has never been clearly defined, a number of synonyms are used to describe the condition including observation hip, transient synovitis and coxitis fugax. The term 'irritable hip' is probably the most frequently used and seems appropriate to present understanding of the condition.

Transient synovitis of the hip presents clinically as a non-specific inflammatory synovitis with a synovial effusion and is of limited duration. There are usually no long-term clinical sequelae. It accounts for a significant number of outpatient consultations and admissions to hospital. Up to 3% of children may be affected at some time. It is approximately twice as common in boys as in girls, both hips are equally affected, and it is rarely, if ever, bilateral.

Aetiology

Approximately one-third of children are in the prodromal period of a viral illness, have an established viral illness, or are recovering from one, one-third appear to have had a recent minor injury, and one-third have no associated factors.

Clinical Features

The most common presentation is of a previously-well child aged 3–8 with an acute onset of pain and limping. Pain is usually felt in the groin, but occasionally in the anterior thigh or knee. Examination confirms the antalgic limp and occasionally the child will refuse to bear any weight. If allowed, the child will usually hold the affected hip in flexion, abduction and external rotation.

On examination there is protective muscle spasm and restriction of movement, particularly adduction and internal rotation. The temperature is sometimes elevated, but rarely above 38°C.

Laboratory Investigations

These are usually within normal limits, although a mild elevation of WCC and ESR is sometimes seen. CRP may be more reliable in differentiating the condition from pyogenic infection.

Joint aspiration is of no therapeutic benefit, but should be performed if there is a suspicion of infection in the hip. It can be carried out under ultrasound control and sedation in the more cooperative child.

Pathology

In the majority of typical cases a synovial fluid effusion is found with a raised intraarticular pressure. Aspiration of the hip reveals 1–4 ml of clear fluid, which is culture negative and non-specific on analysis. Biopsy specimens usually show non-specific synovitis.

Radiology

Plain radiographs of the pelvis and hip are performed to exclude more serious pathology. Ultrasonography of the hip is the most useful investigation and demonstrates the presence of an effusion with great sensitivity. The isotope bone scan is variable and is not useful as a routine investigation.

Differential Diagnosis

The differential diagnosis includes:

- Septic arthritis.
- Proximal femoral osteomyelitis.
- Perthes disease.
- Slipped capital femoral epiphysis.
- Benign tumours such as osteoid osteoma.
- Occult trauma.

Septic arthritis is much less common than irritable hip, but the presentation of the two conditions may overlap and there may be no specific investigation that will clearly differentiate between these two conditions in the early stages. Many patients with irritable hip therefore require admission to hospital for observation and a smaller number require aspiration of the hip.

Management

The principles of management are to rest the affected hip and to exclude other conditions, particularly the insidious development of bone or joint sepsis. Most children can rest at home, but careful follow-up is required. Any suspicion of infection is an indication for admission. Traction is unnecessary and possibly harmful. The most comfortable position is abduction, flexion and external rotation, and it is in this position that the intracapsular pressure is at its lowest. In skin traction the hip tends to lie in extension, adduction and neutral rotation, which can be uncomfortable for the child. If a child requires hospital admission, rest in 'slings and springs' is more appropriate than skin traction.

In the majority of cases it takes about one week for the range of hip movement to return to normal and early mobilization with weight-bearing should be avoided until this time. Failure to rest the hip for an adequate length of time seems to lead to recurrent symptoms and a prolonged recovery.

Outcome

In the majority of cases irritable hip is a short-lived illness from which the child makes a full recovery. However, 5–10% of children will have a second episode. Long-term follow-up studies have shown a number of radiological abnormalities, which are mainly minor and usually asymptomatic.

The relationship between irritable hip and Perthes disease is less clear. One popular theory regarding the aetiology of Perthes disease suggests that raised intracapsular pressure results in occlusion of the epiphyseal vessels and avascular necrosis of the capital epiphysis. However, there is no convincing evidence that irritable hip leads to Perthes disease. In the 1% of children who later present with Perthes disease it is probable that the early symptoms were related to the onset of the Perthes disease and not to a true irritable hip.

FURTHER READING

Carr AJ, Cole WG, Roberton DM, Chow CW. Chronic multifocal osteomyelitis. *J Bone Joint Surg* 1993; **75B**: 582–591.

Cole WG, Dalziel RE, Leitl S. Treatment of acute osteomyelitis in childhood. *J Bone Joint Surg* 1982; **62B**: 218–223.

Gillespie WJ, Mayo KM. The management of acute haematogenous osteomyelitis in the antibiotic era. *J Bone Joint Surg* 1981; **63B**: 126–131.

Gillespie WJ, Nade S. *Musculoskeletal Infections*. Blackwell Scientific Publications, Oxford, 1987.

Grainger RG, Allison AJ *Diagnostic Radiology*. Churchill Livingstone, Edinburgh, 1986

Green NE, Bruno J. *Pseudomonas* infections of the foot after puncture wounds. *South Med J* 1980; **73**: 146.

Menelaus MB. Discitis, an inflammation affecting the intervertebral discs. *J Bone Joint Surg* 1964; **46B**: 16–23.

Nade S. Acute osteomyelitis in infancy and childhood. *J Bone Joint Surg* 1983; **65B**: 109–119.

Nade S. Acute septic arthritis in infancy and childhood. *J Bone Joint Surg* 1983; **65B**: 234–241.

Ozonoff MB. *Paediatric Radiology*, second edition. WB Saunders, Philadelphia, 1992.

Roberts JM, Drummond DS, Breed AL, Chesney J. Subacute haematogenous osteomyelitis in children: a retrospective study. *J Pediatr Orthop* 1982; **2**: 249–254.

Ross ERS, Cole WG. Treatment of subacute osteomyelitis in childhood. *J Bone Joint Surg* 1985; **67B**: 443–448.

Chapter 12

Juvenile Chronic Arthritis

Susan M Randle

Any cause of synovitis can be described as an arthritis in children. It may be infective, traumatic or spontaneous, and its presentation may be acute or chronic. This chapter deals with juvenile chronic arthritis (JCA), which was first described by George Frederick Still in 1896. Further work by Ansell and Bywaters and various colleagues during the last 50 years has helped to define subgroups of JCA (*Table 12.1*). The recognition of subgroups of JCA allows clinicians to recognize the pattern of a particular child's chronic arthritis, provide the most appropriate treatments, and give parents and children an idea of likely complications and possible outcome.

The accepted criteria for a diagnosis of JCA are an onset under 16 years of age and a duration of at least three months. It can be classified according to its onset into pauciarticular arthritis (less than five joints), polyarticular arthritis and systemic illness.

There are two areas of confusion in the nomenclature of JCA.

- The first is that what is called JCA in Australia and the UK is called juvenile rheumatoid arthritis (JRA) in the USA. It is more appropriate to use the term JCA as most of the children with this condition are rheumatoid factor-negative.
- Secondly, JCA of any type is often called 'Still Disease'. This term should now be reserved for the systemic form of JCA, which was the condition Still described originally.

Incidence

Juvenile chronic arthritis affects 1–2 per 10,000 children under the age of 17 years (Cassidy and Nelson, 1988). The incidence of the various types of arthritis is shown in Table 12.2.

Table 12.1 Classification of juvenile chronic arthritis

Arthritic conditions that are mostly unique to childhood
Pauciarticular arthritis
Polyarticular arthritis
Systemic arthritis

Arthritic conditions seen in adult life presenting in childhood
HLA-B27 related spondyloarthritis
Polyarthritis associated with connective tissue diseases
Psoriatic arthropathy
HLA B27-negative spondyloarthropathy and enthesopathy
Rheumatoid factor-positive arthritis
Arthritis associated with chronic inflammatory bowel disease, diabetes mellitus, cystic fibrosis
Gout

Table 12.2 The incidence of the various forms of juvenile chronic arthritis (JCA) seen in the Rheumatology Clinic at the Royal Children's Hospital, Melbourne, 1994–5.

JCA	
Pauciarticular	27%
Polyarticular	21%
Systemic	9%
HLA B27-positive ankylosing spondylitis	15%
Polyarthropathies associated with connective tissue diseases	12%
Psoriatic arthropathy	6%
HLA B27-negative spondyloarthropathy and enthesopathy	6%
Rheumatoid factor-positive arthritis	4%

THE VARIOUS FORMS OF JUVENILE CHRONIC ARTHRITIS

A summary of the clinical features of the various forms of JCA is given in Table 12.3.

Pauciarticular Juvenile Chronic Arthritis

Pauciarticular JCA describes an arthritis in children affecting 1–4 joints in the first three months of the illness. Approximately 50% of children with JCA have a pauciarticular distribution. There is a female predominance.

Clinical Features

These children are usually well at presentation apart from pain, swelling and stiffness of the involved joints. It usually presents in children aged 1–5 years

Table 12.3 Summary of the features of the various forms of juvenile chronic arthritis (JCA)

Pauciarticular JCA
1–4 joints involved in the first three months
Usually aged 1–5 years at onset
Often antinuclear antibody (ANA) positive
Associated with iritis
Incidence greater in females than in males
Usually large joints
Systemic features nearly always absent
Local bony growth abnormalities may develop

Polyarticular JCA
Arthritis of more than four joints in the first three months
All ages at onset
ANA positive in approximately 50% of cases
May develop eye disease
Incidence greater in females than in males
Large and small joints
Systemic features mild
May develop growth abnormalities

Systemic JCA
Usually polyarticular
Systemic features may precede joint features
All ages at onset
ANA and rheumatoid factors rarely present
Incidence equal in females and in males

and affects large joints such as the knees and elbows. The diagnosis may be difficult as young children may not complain until the affected joint is examined or they may present with a limp and irritability. It is often difficult for parents to observe swelling of an arthritic joint in a podgy toddler, and irritability may be thought to be a part of normal toddler behaviour.

Most children with pauciarticular JCA continue to have pauciarticular disease and remain systemically well, but may have persistent problems with the involved joints. With treatment, most do well, with disease remission after months or years. With optimal treatment, many have no long-term loss of joint movement or only minimal loss of function. A few do have long-term sequelae of the disease with a wasted limb, restricted movement of the affected joint and poor function of the limb. Local bony growth abnormalities may occur, with deformities of the lower limb and overgrowth around a joint with chronic synovitis (*Figure 12.1*).

In a few children the condition progresses to polyarticular JCA, psoriatic arthritis or ankylosing spondylitis. Those children progressing to polyarticular JCA have a less favourable outcome with persistent active disease and significant functional disability.

Eye involvement

Chronic iritis, which is asymptomatic until well advanced, is often seen in association with pauciarticular JCA and almost 90% of cases are positive for antinuclear antibody (ANA) if iritis is present. Eye examinations are required three-monthly until the late teens and should continue even if the arthritis has gone into remission. Iritis may develop up to ten years after the onset of JCA.

Laboratory Investigations

Some of these children are ANA positive and some may have an elevated erythrocyte sedimentation rate (ESR). In a monoarticular arthropathy other conditions such as foreign body arthritis, pigmented villonodular synovitis, malignancies of cartilage, bone or synovium, and tuberculosis should be excluded. If the child is ANA positive and has iritis, the diagnosis is most likely JCA, but if the inflamed joint is the only problem, biopsy may be necessary to rule out other important diagnoses.

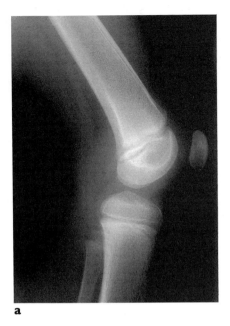 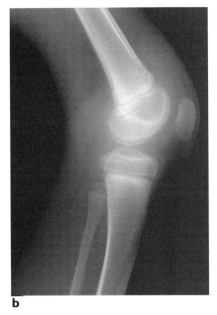

a   b

Figure 12.1 a Normal right knee in an eight-year-old. **b** Monoarthritis of the left knee of four years duration. There is periarticular osteoporosis, soft tissue swelling and overgrowth of the bones.

Polyarticular Juvenile Chronic Arthritis

Polyarticular JCA describes arthritis in children that affects more than four joints in the first three months of the illness, but without systemic involvement. There is a female predominance.

Clinical Features

Children with involvement of more than four joints may present with altered gait and difficulty performing normal everyday tasks such as removing clothing or shoes. They are often a little withdrawn and may not complain of soreness.

The correct diagnosis of the child with polyarticular JCA depends on recognizing the pattern of the child's arthritis. Polyarticular JCA is usually symmetrical and involves small and large joints. Neck, jaw and back involvement may also be present. The presence and severity of growth abnormalities will give clues to the severity and chronicity of the disease (*Figures 12.2, 12.3*).

The child may be thin and pale due to chronic disease, decreased appetite and poor dietary intake. Lack of normal mobility also gives rise to poor muscle bulk. The child may deny pain, but grimace or even cry during examination of the joints.

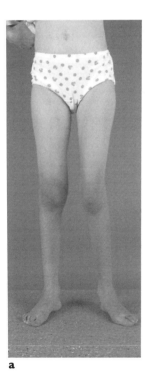 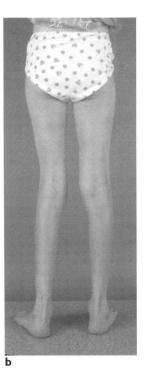

a   b

Figure 12.2 Lower limbs of an eight-year-old girl with polyarticular arthritis of six years duration showing poor muscle bulk and increased left leg length with a valgus deformity at the knee and tibial torsion.

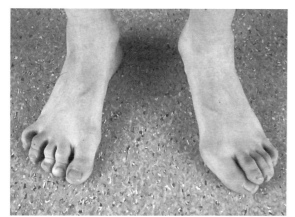

Figure 12.3 These feet show flexion contractures of the proximal interphalangeal (IP) joints, especially of the right foot. There is involvement of the left first metatarsophalangeal and IP joints with hallux valgus and overgrowth of the left foot and great toe compared with the right side.

Children with this form of arthritis usually have persistent disease activity over many years. Untreated, many of these children develop fixed flexion deformities and significant functional disabilities. Because of the early recognition of the disease and improved therapy, many of these children now reach their teens with active disease, but good joint function. In most children, the disease eventually 'burns out'. A small proportion continue to have active disease into adult life.

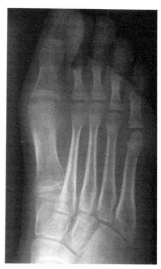

Figure 12.4 The left foot of a nine-year-old girl with rheumatoid factor-positive arthritis of six months' duration. The film shows osteoporosis and focal erosive changes of the proximal phalanx of the first toe and metatarsal head with decreased joint space.

joints as the years go by. Presentation may be at any age and the sex distribution is equal.

Ankylosing spondylitis may present in childhood, but usually after seven years of age. There is involvement of the sacroiliac joint, back and neck pain, and involvement of large joint such as the knees and hips (*Figures 12.5, 12.6*).

Differential Diagnosis

Rheumatoid factor-positive JCA presents as a symmetrical arthritis that often involves the metacarpophalangeal (MCP) and proximal interphalangeal (PIP) joints of the hands as well as the metatarsophalangeal (MTP) joints of the feet. Other joints may be involved and erosions may be present after only a few months of disease, whereas they are usually a later and less frequent finding in rheumatoid factor-negative JCA. The children are usually at least nine years of age and are usually female (*Figure 12.4*).

Psoriatic arthritis is often asymmetrical and may involve large joints as well as cause the appearance of 'sausage digits'. Children with psoriatic arthritis usually have a family history of psoriasis or have psoriasis themselves. It is important to look closely at the skin around the hair line for psoriasis and also at the nails for pitting.

Children with psoriatic arthritis may have a persistent mild arthritis or may develop more inflamed

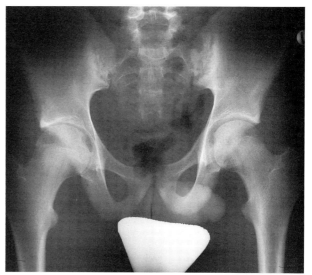

Figure 12.5 Pelvis and hips of an HLA B27-positive teenage boy showing bilateral irregularity of the sacroiliac joints with loss of joint space at the right hip. (Courtesy of Dr Roger Allen.)

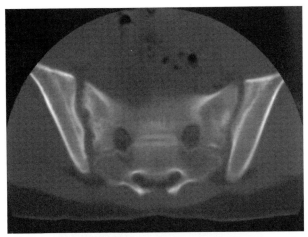

Figure 12.6 Computerized tomographic scans of a 12-year-old HLA B27-positive boy with irregularity of the right sacroiliac joint compared with that of the left side.

Enthesopathy (inflammation of tendon insertion sites) is common, with plantar fasciitis and pain at the insertion of the tendo Achilles and patellar tendon. Polyarthritis without sacroiliac or spinal involvement may be the initial presentation. A history of the onset of large joint arthritis or back pain at a young age in family members is often obtained and the parents of the child may have joint or back and neck pain. HLA B27-related arthritis has been diagnosed in several parents at our clinic after presenting with their similarly-affected child. A group of children with these symptoms may be HLA B27-negative and are described as having the seronegative enthesopathy and arthritis (SEA) syndrome.

Occasionally a child will present with polyarthritis and general ill health in which case the diagnostic possibilities are greatly increased. A thorough physical examination and examination of the blood, urine and occasionally bone marrow, as well as radiological examinations may be necessary to exclude conditions such as systemic lupus erythematosis, leukaemia, vasculitis and chronic recurrent multifocal osteomyelitis.

Very occasionally a child presents with polyarthritis and reasonably good general health, but has other abnormalities typical of various connective tissue diseases such as scleroderma or dermatomyositis (see Chapter 10). It is important in the general physical examination to note the nature of the child's skin and the presence of weakness and purple discoloration over the knuckles and around the eyes, which will lead quickly to the correct diagnosis.

Systemic Juvenile Chronic Arthritis

Systemic JCA describes arthritis in children involving more than four joints associated with inflammation of internal organ systems. The arthritis is usually polyarticular and symmetrical. About 10% of the children with JCA have systemic arthritis. The sex distribution is equal.

Clinical Features

Children with systemic JCA may present in a number of ways. Commonly there is a symmetrical arthritis involving the small joints of the hands and feet, often the distal interphalangeal (DIP) and PIP joints, as well as the large joints. Neck involvement may be particularly severe. Shoulder and back involvement usually occur months to years into the illness. The arthritis may be accompanied at its onset by high swinging fevers and a maculopapular flitting rash, usually on the trunk, volar surfaces of the arms, and insides of the thighs and the face. Its presence is diagnostically very helpful. The rash may be florid or only evident after a bath or during feverish episodes. The fevers and rash may occur for weeks without evidence of the arthritis and the child may be investigated for a pyrexia of unknown origin.

Approximately 50% of cases resolve after one episode. The remainder usually continues as persistent arthritis of one or more joints at any one time, with regular exacerbations of systemic symptoms and polyarthritis over the years. A few children continue to have debilitating fevers, rashes and polyarthritis daily for years, and these children pose a significant therapeutic challenge.

Differential Diagnosis

Children with systemic JCA are often very unwell and the differential diagnosis includes leukaemia, infections, metastatic manifestations of tumours and systemic lupus erythematosus. Children with systemic JCA, although often very stiff and sore, will usually walk at some stage during the day. Beware of the child who will not put his feet to the ground and weight-bear. The diagnosis in this situation is almost always not systemic JCA. A thorough clinical examination, full blood examination, ANA testing and radiology should be performed, and blood culture and bone marrow examination may be necessary.

Children with systemic JCA who present with a painful back may have developed an osteoporotic vertebral crush fracture due to a large intake of oral corticosteroids over the years (*Figure 12.7*).

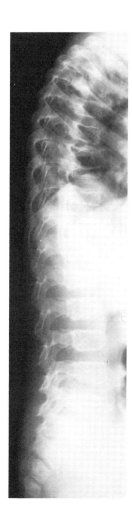

Figure 12.7 Spinal radiograph of a five-year-old boy with a three-year history of very active systemic juvenile chronic arthritis who required prolonged high-dose oral corticosteroids. The thoracic vertebrae are osteoporotic and some show collapse.

Onset of severe pain in a joint may be due to a septic arthritis.

Management

The aims of treatment are:

- To control the disease process.
- To minimize pain.
- To prevent the loss of joint function.
- To prevent growth abnormalities.
- To allow normal physical, intellectual and social maturation.
- To consider the needs of the rest of the family.

Medical management is the key to controlling the disease.

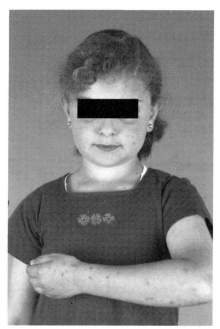

Figure 12.8 Lesions of naproxen-induced pseudo-porphyria on the face and arms of a seven-year-old girl with psoriatic arthritis.

Simple analgesics
Paracetamol is useful as a simple analgesic.

Non-steroidal anti-inflammatory drugs (NSAIDs)
Naproxen, diclofenac, ibuprofen and indomethacin are frequently used. The side-effects common to the NSAIDS are indigestion, headaches (especially with indomethacin), and rashes. Pseudoporphyria is very occasionally seen with naproxen, but is important to recognize because the lesions cause scarring (*Figure 12.8*).

Slow-acting antirheumatic drugs (SAARDs)
Sulphasalazine is useful for mildly aggressive disease and especially for psoriatic and HLA B27-positive JCA. The main side-effects are neutropenia, gastro-intestinal upset with abdominal pain, headaches and skin rashes.

Hydroxychloroquine is effective in children with mild but persistent arthritis that is inadequately controlled on NSAIDS. It is also useful for the arthritis of systemic lupus erythematosus if kidney disease is not a significant problem. It is very well tolerated. There have been reports of maculopathy in adults, so six-monthly ophthalmological examination is necessary.

Gold is very effective for rheumatoid factor-positive arthritis. Children's tolerance to weekly injections limits its use, however, when other SAARDs are available.

Corticosteroids

High-dose intravenous or oral corticosteroids are used, mainly for life-threatening complications of arthritis as seen with systemic JCA and pericarditis, or for severe JCA of any form when the disease is acutely uncontrolled.

Despite their many complications low-dose oral corticosteroids may be used on an alternate day basis when other treatment has not been effective. They should be considered if the child is so poorly controlled that attending school is impossible.

Immunosuppressants

Methotrexate is used for aggressive arthritis early in the course of the disease or later in the disease if the arthritis is progressing despite treatment. It is also useful as a corticosteroid-sparing agent and is probably the most effective and best tolerated disease-modifying agent in use. The main side-effects are neutropenia, mouth ulcers, gastrointestinal upset and altered liver function. Hepatic cirrhosis has very rarely been reported in adults. Toxicity is increased with concomitant administration of sulphamethoxazole and with dehydration.

Azathioprine is used mainly for systemic lupus erythematosus, occasionally for severe iritis and rarely for arthritis resistant to other forms of therapy.

Cyclosporin is used very occasionally for JCA if all other treatments have failed. Availability restricts its use at present.

Injections

Injections of intra-articular corticosteroids can be useful in controlling aggressive disease. Often these have a prolonged effect unexplained by the nature of the corticosteroid, which is administered with a local anaesthetic. In the young child a general anaesthetic is usually necessary and this allows multiple joints to be injected.

Physiotherapy

The use of physiotherapy is most important for children with JCA to control pain, maintain muscle strength and joint movement, prevent deformities and to encourage normal physical maturation.

The techniques used include:

- Provision of exercise programmes.
- Assisted active movements.
- Hydrotherapy.
- Splinting.

Parents should be taught these techniques and encouraged to use simple gentle massage with or without non-steroidal anti-inflammatory creams. The simple application of heat or cold to the painful joints is useful for analgesia.

Painful joints should be rested in splints moulded to a good position to reduce the risk of contracture development. If the joint is painful it should still be taken through a full range of movement two or three times a day. Splints should be supplied early, assessed regularly, and worn temporarily for acutely painful joints, usually at night, to correct growth deformities. An active exercise programme should be undertaken to encourage normal joint movement and prevent contractures. Hydrotherapy is particularly useful because it combines warmth with reduced weight-bearing exercises.

Occupational therapy

The occupational therapist is an important member of the team and can advise the child and the family on ways to help with activities of daily living that are difficult due to pain and stiffness. They can help with the provision of aids for play and school, and also assess hand function and provide special hand splints.

Physical and occupational therapy for children with JCA are best undertaken by specialists, and the skills developed in dealing with the problems of many of these children can benefit similar children treated in the clinic subsequently.

Education

The rheumatologists involved in the care of children with JCA should not only supervise their drug management, but also ensure that normal physical, intellectual and social maturation is facilitated.

The child's growth should be monitored with advice on dietary intake. Endocrine assessment may be required, and in some cases the use of growth hormone.

It is an important time to educate the family about the special needs of the child with JCA. Early morning stiffness and fatigue later in the day at school should be explained. The child may be slow in writing and slow in moving around the school. The pain and stiffness vary from hour to hour and are more commonly due to organic factors than a reluctance to join in activities. An understanding of all these features helps the family and teachers cope with the child's problems.

It is useful to address concerns about the prognosis at the clinic, both in terms of morbidity and mortality. Body image should also be discussed. Parents should be encouraged to voice their specific concerns.

It is important to acknowledge that caring for the child is a part of the family life over many years and that the parent's work and social activities suffer as a result.

Orthopaedic Management

The orthopaedic surgeon is a valuable member of the team involved in the diagnosis and management of the child with JCA. Within the clinic the surgeon is particularly skilled at monitoring the development of deformity and any growth disturbance.

Diagnosis
A biopsy may be required if the child poses a diagnostic problem, particularly if there is single joint involvement. This should be undertaken arthroscopically whenever possible.

Injections
The surgeon may also be called upon to perform intraarticular injections of corticosteroid. Sometimes these can be given in the clinic with the use of local anaesthetic cream, but general anaesthesia is required by some children and is also appropriate if multiple joints are to be injected. Most joints can be injected directly, but assistance from an image intensifier is needed to inject the hips and subtalar and sacroiliac joints. Sometimes contrast material is used to ensure location within the joint.

Synovectomy
Most cases can now be controlled by medical management and the necessity for surgical synovectomy has been greatly reduced over the last 20 years. Synovectomy has no benefit if there is destruction of the articular surfaces and should only be used as a means to cure persistent chronic synovitis. Synovectomy may be required in only a few cases, but particularly if a single joint is involved and medical control is difficult or if there are concerns about the toxic nature of the necessary chemotherapeutic agents. Synovectomy can sometimes be performed arthroscopically, but it is controversial whether this is as effective as an open synovectomy. Continuous passive movement may be used postoperatively, but postoperative stiffness is less of a problem in the child than in the adult.

Soft tissue release
Hip and knee flexion contractures are now less common in children with JCA because of the advances in physical therapy to prevent and treat these problems. Correction of the contracture often leads to dramatic improvements in the gait and a reduction in pain. There is a limited role for soft-tissue release in the upper limb.

At the hip a simple limited exposure has been advocated with division of the psoas tendon, adductors and gracilis. This allows rapid mobilization postoperatively. Although a more extensive procedure with a synovectomy may have more long-term benefit the prolonged recovery can diminish the effectiveness of the procedure.

At the knee soft-tissue release can be performed if there is no posterior subluxation of the tibia on the femur. Through posteromedial and posterolateral incisions the hamstrings are lengthened, the heads of gastrocnemius released and a posterior capsulotomy performed. The release should be as extensive as necessary to achieve correction on table and the capsulotomy may have to be extended anteriorly to divide the retinaculum. A back slab is worn postoperatively and active exercises started out of this after two days.

Bony correction
Osteotomy may be considered for the severe contracture or if there is a failure to respond to a soft-tissue release. Improvement of a severe hip flexion contracture by an extension upper femoral osteotomy can be useful. In the knee with a flexion contracture and posterior subluxation of the tibia on the femur a soft-tissue release is unlikely to correct the subluxation. These cases are probably best treated by supracondylar osteotomy.

Growth abnormalities are common around the knee with a valgus and flexion abnormality. Early control of the disease reduces the risk of this complication. Epiphyseal stapling may have a role for the simple valgus deformity, but the effect is not predictable and a corrective osteotomy may be more appropriate.

Planovalgus deformity of the foot can be a particular problem in some children with JCA. The deformity is usually at the subtalar joint and correction should be obtained by subtalar fusion, or in the older child by a triple arthrodesis.

Joint replacement
In the child with a destroyed joint, a replacement arthroplasty should be considered. This is a major undertaking, and although short-term gains may be considerable the long-term implications may be disastrous.

Custom-made or special small prostheses are often required in the hip and knee. Most of the published results are for cemented prostheses. The results have not been encouraging, particularly for the hip, where there is a high rate of loosening and infection. However, in some children there is no alternative.

Surgery in general

Surgery in children with JCA is often challenging and should only be performed within a specialist unit. The anaesthesia can be difficult with intubation problems because of poor jaw opening and cervical spine instability. Many of these children are on corticosteroids and other immunosuppressants so it is important to consider their medical management, particularly in those with systemic disease. The bone is often osteoporotic, which makes fusions more demanding, and the use of internal fixation should be meticulous. These children are also more susceptible to infection as a result of disease activity and the drugs used.

REFLEX SYMPATHETIC DYSTROPHY

Reflex sympathetic dystrophy (RSD) is a condition included in the differential diagnosis of monoarticular JCA. The affected child usually presents with an extremely painful hand or foot, usually after minor trauma. Often there are personal or family difficulties at the onset of the disorder.

The affected area is usually cool, clammy, purplish and blotchy, and swollen. There is extreme pain when the skin is touched even lightly and there is a refusal to use the limb as it hangs down limply. Although the aetiology of RSD is not fully understood, the signs and symptoms are of local autonomic nervous system dysfunction.

Management

Treatment involves active physiotherapy to the affected part. Passive manipulation aggravates the condition because the limb is touched. NSAID medications and paracetamol are useful for some of the pain, but there is no medication that can help the painful hyperaesthesia of the involved limb. Psychosocial difficulties are often acute and mild and can be remedied by a discussion of the problems during medical consultations. Sometimes the expertise of a child psychiatrist or family therapist can be helpful. With treatment, the pain and physical appearance of the limb usually improves within 3–4 weeks. Return of muscle strength may take weeks to months. The prognosis is good and the condition does not usually return unless the child has significant unresolved emotional difficulties.

HAEMOSTATIC DISORDERS AND THEIR ARTHROPATHIES

Haemophilia (factor VIII deficiency) and Christmas disease (factor IX deficiency) are the hereditary disorders of haemostasis that are most likely to involve the musculoskeletal system. Both conditions are sex-linked recessive, so occur in males. Von Willebrand's disease affects both sexes equally, but only occasionally causes haemarthroses.

In severe haemophilia (i.e. with less than 1% factor VIII) there is spontaneous bleeding into the muscles and joints and this is treated by an infusion of factor VIII. The knee is most commonly involved, followed by the elbow and ankle. In the chronic form these children may present because of the discomfort of repeated bleeding into a joint, which may cause a fixed deformity or a chronic synovitis. The radiograph often shows expansion of the epiphyses, and degenerative change can occur at an early stage. With the backup of a haematologist and adequate factor VIII, a synovectomy can be very useful in preventing repeat bleeds into a joint.

REFERENCES AND FURTHER READING

Ansell BM. *Rheumatic Disorders in Childhood.* Postgraduate Paediatrics Series. General Editor: John Apley. Butterworth, Guildford, 1980.

Ansell BM, Swan M. The management of chronic arthritis of children *J Bone Joint Surg* 1983; **65B**: 536–543.

Cassidy JT, Nelson AM. The frequency of juvenile arthritis. *J Rheum* 1988; **15**: 535–536.

Cassidy JT, Petty RE. *Textbook of Paediatric Rheumatology*, second edition. Churchill Livingstone, Edinburgh, 1990.

Clarke DW, Ansell BM, Swan M. Soft tissue release of the knee in children with juvenile chronic arthritis. *J Bone Joint Surg* 1988; **70B**: 224–227.

Ruddlesdin C, Ansell BM, Arden GP, Swan M. Total hip replacement in children with juvenile chronic arthritis. *J Bone Joint Surg* 1986; **68B**: 218–222.

Rydholm U, Elburg R, Ranstam J, Schroder A, Svantesson H, Lidgren L. Synovectomy of the knee in juvenile chronic arthritis. *J Bone Joint Surg* 1986; **68B**: 223–228.

Swan M, Ansell BM. Soft tissue release of the hips in children with juvenile chronic arthritis. *J Bone Joint Surg* 1986; **68B**: 404–408.

Chapter 13
Osteochrondritic Conditions

D Robert V Dickens

This ill-defined group of conditions characteristically affect the epiphyseal areas of bones. The aetiology is unclear, though trauma, traction or an episode of avascular necrosis appears to be the aetiological factor in some cases. The pathology is often of an avascular necrosis with loss of bone cells, and surrounding increased vascularity and sclerosis in the bone. Excessive activity in the child may account for some of the reaction seen, and in some circumstances these can be thought of as an avulsion stress fracture. Radiological changes are characteristically those of fragmentation followed by healing. This is similar to those seen in Perthes disease, which is considered to be one of the osteochondritides (see Chapter 17).

These conditions usually present during periods of rapid growth, and are most common during early adolescence. They usually affect normal active healthy children. They have been categorized as crushing (Freiberg disease, Panner disease), splitting (osteochondritis dissecans of the knee) and pulling (Osgood–Schlatter disease and Sever disease).

UPPER LIMB

Panner Disease

In 1929 Panner described an osteochondritis of the capitellum. It usually affects children between 4–10 years of age, but can occur up to 14 years. It occurs almost exclusively in boys. The aetiology is unclear.

Clinical Features

The child presents with swelling and tenderness in the region of the elbow and often describes catching or clicking on elbow movement. On examination there is restricted movement of the elbow, and a fixed flexion deformity may be present. The natural history is for a full recovery.

Radiology

There is an irregularity of the capitellar epiphysis with fragmentation (*Figure 13.1*). A slow resolution with recovery of the bony architecture to a more normal appearance takes place over a period of 1–2 years.

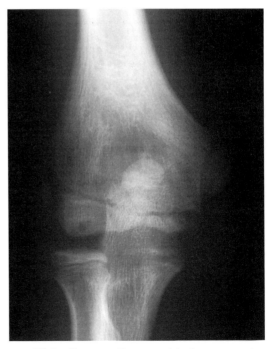

Figure 13.1 Panner disease with fragmentation of the humeral capitellum.

Management

This should be conservative. The child and parents should be reassured that this is a benign self-correcting condition. The child should be encouraged to continue with sport of an appropriate nature, but to avoid overstressing the involved elbow.

LOWER LIMB

Osgood–Schlatter disease

This is a condition involving the tibial tubercle at the insertion of the patellar tendon. The condition was first described in 1903 both by Osgood and Schlatter.

Aetiology

The aetiology of this condition is thought to be either a traction apophysitis or avascular necrosis. It occurs at a time when the child is growing rapidly and may be bilateral. It is more common in boys, but occurs at a younger age in girls. It is not uncommon to find radiological changes affecting both knees and yet symptoms involving only one.

Clinical Features

The clinical features are of a normally-active child with a painful and tender prominence in the region of the tibial tubercle. It is commonly bilateral. Not infrequently the history of symptoms has been present for some months at the time of presentation. The condition is aggravated by activity and improved by restriction of activity. The children are usually enthusiastic participants in sporting activities and often elect to continue playing sport despite their symptoms.

The clinical sign is a prominent tender swelling in the region of the tibial tubercle, which is more obvious when the knee is flexed to 90°. The knee itself is otherwise entirely normal and movements of the knee do not cause any discomfort over the area. The natural history of this condition is for the pain to continue with activity for 1–2 years and then to resolve.

Radiology

Radiographs of the knees demonstrate variable appearances (*Figure 13.2*). There may be quite marked fragmentation and sclerosis of the tibial tubercle. There may also be a tilted appearance to the tubercle epiphysis so that the growth plate

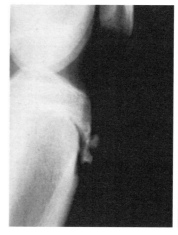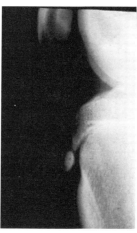

Figure 13.2 Bilateral Osgood–Schlatter disease with fragmentation of the tibial tubercles.

appears widened with a 'fracture' across this tongue of epiphysis. The soft tissues over the area may appear oedematous due to the inflammatory process.

On the plain radiographs there is healing of the fragmentation when the condition resolves and, once the epiphysis is closed, a return to normal appearances.

Management

Since the natural history is for resolution an adequate explanation of this to the child and parents is essential. Management of the acute episode is greatly helped when the natural history is understood. Restriction of activity is advocated if symptoms are unacceptable, but if the the symptoms are acceptable the child can be allowed to participate in normal activities. There is no evidence that immobilization or restriction of sport speeds up resolution or influence the natural history of the condition. Pain can be so severe, however, that immobilization in a plaster or a brace may be required until the inflammation settles.

Although the condition resolves completely in the vast majority of children, a small proportion of patients are left with two residual problems.

- An ossicle may persist within the patellar tendon at its insertion onto the tibia. This can be painful on kneeling. Surgical removal of the bony fragment can be offered, but the patient must be informed that removal of the ossicle will result in a scar. The position of that scar is critical. It must not be placed over the prominence of the tibial tubercle or it may be painful on kneeling.
- There may be overgrowth or bulkiness of the tibial tubercle. This occasionally causes concern because

of its cosmetic appearance in females. The only surgical solution is to reduce the bulk of the tubercle. This is a major undertaking involving reattachment of the patellar tendon, and the results are often less satisfactory than the patient expects. After discussion of the likely outcome and the procedure involved most patients accept the appearance and wear knee pads when kneeling is required.

Recurvatum has been reported as a consequence of Osgood–Schlatter disease, but is a rare complication.

Larsen–Johannson Disease

Larsen in 1921 and Johannson in 1922 described the condition of osteochondritis of the lower pole of the patella at the origin of the patellar tendon. It is another traction apophysitis, but is not as common as Osgood–Schlatter disease.

Clinical Features

The presentation is characteristically with pain on activity, particularly running. There is discomfort and tenderness over the lower pole of the patella, and sometimes a fullness in this area.

Radiology

This reveals irregularity of the lower pole of the patella and some fragmentation of bone. The bone goes through a healing phase with new bone formation.

Management

This consists of rest and reassurance. If the pain is severe it may be necessary to immobilize the knee in a plaster cylinder for a short period of time to promote resolution.

Menelaus–Batten Syndrome

In 1985 Batten and Menelaus described a similar condition to Larsen–Johannson disease affecting the attachment of the quadriceps mechanism to the proximal pole of the patella. The radiological appearances are those of fragmentation with changes in the bone similar to those described for Larsen–Johannson disease (*Figure 13.3*).

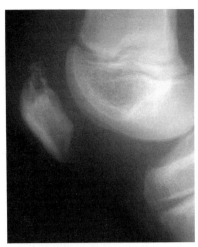

Figure 13.3   Menelaus–Batten disease with fragmentation of the proximal pole of the patella.

The child characteristically presents with tenderness in the upper pole of the patella and resolution can be expected with rest.

Köhler Disease

Köhler described osteochondritis of the navicular in 1908. It usually affects children 3–5 years of age and males more than females. The pathology is of fragmentation followed by healing, suggesting an avascular episode as the aetiology.

Clinical Features

The presentation is variable. In some children it is a coincidental radiological finding, but in others it presents with acute inflammation and can be confused with acute osteomyelitis. More commonly the patient presents with a limp, and examination reveals tenderness and swelling in the region of the navicular.

The natural history of the condition is for resolution within 3–4 months, but the process of radiographic healing takes approximately 1–2 years.

Radiology

This demonstrates density in the navicular as the initial finding with bony sclerosis and often severe flattening of the bony nucleus (*Figure 13.4*). Subsequently fragmentation of the dense bony nucleus occurs, followed by healing. The final radiological appearance shows reconstitution of the navicular

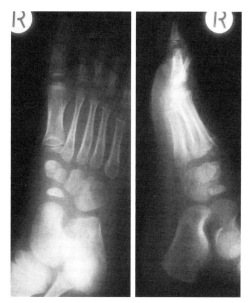

Figure 13.4 Köhler disease with fragmentation of the navicular bone.

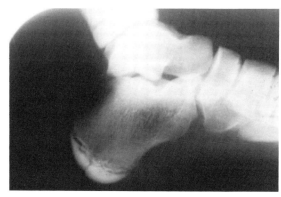

Figure 13.5 A dense sclerotic appearance of the calcaneal apophysis is a common appearance in the growing child.

with little to show for the previous flattening and sclerosis.

Management

This involves reassurance and an explanation of the natural history of the condition. If the symptoms are minimal no treatment is required, but immobilization in a below-knee plaster cast for 3–4 weeks provides relief if the symptoms are troublesome. After removal of the cast most of the patients are able to return to normal activities. There are no long-term consequences.

Sever Disease

In 1912, Sever described osteochondritis of the os calcis, a condition characterized by painful heels in children. It presents most commonly in active children, in boys more than girls, and between the ages of 10–12 years. There is pain and discomfort with activity at the insertion of the tendo Achillis. The condition is regarded as a traction apophysitis and is frequently bilateral.

Clinical Features

There is discomfort at the back of the heel and a limp after activity. Once the limb is rested the complaint and limp settles. The characteristic sign is tenderness over the calcaneal apophysis posteriorly. There is no discomfort on the undersurface of the os calcis. Squeezing the medial and lateral aspects of the os calcis may produce pain. There is no obvious swelling.

The natural history is for resolution with time irrespective of any treatment. Once the epiphyseal line has closed and the os calcis is one single bone the condition can no longer exist.

Radiology

It is now accepted that there are no specific radiological signs in this condition. Sometimes the calcaneal apophysis is densely sclerotic, but this appearance is just as common in those children without heel pain as in those with Sever disease (*Figure 13.5*).

Management

This consists of reassuring the patient and parent and explaining the natural history of the condition. Treatment aimed at relaxing the Achilles tendon such as a heel raise and heel pads inside the shoe can provide some symptomatic relief. Restriction of activity is effective in reducing the patient's symptoms, but there is no evidence that it alters the natural history of the conditon.

Osteochondritis of the Epiphysis of the Base of the Fifth Metatarsal

This condition affects females between 10–13 years of age and is believed to be a traction apophysitis at the attachment of peroneus brevis.

Clinical Features

Presentation is with a painful limp and a swelling at the base of the fifth metatarsal, producing discomfort with shoe wear. The signs are those of a tender lump.

The natural history is of resolution with time. Requests to remove the lumps surgically because of the symptoms as they rub on the shoe should be resisted.

Radiology

Radiographs of the lesion often show a thin flake of bone displaced away from its normal relationship to the base of the fifth metatarsal. There may be some fragmentation of the epiphysis.

Freiberg Disease

In 1914 Freiberg described an osteochondritis of the second metatarsal head. It affects females more than males and is bilateral in about 25% of cases. Less commonly the third metatarsal head is involved.

Aetiology

There has been much debate about the aetiology of this condition and at one stage it was linked to the use of high heels by adolescent girls. However, the incidence of the condition seems to have been unaltered since high heels have become less popular.

Clinical Features

The clinical features are a painful gait with discomfort and swelling in the region of the metatarsal head.

Pathology

The pathology shows an avascular process with collapse of the metatarsal head and a marked synovitis of the joint.

Radiology

Radiographs demonstrate fragmentation of the head of the metatarsal associated with a depression or flattening (*Figure 13.6*). Sometimes a loose body may form.

Management

This consists of weight relief to the area using a metatarsal dome insole, but frequently these are unsuccessful and surgical intervention becomes necessary. The flattened head can be elevated with a bone graft to reconstitute the articular surface. Dorsal closing-wedge osteotomies have been described to rotate the flattened surface out of the joint. When the joint is destroyed salvage procedures may be necessary to restore some movement, such as excision of the proximal portion of the proximal phalanx. Excision of the metatarsal head is no longer acceptable because it affects the weight-bearing ability of the foot.

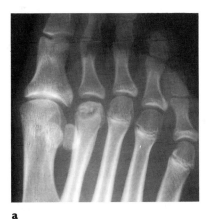
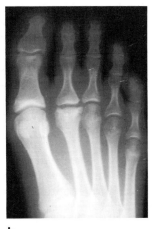

a   b

Figure 13.6 **a** Freiberg disease in the early stages. The affected area is fragmented with a surrounding layer of sclerotic reactive bone. **b** Freiberg disease at a later stage with collapse and distortion of the joint.

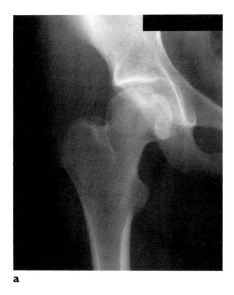
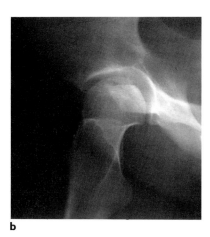
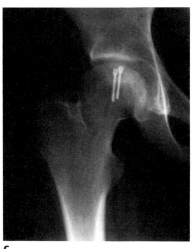

a
b
c

Figure 13.7 a,b Osteochondritis of the hip. There is fragmentation of a small segment in the weight-bearing area. **c** The fragment has been internally fixed with two Herbert screws.

Osteochondritis Dissecans of the Talus

Osteochondritis of the talus is a splitting form of osteochondritis that occurs in both adults and children. It affects the superior medial or lateral corner of the talus. In children it is most common in boys aged 10–14 years. It is often associated with trauma, and sometimes presents as a non-union of an osteochondral fracture. The pathology is similar to that of osteochondritis dissecans of the knee (Chapter 20).

Clinical Features

The presentation is with pain and a limp, and there may be some synovitis around the ankle. There is tenderness on direct palpation of the affected area and there may be restricted movement of the ankle. The lesion is best seen on an anteroposterior radiograph of the ankle. In children it is unusual for the fragment to detach and form a loose body within the joint.

Management

In this age group, management involves restricting activity, and most will heal over a few months. If the symptoms are severe or persistent, arthroscopic or open exploration can be undertaken. If the articular cartilage is intact and the fragment is not mobile, the abnormal area of bone is drilled through the articular cartilage. This encourages healing between the underlying healthy bone and the abnormal soft bone of the fragment. If the fragment is loose or mobile it should be removed and the crater drilled to encourage the development of fibrocartilage to fill the defect.

Osteochondritis Dissecans of the Hip

This is not common and can be a consequence of Perthes disease of the hip. It may be part of a rare generalized condition of osteochondritis dissecans of multiple epiphyses.

Clinical Features

The condition presents in adolescents with pain and a limp, and may be discovered when a slipped upper femoral epiphysis is suspected.

Management

The rationale for management is outlined in the section on osteochondritis dissecans of the knee. In the hip, arthroscopic treatment is difficult, but open treatment necessitates dislocation of the hip with the risk of avascular necrosis (*Figure 13.7*). Treatment is therefore delayed until it is clear that natural resolution will not take place. Some have healed after drilling of the fragment from below along the femoral neck. Other options include upper femoral osteotomy to rotate the affected part of the head out of the weight-bearing area.

REFERENCES AND FURTHER READING

Batten J, Menelaus MB. Fragmentation of the proximal pole of the patella. Another manifestation of juvenile traction osteochondritis. *J Bone Joint Surg* 1985; **67B**: 249–251.

Glynn MK, Regan BF. Surgical treatment of Osgood–Schlatter disease. *J Pediatr Orthop* 1993; **3**: 216–219.

Ippolito E, Ricciardi Pollini PT, Falez F. Köhler's disease of the tarsal navicular: Long-term follow-up of 12 cases. *J Pediatr Orthop* 1984; **4**: 416–417.

Krause BL, Williams JPR, Catterall A. Natural history of Osgood–Schlatter's disease. *J Pediatr Orthop* 1987; **10**: 65–68.

Micheli LJ, Ireland ML. Prevention and management of calcaneal apophysitis in children: an overuse syndrome. *J Pediatr Orthop* 1987; **7**: 34–38.

Chapter 14

Normal Variants: Intoeing, Bow Legs and Flat Feet

H Kerr Graham

Many children who are referred to orthopaedic clinics are normal and have no specific disease or deformity. They are referred with a variation of normality such as flexible flat foot, intoeing, outtoeing, knock knees or bow legs. It is essential to recognize that there can be just as much parental anxiety in these circumstances as there is about a child with a definable pathological condition. If the clinician fails to address parental concern appropriately and to explain the natural history of the condition, the parents of these children may be more concerned, more aggressive and demand more second opinions than the parents of a child with a specific pathological process.

The general principles of the management of these children are as follows:

- These conditions are common because they are normal variations.
- A reasonable description of normal is the mean value of the measurement plus or minus two standard deviations. This is of value to surgeons, not to parents (*Figure 14.1*).
- These conditions generally resolve spontaneously and there is little evidence that intervention changes the natural history.
- Overinvestigation of these children should be resisted.
- Overtreatment should be resisted.
- Within the large group of normal children with physiological variants, there are a small number with specific pathology. These children should be identified, investigated, diagnosed and treated appropriately.

Examination

The examination of this large group of children with normal variations is very important. A thorough examination reassures parents and within the group of apparently normal children, there will be the occasional child with a dislocated hip or hemiplegia. Although much of this has been described in Chapter 1, it is very helpful to have a routine for these children.

- Check the history: who is worried and about what? This frequently does not coincide with the referral letter.
- Watch the child playing on the floor, standing up (look for Gowers sign), walking and running. A mild hemiplegia may only be noticed by a paucity of arm movements when the child runs.
- Ask the child to walk on heels, walk on toes and hop on either foot. Frequently this has to be in the form of a game with the examiner leading the dance!
- When standing measure the intercondylar separation in bow legs and the intermalleolar separation in knock knees in fingerbreadths. A polaroid photograph may be useful for future comparisons.
- In walking estimate the 'foot progression angle;' imagine that the child is walking along a straight line on the floor. What angle does each foot make with the line?
- On the examination couch with the child prone assess the torsional profile. This is a game of 'show and tell.' Explain each step to the parents, what you find and what it means. (a) Check the alignment of the forefoot on the hindfoot. It may be

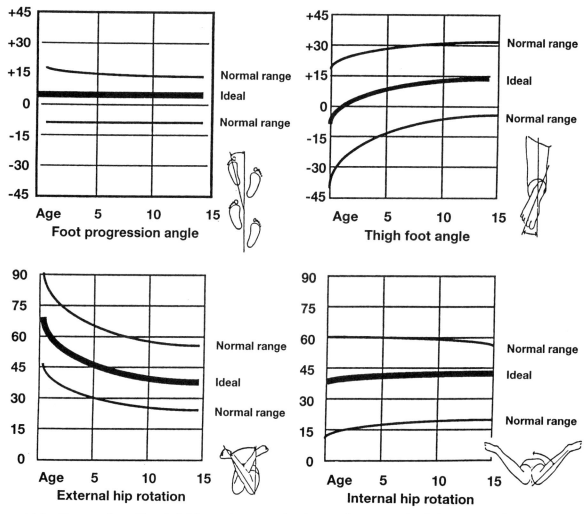

Figure 14.1 Torsional profile of children: the normal values and two standard deviations. These charts were prepared by Dr Mercer Rang based on data provided by Dr Lynn Staheli. They can be used to record findings and then be shown to parents. They provide some scientific basis to show that their child is normal and that the twists will disappear. The shape of the leg gradually changes as the child grows and twists tend to disappear. (Reproduced with permission from Raven Press.)

straight, adducted (infants with metatarsus adductus) or abducted (children with cerebral palsy). (b) In the same position check the 'thigh foot angle' (TFA). This is a measure of the alignment of the femur/thigh with the foot. In between these segments is the leg/tibia; the TFA therefore gives an estimate of tibial torsion. (c) Measure internal and external rotation of the femur with the knees flexed to 90°. Children with intoeing because of inset hips will frequently have 80° of internal rotation and only 20° of external rotation.

- Because many of these variants are accompanied by or modified by joint laxity, perform the Wynn–Davies tests for joint laxity. (a) Hyperextension at the elbow. (b) Hyperextension at the knee. (c) Thumb can touch the volar surface of forearm.

(d) Fingers hyperextend to lie parallel to forearm.
(e) Ankle dorsiflexion above 45°.

Rang's charts of torsional profiles are very useful to check the findings against. They can be used for education and reassurance.

INTOEING

Intoeing is one of the commonest presenting symptoms at paediatric orthopaedic clinics. The reason for the referral is usually the appearance and parental concern about long-term sequelae. Sometimes the concern is from the grandparents or nursery school teacher. There may also be a complaint that the child is clumsy or trips frequently. There is often a marked contrast between the parent and the child. The parent is anxious about the 'deformity' whereas the child runs around the consulting room in a carefree fashion, frequently not demonstrating as much intoeing as the parents claim is the case at home.

There are three causes of intoeing due to problems at different levels (i.e. the foot, the tibia and the femur). These problems tend to present in different age groups and the assessment, management and natural history of each is quite different.

Metatarsus Adductus

Metatarsus adductus presents either at birth or in the early months of life. The forefoot (in particular the first ray and hallux) is adducted and the sole of the foot may have a 'kidney shape.' The deformity is often bilateral, but not usually symmetrical (*Figure 14.2*). It is usually mobile and is a typical 'packaging defect.' It probably arises from intrauterine positioning and there is some evidence that it is perpetuated by the infant sleeping in the prone position. The publicized association between sudden infant death syndrome (SIDS) and prone nursing has now reduced the frequency of this condition in most orthopaedic clinics.

It is important to distinguish metatarsus adductus from congenital talipes equinovarus (CTEV) by examination of the position of the heel and the range of dorsiflexion at the ankle. In true CTEV, there is restriction of dorsiflexion at the ankle and the

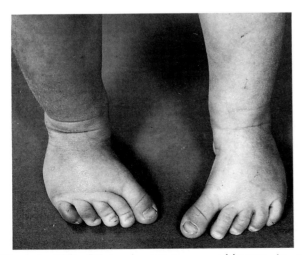

Figure 14.2 Bilateral metatarsus adductus in a toddler. (Reproduced with permission from Williams PF, Cole WG. *Orthopaedic Management in Childhood*. Chapman & Hall, London.)

heel is in varus. In metatarsus adductus the heel is neutral or in valgus and there is a normal range of ankle dorsiflexion.

A significant number of children with metatarsus adductus also have developmental dysplasia of the hip (DDH). It is important that all children presenting with metatarsus adductus have their hips examined and either an ultrasound or X-ray examination to look for acetabular dysplasia.

Management

Observation
The natural history of the condition is spontaneous resolution in the majority of children. However, in about 15% of children, resolution of the deformity is either slow or incomplete. For children up to three months old, advice against prone nursing should be given, but no specific treatment is necessary.

Splintage
If there is a delay in resolution, simple conservative treatment with corrective serial casts can be considered. The majority of feet will be corrected by the application of serial plasters (three casts, applied at two-week intervals) followed by straight or reversed-last shoes for several months. It is important to avoid excessive valgus of the heel by inappropriate casting. The use of corrective night splints is advocated by some.

Medial release
If there has been no improvement by the age of five years then prolonged conservative treatment is unlikely to be beneficial. A very small number of all children who originally present with metatarsus adductus require a simple medial soft tissue release of the foot.

Bony procedures
If the child presents late, surgical correction by metatarsal osteotomies can be considered at about seven years of age.

Other Causes of Adducted Feet

Relapsed Club Feet

These are more rigid and do not follow the natural history of metatarsus adductus. They do not resolve spontaneously and are resistant to cast treatment. Surgery is usually necessary to achieve any improvement.

Metatarsus Varus

The term metatarsus varus is used by some authors synonymously with metatarsus adductus; others reserve it for a more rigid deformity that includes forefoot supination and cavus deformity, which is more likely to need surgical release.

The Serpentine (Z-Shaped) Foot

This may be seen in either normal children or children with generalized problems such as Larsen syndrome. There is a severe and rigid metatarsus adductus combined with severe hind foot valgus. The orthotic and surgical management of this deformity is complex and generally unsatisfactory. Options include a Grice subtalar fusion to control the hindfoot and metatarsal osteotomies to correct the adductus deformity.

Internal Tibial Torsion

Internal or medial tibial torsion is very common in toddlers and usually presents as intoeing at 1–3 years of age. It is probably a packaging defect and the result of intrauterine positioning. It frequently coexists with, and may be confused with, bowing of the tibia (physiological genu varum).

Management

The natural history is for spontaneous resolution. A number of orthotic devices have been used: principally boots on a curved metal bar with the feet turned outwards (Denis Browne splint). This is used as a night splint, often leading to disturbed sleep and family distress. It may speed resolution of the deformity, but this has never been proven. Surgery is almost never required in normal children. In pathological conditions such as spina bifida it can be treated by derotation tibial osteotomy at the supra-malleolar level.

Internal Femoral Torsion (Inset Hips)

This is frequently seen in children between 3–10 years of age. The intoeing is symmetrical. Parents complain that their children look awkward and trip frequently, but the degree of disability is not great. The child often has signs of generalized joint laxity and may have associated features such as flexible flat feet. Examination reveals a characteristic shift of the arc of hip rotation inwards, hence the synonym 'inset hips.' A typical finding is internal rotation of 80–90° and external rotation of 0–10°. This is the reason why the children can sit comfortably in the 'W' position (*Figure 14.3*). It is doubtful if sitting in this position causes the condition, but there is some evidence that

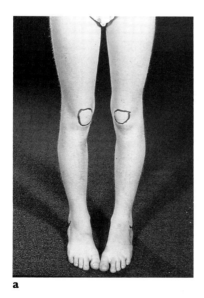
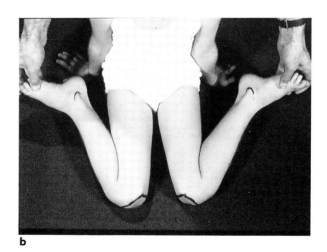

a   b

Figure 14.3   a Inset hips in an eight-year-old girl. Note the position of the patellas and the intoed posture. **b** The same girl sitting in the W position (reproduced with permission from Williams PF, Cole WG. *Orthopaedic Management in Childhood*. Chapman & Hall, London).

habitually sitting in this posture slows down the natural tendency to spontaneous recovery.

Management

The natural history of the condition is for spontaneous resolution during the growing years. There is no evidence that any form of exercises or orthotic devices influences the resolution.

The condition can be treated surgically by an external rotation osteotomy of the femur, but the vast majority of children improve spontaneously and do not require intervention. As a rule the child who has more than 10° of external rotation rarely requires surgery, whereas those who do not develop any arc of external rotation may. Surgery should not be performed at an early age because the degree of natural recovery cannot be predicted. There is also a significant risk of recurrence. Improvement probably stops at the age of about 8–10 years. The surgical options include external rotation osteotomy of the femur at the intertrochanteric level with blade plate fixation or distal with plate fixation. In adolescents, a closed intramedullary osteotomy with a cam saw and intramedullary nailing may be preferable.

In some children, natural correction of the intoeing occurs by compensatory external tibial torsion. In these children the feet no longer turn in, but on standing and walking the patellas face inwards or 'squint' (*Figure 14.4*). This combination of deformities looks unattractive. Surgical improvement of 'squinting patellas' requires an external rotation osteotomy of the femur and an internal rotation osteotomy of the tibia. This combination of complex procedures is rarely indicated in the otherwise normal child. A small number of patients with neuromuscular disease such as hemiplegia can occasionally benefit from the combined procedure.

CORONAL PLANE DEFORMITIES

Coronal plane angular deformities in the lower limbs are common in normal children. There is a normal sequence of maturation in which infants and toddlers start life with bowed legs, have a short period in which the legs are straight before they become knock kneed between 3–8 years of age. They then straighten up to the normal adult configuration with straight lower limbs. It is very important therefore to realise that it is unusual for toddlers and children to have absolutely straight legs: mild bowing in the toddler and mild knock knee in the child is normal. Of every

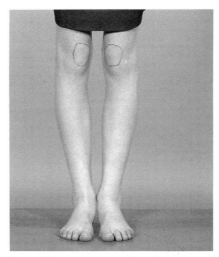

Figure 14.4 This girl has medial femoral torsion and lateral tibial torsion. She has a neutral foot progression angle, but with her feet pointing forwards her patellas face inwards (i.e. squinting patellas).

100 children who attend orthopaedic clinics with bow legs or knock knees perhaps two have a definable disease causing the deformity and probably only one requires operative correction.

Bow Legs

When the toddler first begins to walk bowing is common. It is frequently accompanied by some degree of internal tibial torsion, and the one deformity accentuates the other (*Figure 14.5*). Bowing seems to be pronounced in overweight children.

Physiological bowing is characterized by being symmetrical, not excessively severe, and improving with time. Measurement of the distance between the knees in the standing child provides a simple means of follow-up to assess whether the condition is improving or not. Often this is all that parents wish for reassurance. Many of these children used to be managed in night splints, but this treatment has now been abandoned with the recognition that it does not influence the natural resolution of the condition.

Pathological bowing may be asymmetrical, is often more severe, and deteriorates with time. Causes of pathological bowing include Blount disease, rickets, trauma and skeletal dysplasia.

Radiology

Radiological examination should be reserved for children who appear to be outside the normal range

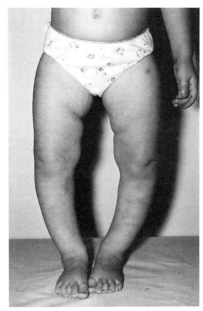

Figure 14.5 A toddler with symmetrical bowing and mild internal tibial torsion.

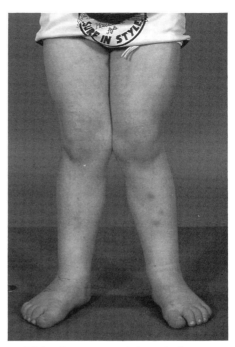

Figure 14.6 Symmetrical knock knees in a four-year-old child.

or in whom there are reasonable grounds to suspect a specific pathology, for example if:

● The deformity is unilateral or asymmetrical.
● The child has short stature and may have a syndrome.
● The child is over 3 years of age.

The radiograph should be a standing anteroposterior view of the lower limbs, which is not easy to obtain in the younger child. The metaphyseal–diaphyseal angle is a useful means for differentiating between physiological and pathological bowing. More than 11° indicates pathological bowing such as Blount disease (Chapter 20).

Knock Knees

Physiological genu valgum or knock knee deformity is common in children aged 3–8 years (*Figure 14.6*). The majority of children straighten spontaneously. The deformity is symmetrical, not excessive and improves with time.

Pathological genu valgum is usually more severe, asymmetrical and increases with time (*Figure 14.7*). Causes include trauma (proximal metaphyseal greenstick fracture of the tibia or growth plate injury), rickets, skeletal dysplasias and congenital limb deficiencies.

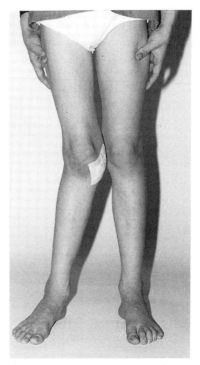

Figure 14.7 Asymmetrical genu valgum as a result of trauma (proximal medial greenstick fracture of the tibia). Staples have been inserted across the proximal medial tibial physis.

Management

There is no evidence that the natural history of the condition is affected by exercises, shoe inserts or night splints.

A small number of children with physiological genu valgum do not correct completely. The reasons to consider surgery are discomfort from 'knee-swishing' while running, concern about the appearance, and progression of the deformity in pathological cases. In order to assess the degree and site of deformity a standing radiograph of the lower limb should be obtained.

Correction can be achieved by restricting growth in the distal femoral or proximal tibial growth plates on the medial side of the knee. This may be accomplished by hemiepiphyseal stapling or by a hemiepiphyseodesis using the Phemister technique. The timing of this procedure is crucial and depends principally on the degree of deformity and bone age of the child (*Figure 14.8*). There are some published guidelines to help in timing and whether to do distal femur, upper tibia or both. However, these should not be considered as precise or foolproof. Careful follow-up is required to avoid undercorrection or overcorrection, and stapling has the advantage that the staples can be removed to allow further growth to take place at the medial physis.

When the growth plates are fused, an osteotomy of the distal femur or proximal tibia is required.

Flat Feet

Almost all infants have flat feet and in the majority an arch will develop by the age of six years. The clinical findings of a flexible flat foot include absence of the medial longitudinal arch and a variable degree of hind foot valgus. When the child stands at ease the only supports to the medial arch are the interosseus ligaments and intrinsic muscles of the foot, which are not continuously active. When the child stands on tip toe, the long flexor and extensor muscles are recruited into continuous activity. In the correctable flat foot the medial longitudinal arch usually appears and the heel tilts into neutral or varus. This 'tip-toe test' can be used to explain the nature of the condition to parents and to reassure them that the internal structure of the foot is normal. In the flexible flat foot the medial arch is also reformed on weight-bearing when the hallux is passively dorsiflexed. This is referred to as the 'toe-raising test of Jack.'

Pathological causes of flat foot include hypermobility syndromes and cerebral palsy (see Chapter 8). These usually present later and are stiff and painful. There is also a phenomenon of 'valgus ex-equino' in which attempted dorsiflexion of the foot against a slightly tight tendo Achillis results in a plano valgus deformity of the foot. The range of dorsiflexion of the foot should therefore be checked with the heel held in neutral or slight varus.

Management

Most of the enthusiasm for treating flat foot has probably been based on the observation that using any of the popular forms of treatment the majority of children are noted to get better.

Orthotics

There have been few studies in which treatment options have been compared and almost none in which a control group has been included. The recent study by Wenger *et al.* (1989) is therefore of great importance in defining the natural history of flat foot and the influence of treatment. In a prospective study, children who were aged 1–6 years and who presented with flexible flat feet were randomized to one of the following four treatment groups:

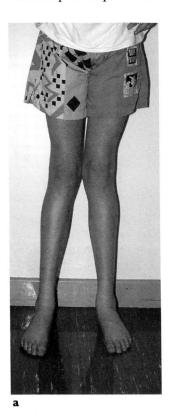
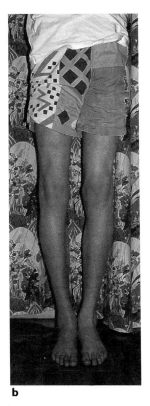

a   b

Figure 14.8 a A 14-year-old boy who presented with genu valgum. **b** The medial distal femoral and proximal tibial growth plates were stapled and overcorrected to mild varus.

- Control group in ordinary shoes.
- Corrective shoes.
- Shoe plus Helfet heel cup.
- Shoe plus University of California Biomechanics Laboratory (UCBL) insert.

Photographs and standing radiographs were taken every six months and the majority of patients were followed for 4–5 years. The results showed that in each of the four groups the radiological parameters of flat foot improved. There was no significant difference between the three 'treatment groups' and the control group. The conclusion from this study is that there is a natural tendency for the physiological flexible flat foot to improve with growth and development and that this is not influenced by the most popular forms of treatment.

Although shoe modifications and inserts do not change the shape of the foot in the long term, there is some evidence that orthotics may prolong the life of the shoe by decreasing deformation and wear. If excessive shoe wear and cost of replacements are important to the parents or pain is a problem, the Helfet or UCBL heel cup or a simple medial arch support may be helpful.

Surgery

Surgery is very rarely required for children with a normal flexible flat foot and the results are frequently indifferent.

In the child over 12 years of age who has a significant deformity and pain not improved by orthotics there may be an indication for surgery. If the valgus heel is the more important deformity, a calcaneal osteotomy should be performed. If on a weight-bearing lateral radiograph of the foot the abnormality is at the navicular–medial cuneiform joint, a Miller procedure can be considered. This involves arthrodesis of the navicular–medial cuneiform joint with advancement of tibialis posterior on an osteoperiosteal flap. It is sometimes necessary to add an arthrodesis of the medial cuneiform–first metatarsal joint.

TOE WALKING

When children are learning to walk, a short period of intermittent toe walking is common. It is then followed by a period of 'flat foot' strike before the gait matures to the adult pattern in which a heel strike is normal. In some children the period of toe walking is prolonged and pronounced, causing parental concern and referral to the orthopaedic surgeon.

Differential Diagnosis

The majority of these children are otherwise normal and are then diagnosed as 'idiopathic toe walkers.' Pathological causes of 'toe walking' are diplegic cerebral palsy, Duchenne muscular dystrophy, the hereditary motor and sensory neuropathies, and spinal dysraphism. Unilateral toe walking is almost always pathological and the most common causes are hemiplegic cerebral palsy and unilateral developmental dysplasia of the hip.

Laboratory Investigations

Idiopathic toe walking is a diagnosis of exclusion, and the history and examination should be considered carefully to decide whether to investigate for a pathological cause. Investigation should be directed by any concerns raised by the examination. In the standard case it is wise to test creatinine phosphokinase for muscular dystrophy and to obtain a radiograph of the spine to exclude spinal dysraphism before any surgery. A neurological opinion may be sought.

Recent studies have shown some abnormal findings in muscle biopsies in idiopathic toe walkers and in some of these children there may be a subtle myopathic process.

Management

Management is by observation, casting, splinting or surgery. If the pattern of toe walking is mild and intermittent, observation until resolution may suffice. If the pattern persists, casting or ankle–foot orthoses may help. If the gait pattern persists or there is a significant calf contracture, surgical lengthening of the tendo Achillis should be considered.

The timing of the various forms of treatment is not easy. Most clinicians would delay any treatment until the age of four years because spontaneous resolution is so common. Many children grow out of the condition by ten years of age, so if surgery is delayed it may prove to be unnecessary. Some children are, however, so severely affected that surgery may be undertaken at a younger age. A surgical approach can be so effective that most parents wonder why the operation was delayed.

GROWING PAINS AND NIGHT CRAMPS

About 15% of children go through a period where they wake up at night crying because of pains in their legs. The child goes to sleep after an energetic day only to awaken in pain and misery, but the following day all is well. Presentation is often delayed until there have been many disturbed nights.

Clinical Features

The child has no day time pain and no limp. The pain at night is relieved by rubbing, heat and simple analgesics. Examination reveals no abnormalities.

Differential Diagnosis

Night pains are a feature of osteoid osteoma, but this is always unilateral and often reasonably well localized. One cause of bilateral leg pains is leukaemia, which can be excluded in most children by a full blood count. There are usually other features in leukaemia or an atypical story, so investigation is not necessary in all children with bilateral nocturnal leg pain.

Management

Taking a full history and carrying out a thorough examination excludes pathological causes and allays parental anxiety. Reassurance is very important, and most parents can accept this. There may be a role for a programme of stretching exercises.

REFERENCES AND FURTHER READING

Baxter A, Dulberg C. Growing pains in children. *J Pediatr Orthop* 1988; **8**: 402–406.

Bowen JR, Leahey JL, Zhang ZH, MacEwen GD. Partial epiphysiodesis at the knee to prevent deformity. *Clin Orthop Rel Research* 1985; **198**: 184–190.

Fraser RK, Menelaus MB, Williams PF, Cole WG. The Miller procedure for flexible flat feet. *J Bone Joint Surg* 1995; **77B**: 396–399.

Griffin PP, Wheelhouse WW, Shiavi R, Bass W. Habitual toe walkers. A clinical and EMG gait analysis. *J Bone Joint Surg* 1977; **59A**: 97–101.

Hensinger RN. *Standards in Pediatric Orthopedics*. Raven Press, New York, 1986.

Kling TF, Hensinger RN. Angular and torsional deformities of the limbs in children. *Clin Orthop Rel Research* 1983; **186**: 136–142.

Pistevos G, Duckworth T. The correction of genu valgum by epiphyseal stapling. *J Bone Joint Surg* 1977; **59B**: 72–76.

Staheli L. Lower positional deformity in infants and children: a review. *J Pediatr Orthop* 1990; **10**: 559–563.

Svenningsen S, Terjesen T, Apalset K, Anda S. Osteotomy for femoral anteversion. *Acta Orthop Scand* 1990; **61**: 360–363.

Wenger D, Maudlin D, Speck G, Morgan D, Leiber R. Corrective shoes and inserts as treatment for flexible flat feet in infants and children. *J Bone Joint Surg* 1989; **71A**: 800–810.

Chapter 15
The Upper Limb

Andrew J Herbert and Nigel S Broughton

UPPER LIMB BIRTH PALSIES

Incidence

Obstetric brachial plexus injuries are the most common type of birth palsy, occurring in about one per 1000 live births. One in ten of these goes on to develop a significant permanent impairment. Although improved obstetric technique would have been expected to reduce this number, this has not been demonstrated. High birth-weight, prolonged labour, breech position, and shoulder dystocia are recognized risk factors.

Aetiology

Excessive lateral flexion of the head on the trunk during delivery of the shoulders (vertex presentation) or delivery of the head (breech presentation) results in a traction injury to one or more components of the brachial plexus. Forceps may contuse the brachial plexus directly and the problem is also seen after delivery by caesarean section.

Pathology

Most nerve disruptions occur at the level of the neural foramen or the groove of the transverse process. The effect ranges in severity according to the force applied and the level injured. The lower plexus is injured with about half the force required to damage the upper plexus. This has been attributed to the protective role of the surrounding soft tissue in upper plexus injuries. Changes can be:

- Mild with perineural oedema and haemorrhage. Cicatricial fibrosis may slow what is usually a rapid and complete recovery.
- Moderate if some nerve fibres are ruptured. Intraneural and extraneural bleeding may occur and recovery is slow and incomplete.

- Severe with avulsion of the trunks from the plexus or the roots from the spinal cord. This carries the worst prognosis, but there have been reports of recovery from even this type of injury.

Incomplete recovery may result in muscle contractures and secondary skeletal changes. The most common residual deformity is that of medial rotation and adduction contracture of the shoulder associated with contracture of the pectoralis major, subscapularis, teres major and short head of biceps (*Figure 15.1*). Severely affected children demonstrate posterior subluxation or dislocation of the glenohumeral joint, flattening of the humeral head and retroversion of the humeral neck. The glenoid fossa is shallow and the scapula high.

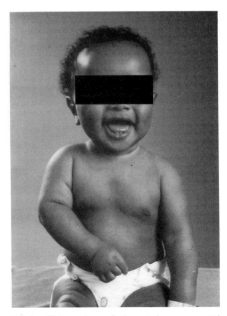

Figure 15.1 Erb palsy of the right arm with medial rotation of the arm and adduction contracture. Flexion deformity of the elbow is common.

Classification

Upper root injury (C5 and C6)
Also known as Erb–Duchenne paralysis, this is the most common upper limb birth palsy. The deltoid, lateral rotators of the shoulder, biceps, brachialis, supinator and brachioradialis are involved, so the shoulder is held adducted and internally rotated. A fixed flexion deformity of the wrist and pronation contracture of the forearm contribute to the porter's tip posture these babies develop. Sensory loss is mild if present. A flexion deformity of the elbow often develops later in childhood.

Complete injury
Complete injury is the second most common form of upper limb birth palsy and results in flaccid paralysis of the entire upper limb. Vasomotor abnormality may give a marbled appearance and the hand is often clutched.

Lower root injury (C8 and T1)
Also known as Klumpke paralysis, this is the least common form of upper limb birth palsy. It affects the wrist flexors, long finger flexors and intrinsic muscles of the hand. Hand function is poor and the hand is held with the fingers flexed, but shoulder and elbow function is good.

Diagnosis

An absence of active movement is noticed in the affected upper limb of the newborn child despite the presence of a full range of passive movement. The Moro reflex is absent in the affected limb. The grasp reflex may also be absent in the lower and complete types of injury. Injury to the cervical sympathetic fibres at the T1 level is often present in the complete injury, causing a Horner syndrome (ipsilateral enophthalmos, miosis and ptosis), which is a bad prognostic sign. Phrenic nerve palsy can occur and is recognized by a raised hemidiaphragm on the chest radiograph. Haematomyelia associated with nerve root avulsion causes spasticity of the other limbs if it occurs and should be differentiated from cerebral palsy.

Differential Diagnosis

Pseudoparalysis of the upper limb may be present in the newborn for the following reasons.

Delivery fractures
An isolated fracture of the clavicle is common and may present at birth or at about two weeks of age when the fracture callus presents as a mass. Approximately 5% of clavicular fractures are associated with an obstetrical palsy. Treatment other than careful handling is unnecessary. A mid-shaft humeral fracture should be treated by bandaging to the body for two weeks. Dislocation of the shoulder or elbow at delivery is extremely rare, but often radiographs suggest this diagnosis because of a disruption through the growth plate before the upper or lower epiphyses of the humerus have started to ossify. Arthrography or ultrasound can confirm the diagnosis. Reduction of the upper humeral epiphyseal injury is unnecessary, but a displaced distal humeral epiphyseal injury should be reduced.

Osteomyelitis and septic arthritis of the shoulder
These conditions are also seen in the neonatal intensive care unit and present with pseudoparalysis. Unusual organisms may be the cause in this setting, for example, *Escherichia coli* or group B beta haemolytic streptococci, and their management is discussed in Chapter 11.

Arthrogryposis
This may present with poor movement of the arm due to the contractures about the shoulder.

Management

Most upper limb birth palsies recover in the first three months of life. A full range of joint movement is obtained 3–4 times a day to prevent muscle contractures. Complications associated with abduction–external rotation splints have resulted in a decline in their use. Supination splints may be used at night to prevent pronation contractures of the forearm while recovery is progressing.

Surgical exploration of the brachial plexus
Recently there has been great interest in the early surgical exploration of these injuries. Spontaneous recovery will usually begin within three months of injury, therefore surgery is not indicated before this. Early return of biceps function is considered a good prognostic sign. Electromyography (EMG) is poorly tolerated, but may indicate a return of function one month before there is any clinical evidence of this. The goals of surgery are to restore the best possible function, and the family must understand that this may not represent normal function. If there is no sign of any improvement clinically or by EMG by the age of three months surgical exploration is recommended.

The plexus is exposed by a supraclavicular approach. The pathology is a mixture of nerve root avulsions and total ruptures: injuries are usually avulsions to the lower roots and ruptures to the upper roots.

- Nerve reconstruction (grafting or repair): any neuroma is resected back to healthy nerve tissue and the gap grafted by a harvested sural nerve. Grafting of upper root lesions results in nearly normal shoulder function in over 50% of cases.
- Neurotization is used for nerve root avulsion. For example, an intercostal nerve may be re-routed to take over the function of the musculocutaneous nerve providing reinnervation of the biceps. The C7 root may be linked to the upper trunk. Children seem to adapt well to these neurotizations, though individual cases present different dilemmas and solutions.

The results of grafting for upper root lesions have been encouraging, but restoration of hand function when the lesions are complete has been less successful. However any improvement in hand function in these circumstances is worthwhile.

Management of late deformity

Late deformity at the shoulder as a result of muscle contractures results in fixed internal rotation deformity and restricted abduction. This restricts any hand function the child may have. The internal rotation contracture results in poor glenoid development and posterior dislocation of the humeral head. Surgical options to improve the restricted movement include the following.

- Sever release to release or lengthen pectoralis major and subscapularis. This improves the range of lateral rotation and abduction and allows the weakened muscles producing this movement to work more effectively.
- Open reduction of the dislocated humeral head. The release can be combined with reduction of the dislocated humeral head and held reduced by a temporary K wire and shoulder spica. It should be performed in the first year or two of life.
- External rotation osteotomy of the upper humerus to improve lateral rotation. This ignores any upper humeral abnormality and is best carried out at about the age of six years.
- L'Episcopo procedure, in which the transfer of teres major to a lateral position together with latissimus dorsi improves lateral rotation and abduction power.

The external rotation osteotomy of the upper humerus at about the age of six years was commonly carried out in our institute. However, we now recognize that there is an approximately 40% incidence of posterior dislocation of the shoulder as a consequence of the internal rotation contracture and so now perform more open reductions at an early stage. Early release of the contractures has reduced the need for muscle transfer and there seem to be few problems from late internal rotation deformities (Dr IP Torode).

Fixed flexion deformity of the elbow may compensate for residual deformity at the shoulder, so careful judgement is needed when considering any correction of elbow deformity. Surgical correction is by lengthening of the brachialis and biceps.

A fixed pronation deformity of the forearm is corrected by pronator teres tendon lengthening, but if the deformity is not responsive to soft-tissue surgery, osteoclasis of the radius may be required. A supination deformity of the forearm is treated by a distal release of the biceps and reattachment to the tendon of brachioradialis with an extensive release of the interosseous membrane.

The Green transfer re-routing flexor carpi ulnaris to extensor carpi radialis longus may have some application in the management of wrist flexion deformity. However, the effect of tendon operations and transfers on improving hand function in these children has proved disappointing.

CONGENITAL PSEUDARTHROSIS OF THE CLAVICLE

Congenital pseudarthrosis of the clavicle is a rare condition that presents at birth as a non-tender swelling in the middle of the clavicle. Although it has been stated in the past that these are all right-sided except when bilateral or in the presence of dextrocardia, doubts have recently been raised about this.

Aetiology

The clavicle normally has a medial and a lateral ossification centre. Congenital pseudarthrosis of the clavicle is probably a consequence of their failure to fuse. The pulsation of an abnormally high subclavian artery has been suggested as a cause.

Differential Diagnosis

Trauma at this age is usually associated with massive callus formation and a history of pseudoparalysis of

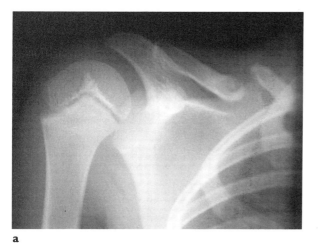

a

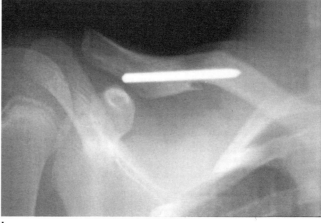

b

Figure 15.2   a Pseudarthrosis of the clavicle.   **b** Pseudarthrosis of the clavicle following internal fixation with an intramedullary wire.

the involved upper limb. Non-union is usually atrophic. Cleidocranial dysostosis is bilateral and associated with other skeletal abnormalities and there is no palpable lump on the clavicle.

Management

The condition is painless and produces little functional abnormality, but presents because of parental concerns about the unsightly lump. Excision of the pseudarthrosis, curettage of the bone ends, and intramedullary fixation are recommended. Autogenous bone grafting may be required. Surgery is usually advised by four years of age, but early surgery, at about one year of age, may improve the final appearance (*Figure 15.2*).

SPRENGEL SHOULDER

Sprengel shoulder is a condition characterized by congenital elevation of the scapula. It is more common in girls and in the left shoulder (*Figure 15.3*).

Aetiology

The condition usually occurs sporadically but can be transmitted as an autosomal dominant trait.

The upper pole of the scapula appears adjacent to the fifth cervical vertebra during the fifth week of embryonic development. It is small and has an increased width to height ratio compared with the adult. It normally descends to the adult position by the third fetal month. However, in Sprengel shoulder

the embryological state persists and the scapula fails to descend. An omovertebral bone is frequently present connecting the vertebral border of the scapula to the adjacent laminae or spinous processes. The supraspinatus portion of the scapula is curved forwards around the upper thorax. The pectoral girdle is usually hypoplastic, with trapezius being the most severely affected.

Sprengel shoulder is associated with spinal deformities such as scoliosis, kyphosis and diastematomyelia. The Klippel–Feil syndrome is a congenital fusion of two or more cervical vertebrae and is often associated with bilateral Sprengel shoulder. A low

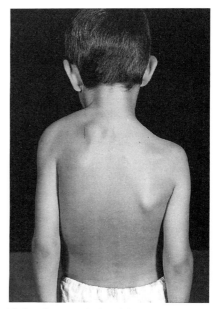

Figure 15.3   Sprengel shoulder.

hairline and associated webbing of the neck give the characteristic 'no neck' appearance.

Clinical Features

Sprengel shoulder usually presents at birth with asymmetry of the shoulders. However, there is a range of severity and milder cases may present at a later stage. Combined abduction is limited due to decreased scapulothoracic motion.

Radiology

Anteroposterior radiographs that include both shoulders on the same film in active and passive abduction demonstrate the fixed position of the scapula, which is obvious clinically. A plain radiograph of the cervical spine will show any associated anomalies, and a lateral oblique radiograph may demonstrate an omovertebral bone.

Management

The best results of surgery are seen in children who are operated on when less than eight years of age, but intervention as early as 6–9 months of age is recommended by some authors.

Surgical correction may be considered to improve the cosmetic appearance, but shoulder function is unlikely to be improved by any of the available procedures. After discussion many of the mild cases are observed and surgery is unnecessary.

Resection of the upper pole of the scapula and the omovertebral body

This improves the cosmetic appearance, but does not alter the position of the scapula.

The Woodward procedure

The trapezius and rhomboids are detached from their origin on the spinous processes of the vertebrae through a long midline approach. The omovertebral bar is excised. The scapula can then be everted, and serratus anterior and subscapularis detached from their vertebral and deep surfaces. Supraspinatus is elevated, and the supraspinous portion of the scapula is excised. The scapula is then held in its corrected position and the muscles are reattached to the scapula and to the spinous processes to maintain this position. Excessive correction may result in brachial plexus lesions, but this type of approach is often advocated for the more severe deformity.

The Green procedure

This is a similar muscle release procedure to that of the Woodward procedure, but a clavicular osteotomy is performed first to bring the point of the shoulder down. Trapezius, levator scapula and the rhomboids are detached from the scapula rather than from their spinal origin. The omovertebral bar and the part of the scapula above the scapular spine are excised. The muscles are reattached in the corrected position.

Scapular osteotomy

This is carried out in a vertical direction 2 cm from the vertebral border. The main part of the scapula is rotated down and reattached through drill holes.

DISLOCATION OF THE SHOULDER

Congenital Dislocation of the Shoulder

This is exceptionally rare and usually associated with other abnormalities of the upper limb and glenoid hypoplasia. There is a global instability and no pain. Function is surprisingly good and unlikely to be improved by surgery.

Congenital Glenoid Hypoplasia

This is rare and usually presents in late childhood with a posterior dislocation of the shoulder. It may be associated with other congenital abnormalities such as Apert syndrome or Hurler syndrome.

Traumatic Dislocation of the Shoulder

This is uncommon in the under-16 year age group. It is usually anterior and almost always progresses to recurrent dislocation.

Habitual Dislocation

This is seen in conditions with ligamentous laxity such as osteogenesis imperfecta, Larsen syndrome and Ehlers–Danlos syndrome. It may present in a child under two years of age with parents concerned about the clunking they experience when dressing the child. It is also seen in Down syndrome. Treatment is

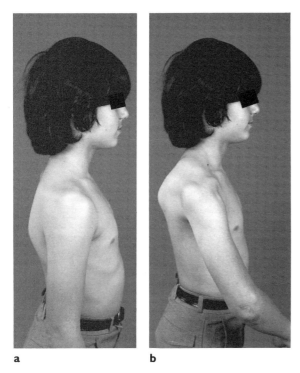

a   b

Figure 15.4 a Voluntary dislocation of the right shoulder in a boy: normal position. **b** After posterior dislocation. The humeral head is easily seen as a prominence posteriorly.

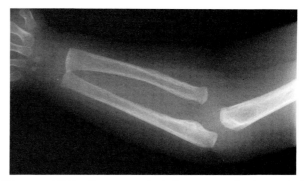

Figure 15.5 Congenital dislocation of the radial head. If a line is drawn along the axis of the radius it does not pass through the capitellum, but passes anteriorly.

difficult. Often there is little functional impairment, and surgery is unnecessary, but anterior and posterior capsular reefing has been tried.

Voluntary Dislocation

This is seen in adolescents particularly in girls (*Figure 15.4*). It may be performed as a 'party trick' or as a mechanism to attract attention or avoid situations. Patients should be discouraged from performing the manoeuvre. Surgery is likely to fail. The best approach to treatment is a combination of muscle retraining and psychological help.

DISLOCATION OF THE RADIAL HEAD

Classification

Differentiation between congenital and acquired dislocation of the radial head (see below) is often difficult. The radial head in the congenital form is

dome-shaped rather than having the normal central depression and there are capitellar abnormalities.

Congenital dislocation of the radial head
This is rare. The dislocation may be anterior or posterior and less commonly lateral (*Figure 15.5*). It is often bilateral.

Acquired dislocatioin of the radial head
This is most often seen after an unrecognized Monteggia fracture (see Chapter 22).

Skeletal dysplasias
Skeletal dysplasias such as nail–patella and Klinefelter syndrome can present with a dislocation of the radial head, which may also occur if the ulna is relatively short, as in hereditary multiple exostoses.

Clinical Features

The elbow is usually asymptomatic and the abnormality is often identified following some minor injury to the elbow. There may be limited flexion (anterior dislocation) or extension (posterior dislocation), and the affected radial head can be palpated. In the congenital or skeletal dysplasia type there is usually little pain or loss of function. Pain may develop in the adult as a result of degenerative change.

Radiology

A line drawn along the long axis of the proximal radius fails to bisect the capitellum in all planes. The ulna bows in a direction opposite to that of the dislocation.

Management

Surgery for the acquired case is discussed in Chapter 22. Surgical correction for most congenital cases is probably not necessary as there is little to be gained in terms of pain or improvement in function. Some units perform open reductions with reconstruction of the annular ligament from triceps with a temporary wire fixation of the radial head to the capitellum and ulnar osteotomy. However, this commonly fails and we feel that surgery should not be carried out in childhood; the radial head can be excised after skeletal maturity to improve the appearance and relieve pain, which may develop at this time.

RADIO-ULNAR SYNOSTOSIS

Congenital radio-ulnar synostosis is often bilateral and inherited as an autosomal dominant trait. It is thought that the cartilaginous rods that are the precursors of the radius and ulnar either fail to separate at their proximal ends or the intervening mesenchymal tissue ossifies (*Figure 15.6*). The distal ends are nearly always separate.

Clinical Features

The forearm is fixed in varying degrees of pronation, or less commonly, supination. There may be difficulty turning door knobs, buttoning shirts and using eating utensils. There are greater difficulties if there is hyperpronation of the forearm and the condition is bilateral. However, some go unnoticed because of compensatory movements at the glenohumeral joint and the wrist. One of our surgical colleagues has bilateral radio-ulnar synostoses: he noticed difficulties in the use of a screwdriver during his orthopaedic training, but otherwise has little functional deficiency.

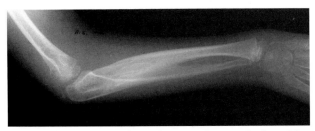

Figure 15.6 Synostosis of the radius and ulna. The amount of synostosis is often not as extensive as in this impressive example.

Management

The results of operations to excise the synostosis and regain supination have been poor and associated with a high rate of recurrence. Fortunately most are fixed in a slight pronation position, which is functional for writing and keyboard use, but may be difficult for receiving coins. If the deformity is in an unacceptable position this may be improved by osteotomy of the proximal one-third of the radius and ulna.

Acquired Radio-Ulnar Synostosis

This is seen occasionally after severe trauma to the proximal forearm, sometimes with a compartment syndrome. Excision of the synostosis with postoperative continuous passive movement machines and non-steroidal anti-inflammatory drugs to prevent recurrence of the heterotopic ossification has been tried, but the results are poor. Radiotherapy should not be used in the growing child.

RADIAL CLUB HAND

Radial club hand is a preaxial deficiency of the forearm. There is a congenital longitudinal deficiency of the radius and the thumb is usually absent (*Figure 15.7*).

Incidence

The incidence of radial clubhand is approximately 1 in 100,000 live births. Approximately 50% of the cases are bilateral, and when unilateral the right side is affected twice as often as the left. It is usually sporadic.

About 50% occur in association with various syndromes, for example:

- Thrombocytopenia absent radius (TAR) syndrome. The thumb is present and almost normal.
- Fanconi syndrome. There is a pancytopenia and the radius is absent.
- Holt–Oram syndrome. There is an atrial septal defect associated with the absent radius. This can be transmitted as an autosomal dominant trait.
- Vater syndrome. There are vertebral, anal, tracheo-oesophageal, renal and radial abnormalities.

Many other associations have been described.

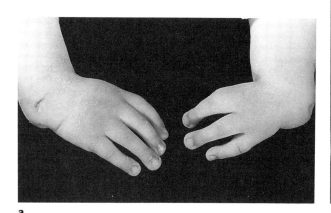
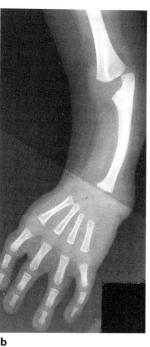

a   b

Figure 15.7 a Bilateral radial club hands. **b** Radiological appearance of radial club hand.

Pathology

Structures along the preaxial border of the forearm are most severely affected. The radius may be hypoplastic, partially absent at its distal end, or completely absent. The ulna is shortened by one-third to one-half and bowed, with its concavity towards the radius. The carpus is connected to the distal ulna by either fibrous tissue or a small synovial joint and is deviated in a radial and volar direction. This progresses with growth. There are also abnormalities of the finger joints, which are most marked in the radial digits and muscle deficiencies on the radial side of the forearm. The median nerve is thickened because it carries the sensory fibres normally found in the radial nerve. It is located deep to the deep fascia on the most radial side of the wrist and is therefore at risk from the surgeon's knife.

Clinical Features

One or both forearms are short with radially-deviated wrists at birth. The ulnar styloid is prominent, and there is an extension contracture of the elbow in about 25% of cases. Radial deviation at the wrist may allow satisfactory hand-to-mouth function. Any treatment must ensure that this important function is maintained.

Management

The objective of treatment is to improve appearance and retain function. Treatment is started as early as possible by passive stretching of the preaxial soft tissues while systemic disorders are sought and treated.

Operative treatment is performed between the ages of six months and three years. By soft-tissue release the carpus is centralized and secured to the distal end of the ulna. Tendon transfers may be used to help prevent postoperative recurrence of deformity. Other centres advocate radialization or overcorrection of the deformity in order to place the ulna where the radius would normally be (Buck–Gramcko procedure). It is claimed that this provides a better balance between the opposing forces of radial and ulnar deviation and recurrence is less likely. Correction is maintained using moulded splints until distal ulna hypertrophy is seen. Some centres have reported success using the Ilizarov principles of gradual correction of the deformity and staged lengthening of the bone.

Pollicisation of the index finger is usually indicated before the age of two years. An active long flexor tendon to the index finger is a prerequisite.

Arthrodesis is a salvage procedure for the skeletally-mature patient with recurrence. The late-presenting child should be examined very carefully because functional patterns developed over the years may be destroyed by attempts at arthrodesis.

MADELUNG DEFORMITY

Madelung deformity is a result of premature fusion of the volar and ulnar aspects of the distal radial growth plate. It presents after eight years of age with a volar and ulnar angulation of the distal radius. The ulna continues growing straight in its normal way and becomes prominent (*Figure 15.8*). Wrist dorsiflexion, ulna deviation and supination are reduced. Pain develops slowly in severe deformity as the carpus impinges on the distal ulna.

Aetiology

Madelung deformity is inherited as an autosomal dominant trait with incomplete penetrance. Females are more commonly affected than males, and the condition is frequently bilateral. It is also associated with various syndromes including dyschondrosteosis (Leri–Weill disease) and Turner syndrome. A similar picture can be seen after trauma or infection.

Radiology

Radiographs demonstrate dorsoradial bowing of the distal radius and volar–ulnar tilt of the distal radial

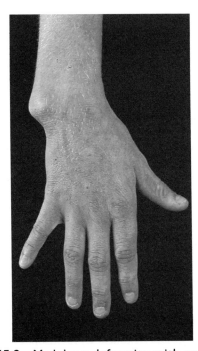

Figure 15.8 Madelung deformity with prominence of the distal ulna and volar ulnar deviation of the distal radial articular surface.

articular surface. The proximal carpal row becomes wedge-shaped with the lunate at its apex. This 'falls into' and then becomes wedged in the widened interosseous space between the radius and the ulna. The carpus is shifted to the ulna and volar side of the wrist.

Management

The severity of the deformity is variable and many children function well with few concerns about the appearance. Surgical options include the following and are often used in combination.

- Epiphyseolysis of the fused growth plate and interposition with a fat graft. Good results have been described by Vickers (1980).
- Complete epiphyseodesis of the distal radial growth plate to prevent progression of the deformity.
- Osteotomy of the distal radius to correct the volar and ulnar tilt by opening wedge with bone graft interposition.
- Epiphyseodesis of the distal ulna growth plate to prevent overgrowth of the ulna.
- Shortening of the ulnar by excision of a section at the distal end of the diaphysis.
- Excision of the distal ulna (Darrach procedure) after maturity for prominence of the ulna or pain from carpal impingement.
- Wrist arthrodesis for pain and instability in the skeletally mature.

We would fuse the radial growth plate if still open and correct the deformity with an osteotomy. At the same time the distal ulna growth plate is fused if still open and the ulna is shortened if unduly long.

TRIGGER THUMB

The trigger thumb of childhood presents with the interphalangeal joint of the thumb locked in flexion, and the snapping or triggering seen in adults is unusual. There is always doubt as to when the deformity developed and whether it was present at birth. The true congenital trigger thumb presenting at birth is bilateral in 50% of cases and resolves in 35% of cases. The more common type presents between 6–30 months of age, is bilateral in 25% and resolves in 12% (Dinham and Meggitt, 1974).

Trigger thumb is due to a constriction in the sheath of flexor pollicis longus at the A1 pulley. The tendon develops a nodule, which cannot enter the pulley, and so the thumb is locked in flexion.

202 Paediatric Orthopaedics

Clinical Features

The parents bring the child to see the surgeon because the thumb is locked in flexion at the interphalangeal joint. A non-tender nodule on flexor pollicis longus is palpable on the volar aspect of the metacarpophalangeal joint of the thumb. Trigger thumb is often misdiagnosed by referring doctors as a dislocated thumb, and there may have been attempts to 'reduce it.'

Management

Surgery is deferred in the first year of life because the condition may resolve. Fixed deformity may develop if correction is delayed until after four years of age. A transverse incision is made at the flexion crease of the metacarpophalangeal joint, the digital nerve is pushed to one side, and the stenosed tendon sheath is released. Recurrence is unlikely.

CAMPTODACTYLY

Camptodactyly is a flexion deformity of the proximal interphalangeal joint of a finger, and most commonly affects the little finger. There is an infantile type and an adolescent type, which occurs at 12–14 years of age. The latter is more common in females, and deformity increases during the adolescent growth spurt. It is familial and often bilateral. Radiographs show that the base of the middle phalanx has subluxed volar to the head of the proximal phalanx, which is flattened.

Aetiology

The deformity has been attributed to the following abnormalities: flexor and extensor tendon imbalance, ischaemic fibrosis or abnormal insertion of the intrinsic muscles of the hand, and contracture of the collateral ligaments of the digits. Malformation syndromes are frequently associated with this deformity.

Management

Mild cases require no treatment. If progression is expected a night splint can be tried. In severe cases surgery should be performed at a young age. Flexor digitorum sublimis is lengthened if there are no bony changes. When bone remodelling has occurred the position of the range of movement can be altered by extension osteotomy of the proximal phalanx.

CLINODACTYLY

Clinodactyly is a bowing deformity of the little finger. It is common and is an autosomal dominant trait. There is an increased incidence in Down syndrome. The problem is cosmetic. Surgery is only indicated if the little finger overlaps the ring finger on forming a fist, and a closing wedge osteotomy of the phalanx proximal to the affected joint is then performed.

KIRNER DEFORMITY

Kirner deformity refers to a volar–radial deviation of the distal phalanx of the little finger, which is inherited as an autosomal dominant trait.

The deformity becomes clinically apparent at about ten years of age. It is almost always bilateral. The differential diagnosis includes frostbite, which can damage the distal phalanx growth plate. Surgery is generally for cosmetic reasons only.

REFERENCES AND FURTHER READING

Buck–Gramcko D. Radialisation as a new treatment for radial club hand. *J Hand Surg* 1985; **10A**: 964–968

Carson WG, Lovell WW, Whitesides TE. Congenital elevation of the scapula. *J Bone Joint Surg* 1981; **63A**: 1199–1207.

Cavendish ME. Congenital elevation of the scapula. *J Bone Joint Surg* 1972; **54B**: 395–408.

Dinham JM, Meggitt BF. Trigger thumbs in children. A review of the natural history and indications for treatment in 105 patients. *J Bone Joint Surg* 1974; **56B**: 153–155.

Gibson DA, Carroll N. Congenital pseudarthrosis of the clavicle. *J Bone Joint Surg* 1970; **52B**: 629–640.

Hardy AE. Birth injuries of the brachial plexus: incidence and prognosis. *J Bone Joint Surg* 1978; **60A**: 691–695.

Hentz VR, Meyer RD. Brachial plexus microsurgery in children (review). *Microsurgery* 1991; **12**: 175–185.

Lamb DW. Radial club hand, a continuing study of eighty six patients with one hundred and seventeen club hands. *J Bone Joint Surg* 1977; **59A**: 1–13.

Lloyd-Roberts GC, Apley AG, Owen R. Reflections upon the aetiology of congenital pseudarthrosis of the clavicle. *J Bone Joint Surg* 1975; **57B**: 24–29.

Vickers DW. Premature incomplete fusion of the growth plate: causes and treatment by resection (physiolysis) in fifteen cases. *Aust NZ J Surg* 1980; **50**: 393.

Chapter 16
Developmental Dysplasia of the Hip

Nigel S Broughton

Developmental dysplasia of the hip (DDH) is the term now used for what used to be called congenital dislocation of the hip. The name change recognizes that not all cases are present or detectable at birth, but some develop over the first few months of life. It also recognizes that there is a spectrum of the disorder ranging from hips that are dislocated and cannot be reduced, through hips that are dislocated but can be reduced and hips that can be dislocated but at rest are enlocated to hips which cannot be dislocated, but have some abnormality of development of the acetabulum.

Incidence

The incidence of significant DDH is approximately two per 1000 live births. At birth, the incidence of unstable hips is 5–20 per 1000, but most of these settle and stabilize in the first few weeks of life and would do so even without treatment.

The condition is seven times more common in females than in males, and is more common following a breech presentation, particularly the frank breech presentation with extended knees, by a factor of about 10. Often there is a family history of hip dislocation. It is associated with oligohydramnios and is more common in babies delivered by caesarean section and the first born of the family.

There is a high incidence in certain races. This would appear to be genetic in the northern Italians, but environmental in North American Indians due to the binding of the baby's legs in extension. It has been suggested that DDH is more common where there is ligamentous laxity. This may be a temporary phenomenon after transplacental passage of maternal relaxin.

Table 16.1 Causes of hip dislocation in the child

Developmental dysplasia of the hip
Neurological (e.g. cerebral palsy and spina bifida)
Septic arthritis (Smith arthritis)
Habitual (e.g. Down syndrome) where there is ligamentous laxity
Trauma (unusual)

There is a higher incidence of DDH in children with other congenital deformities such as torticollis, plagiocephaly and foot deformities including metatarsus adductus and calcaneovalgus.

In about 20% of cases it is bilateral, and when unilateral the left hip is affected more often than the right.

Dislocation of the hip is also observed at birth in neuromuscular conditions such as arthrogryposis, and may develop in the early years of life in cerebral palsy and spina bifida. It may also be a result of septic arthritis. All these conditions are dealt with in the respective chapters (*Table 16.1*).

Pathology

Stability of the hip in the newborn depends on the presence of a well-formed acetabulum with a normal labrum and a stable capsule. In DDH there is excessive capsular laxity, a shallow acetabulum and a labrum that is poorly developed and pushed out of the way by the femoral head. It is unclear whether the capsular laxity leads to the shallow acetabulum or whether the shallow acetabulum is primary and allows the development of capsular laxity.

If the hip is not reduced and is allowed to develop in this position, the pressure on the femoral head leads to abnormal growth and excessive femoral anteversion. The acetabulum fails to develop and persists in being dysplastic. Both these are secondary effects and can be reversed if the hip is reduced at an early stage.

In established cases the capsule of the hip becomes plastered across the mouth of the normal acetabulum. An hourglass constriction of the capsule develops and this prevents the hip from being reduced into the normal acetabulum. This hourglass constriction appears to be exacerbated by the psoas tendon, which runs across the front of the capsule at this point. This constriction can be felt in the inferior aspect of the joint from the anterolateral open reduction. The labrum may be inverted into the hip blocking reduction of the femoral head. The ligamentum teres elongates and can become bulky, again preventing reduction of the hip.

The femoral head lies superior to the normal acetabulum and eventually develops a false acetabulum at this point. The superior capsule stretches to accommodate the femoral head.

Diagnosis

Screening

All babies are screened for DDH by clinical examination at birth, but many centres select high-risk groups for screening by ultrasound in an attempt to reduce the number of children who present late. We would advocate ultrasound screening for all breech deliveries, where there is a significant family history and where there are associated congenital abnormalities.

Examination

The hips of all newborn babies should be examined and this examination should be repeated at six weeks and six months as part of the routine examination of the child in the community. The baby must be relaxed and warm and handled gently because crying and wriggling can make it difficult to assess the hip. As always the examination starts by simple observation, looking particularly for asymmetry of the hips with extra skin creases, abnormal posture of the hips, and any apparent shortening of the limb.

Barlow test

In the newborn and in the first few months of life the pelvis is held with a thumb on the pubic symphysis and the fingers on the sacrum. In this way the hand of the examiner cradles the perineum of the baby so that the pelvis can be held firmly but comfortably (*Figure 16.1a*). The examiner's other hand then grips the baby's leg with the knee flexed at 90°, the examining thumb on the medial aspect of the thigh, and the fingers on the lateral aspect of the thigh with the tip of the middle finger on the greater trochanter. In this position with the hip flexed to 90° but in neutral abduction, longitudinal pressure is exerted in an attempt to sublux the femoral head over the posterior acetabular rim. The hip is then abducted and if the hip is unstable and has been subluxed by the longitudinal pressure there is a clunk as the hip re-enters the acetabulum.

The test relies on the presence of a posterior acetabular wall for the femoral head to clunk over; it is exceptionally rare for the acetabular wall to be so poorly developed that this does not occur.

Ortolani test

Ortolani worked in northern Italy in the 1930s and was the first to popularize a test for the early

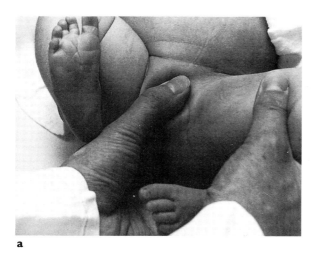

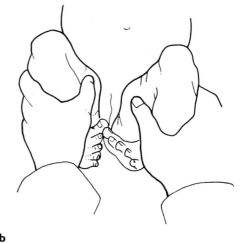

a   b

Figure 16.1 **a** Barlow's test: one hand stabilizes the pelvis and the other abducts the leg. **b** Ortolani's test: the legs are abducted simultaneously. (Reproduced with permission from Williams PF, Cole WG. *Orthopaedic Management in Childhood*. Chapman & Hall, London.)

detection of DDH in children aged 6–12 months of age. In this test both legs are flexed to 90° at the hip and knee, and the knees are grasped with a thumb on the medial aspect and fingers on the lateral aspect. Abduction of both hips is performed at the same time. A positive test is produced when there is a clunk as the dislocated hip reduces. The English translation of Ortolani's original description is a 'jerk of re-entry.' The test is most useful in older children in whom it is difficult to stabilize the pelvis with the examiner's hand (*Figure 16.1b*).

Often the hip does not clunk into place, but there is a click on abducting the hip without any sense of movement. Many of these clicks are benign and may be due to a vacuum effect, rather than hip instability. However, they should be followed up as they are associated with a high incidence of DDH. It is

unclear whether this is because of capsular laxity or misinterpretation of the sign. Any reduction in the range of abduction should be noted because a dislocated hip that cannot be reduced will have restricted abduction in this position.

Radiology

Ultrasound

Ultrasound is useful in the first six months of life when much of the hip anatomy is only a cartilage analogue. It provides a clear indication of the position of the femoral head and the shape of the acetabulum before the upper femoral ossific nucleus forms (usually at the age of three months). A linear probe is used, the baby should be warm and comfor-

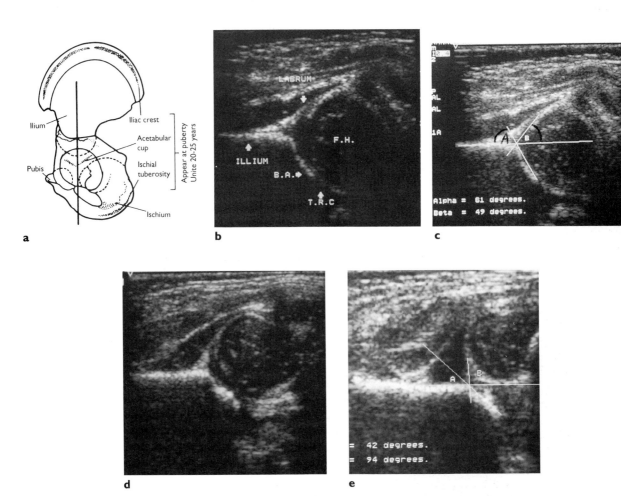

Figure 16.2 a Ultrasound of the hip. The mid-coronal plane of the femoral head and acetabulum. **b** The mid-coronal ultrasound image of the hip (F.H., femoral head; T.R.C., triradiate cartilage; B.A., bony acetabulum). **c** Using lines drawn by the computer, the alpha and beta angles are calculated. **d** Ultrasound of a type 2C hip. The femoral head is poorly covered, the beta angle is more than 77° and the alpha angle less than 45°. **e** Ultrasound of a type 3 hip with alpha angle (A) of 42° and a beta angle (B) of 94°. The femoral head is not covered by any part of the bony acetabulum.

Table 16.2 Graf's classification of ultrasound findings in a child's hip (Graf, 1984)

Type	Alpha angle (°)	Beta angle (°)	Conclusion
I	>60	–	Normal
2A	50–59	–	Under three months of age, physiological immaturity, *head is contained*.
2B	50–59	–	Delayed ossification in a child over three months of age, *head is centered, over 3/12 old*.
2C	43–49	<77	
2D	43–49	>77 (i.e. labrum everted)	
3	<43	>77	Dislocated
4	<43	>77	Dislocated but labrum interposed between the femoral head and acetabulum

table, and warm gel should be used to avoid irritating the baby.

Graf (1984) has developed the use of ultrasound in the management of DDH. The examination starts with a static mid-coronal view of the femoral head and acetabulum (*Figure 16.2*). This equates to the anteroposterior view on a radiograph, but conventionally the straight line of the ilium is placed horizontally on the image. The ilium must be straight on the image so that the scan plane is taken through the centre of the acetabulum. The femoral head can be well seen, together with the bony acetabulum and the cartilaginous labrum. This allows the depth of the bony acetabulum and the cover of the cartilaginous labrum to be calculated by describing the alpha and beta angles according to the technique of Graf (1984). Graf has defined categories using the alpha and beta angles, and decisions for treatment can then be made (*Table 16.2*). In this position the percentage of femoral head cover is also useful.

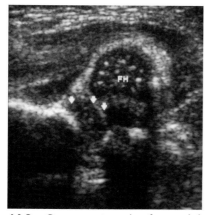

Figure 16.3 On stressing the femoral head in an unstable hip the femoral head becomes visible on this coronal plane ultrasound through the posterior lip of the acetabulum. Arrows indicate posterior hip of acetabulum; F.H., femoral head.

It should always be remembered that the Graf category is a static representation and does not take into account the degree of instability or any movement between the femoral head and acetabulum when the hip is stressed.

The next stage of the examination is to perform a dynamic stress test as described by Harcke *et al.* (1984). With the baby on its side the sonographer positions the probe in a coronal plane on the posterior lip of the acetabulum (*Figure 16.3*). The fingers of the hand holding the probe are placed behind the sacrum to stabilize it. With the hip and knee flexed to 90° the other hand then pushes on the knee posteriorly, and the ultrasound can detect if the femoral head is pushed over the posterior lip of the acetabulum, indicating instability. This has been described as a visual Barlow test.

An axial view of the femoral head and neck can also be obtained and the hip can be stressed to look for any hip instability.

It is important to realise that there is no specific recipe for treatment or non-treatment based on one particular classification. Any decision for treatment is based on the clinical examination of the child together with appraisal of not only the static Graf classification, but also of the static femoral head cover percentage and the dynamic assessment of hip instability. Ultrasound is useful for confirming adequate reduction in an abduction device and also for monitoring the progress of acetabular development during treatment.

Radiographs

A radiograph in the first three months of life is unreliable because of the large amount of cartilage in the femoral head and acetabulum. Even after the age of three months when the ossific nuclei develop, interpretation can be difficult. It is after the age of six

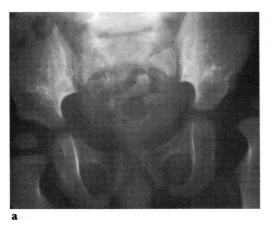
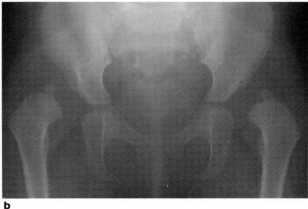

a   b

Figure 16.4 **a** Radiograph showing left-sided unilateral DDH in an 18-month-old child. **b** Radiograph showing bilateral DDH in a 15-month-old child.

months that radiographs are the imaging technique of choice (*Figure 16.4*).

The pelvic radiograph is a static examination, but in the young child allows a useful assessment of the relationship between the metaphysis of the femur and the acetabulum. The pelvis is X-rayed with the legs in neutral. If the ossific nucleus of the femoral head has formed, it should be below a projection of the Hilgenreiner line and the major part medial to the Perkin line, in the inferomedial quadrant. The dislocated hip shows the ossific nucleus in the superolateral quadrant. If there is no ossific nucleus the metaphyseal edge (ME) angle, which assesses the relative position of the medial edge of the metaphysis to the edge of the bony acetabulum can be useful. The hip is probably dislocated if the medial edge of the upper femoral metaphysis lies lateral to the outer edge of the acetabulum. Von Rosen views can also be helpful if there are no ossific nuclei. The legs are abducted to 45° and a line is drawn along the axis of the femoral shaft. This should project

through the centre of the acetabulum. Disruption of the Shenton line should be sought. The acetabular index has some value in the interpretation of acetabular dysplasia; however, it is subject to marked interobserver error (*Figure 16.5*).

In the older child assessment of any ongoing acetabular dysplasia is carried out by examining a series of pelvic radiographs and looking at the shape of the acetabulum, which may involve measuring the acetabular index. The centre–edge (CE) angle, Shenton line and Moses concentric rings are also useful in the older child.

Arthrography

In the young child in whom there is only a small ossific nucleus and much of the hip is cartilage, arthrography is useful for defining the relationship between the femoral head and the acetabulum. This requires a general anaesthetic. It can define an hourglass constriction of the capsule, and the inverted limbus may show up as the 'rose thorn' sign.

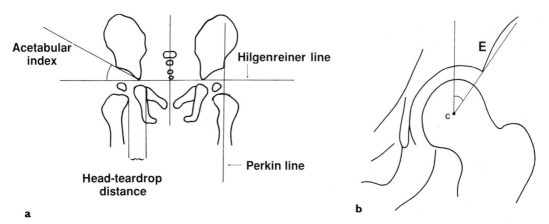

a   b

Fig 16.5 **a** Diagram showing the acetabular index, Hilgenreiner line and Perkin line. **b** The centre–edge angle. This becomes useful at about eight years of age.

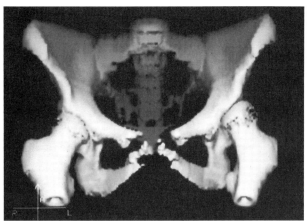

Figure 16.6 Three-dimensional reconstruction of a computerized tomographic scan of the pelvis.

Computerized tomography

Following the reduction of DDH in the young child a computerized tomographic (CT) scan may be useful for confirming reduction within the hip spica and may reveal the eccentric nature of the ossific nucleus. CT scanning is also useful when considering reconstruction procedures for the adolescent child with persistent acetabular dysplasia and femoral abnormalities. The images can be built up into a three-dimensional picture, and then the image can be rotated to give a view of the anatomy from different areas. It is also possible to remove the image of the femoral head to obtain a picture of the underlying acetabulum. This type of image is very useful when considering the type of acetabular reconstruction and inter-trochanteric femoral osteotomy required to reproduce normal anatomy (*Figure 16.6*).

Magnetic resonance imaging

Magnetic resonance imaging (MRI) is becoming increasingly useful in the management of the child as the scan times are reduced. It is now possible to perform an MRI scan without having to anaesthetize the child, and it is particularly useful if there are metal implants, which produce scatter on the CT scan. It can be performed with the child in a spica. It is also useful for assessing avascular change in the femoral head, and has a similar application to CT for providing three-dimensional images.

Management 0–6 months

All babies should be clinically examined within 48 hours of birth. Any hips that are unstable should be examined by ultrasound. Each institution should decide on an ultrasound screening policy to decide how far to 'cast the net.' This varies from no selective screening to carrying out ultrasound on all babies. A reasonable approach is to screen all breech deliveries, hip clicks and babies with a significant family history or associated congenital abnormalities such as torticollis and talipes. Many of the unstable hips stabilize within the first ten days of life so it is usual to examine the children again at ten days to prevent the unnecessary treatment of children with rapidly resolving unstable hips.

Unstable hips

If the hip remains unstable at ten days it should be treated by an abduction brace whatever the ultrasound findings. If the ultrasound shows the hip to be Graf type 3 or 4 and there is instability on the dynamic views, most of these will be unstable on clinical examination. Crying and wriggling can make interpretation of the clinical sign very difficult; any abnormality on the ultrasound should result in repeated examinations of the child until an accurate test with the baby relaxed and comfortable has been achieved.

Stable hips

If the hip is stable, the ultrasound has been carried out for screening purposes and the hip is Graf type I, there is no need for any further follow-up or management.

If the hip is stable on clinical examination, but is a Graf type 2 on the ultrasound, the management usually comprises follow-up and observation rather than abduction splintage. An ultrasound is repeated at 4–6 weeks and a plain radiograph at four months. If both of these are normal the child can be discharged. Some centres advocate treatment with abduction braces for hips that are 2C or 2D on ultrasound but stable clinically; however, the role of this management has not yet been established.

The unnecessary use of abduction bracing should be avoided because avascular necrosis and subsequent growth plate abnormalities in the femoral head have occasionally been described, both in the treated hip and in the contralateral normal hip.

Abduction braces

Various types have been described (*Figure 16.7*). The Pavlik harness is very popular. The Von Rosen malleable splint has also been used and the Freijka pillow is popular in eastern Europe. Double or even triple nappies should never be used as an effective abduction device. Their use in the early stages when it is not clear whether the hip is unstable indicates a lack of precision in the diagnosis, which should not occur if good ultrasound facilities are available. The

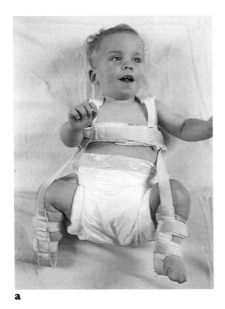
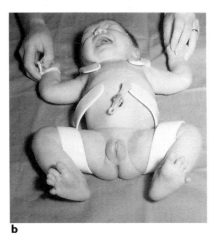
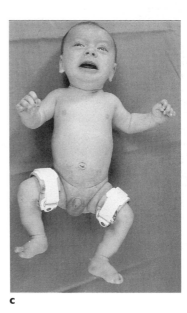

a   b   c

Figure 16.7 a The Pavlik harness. **b** The Von Rosen splint. **c** The Denis Browne abduction splint. All abduction devices for DDH.

Denis Browne bar is an effective and safe abduction device. It is sometimes difficult to fit on the newborn because of the size of the thighs, but can be easily used after the age of about two months.

The fitting of an abduction device is usually a traumatic event for the parents. This is often their first born child who is then prevented from having baths and being dressed in clothes which have been provided by the extended family. Being able to chat to mothers who have had the same experience is very helpful for these parents.

The adequacy of reduction in an abduction device should be checked with an ultrasound at four weeks. If the reduction is inadequate consideration should be given to changing the type of orthosis.

If the hip is adequately reduced on the follow-up ultrasound the abduction brace is worn for three months. At the end of this time the brace is removed, the hips are re-examined, and an ultrasound or radiograph is taken to confirm the adequacy of reduction. If there is significant acetabular dysplasia a brace may be advocated to speed up its improvement, although there is little evidence that this is effective. Once the clinician is happy with the appearance of the acetabulum the brace is discarded. Follow-up should continue until skeletal maturity to monitor the development of the acetabulum and to correct any acetabular dysplasia that does not improve with time.

If the hip remains dislocated after four weeks of treatment in an abduction device it is unlikely that it will reduce with further abduction splintage and abduction in the dislocated position may predispose to the additional risk of avascular necrosis of the femoral head.

Examination under anaesthetic

If it has been decided that the hip is inadequately reduced it should be examined under a general anaesthetic. It is important under the anaesthetic to establish whether there is an adequate concentric reduction. This may be assessed by feel, image intensifier, arthrography or ultrasound. It is also important to assess the safe zone of reduction. The hip should not be placed into extremes of position to ensure a reduction. If the hip has to be placed in 90° of abduction to feel stable the risk of avascular necrosis is high. It is ideal that there should be a safe zone of reduction between 40–60° of abduction, but if in this position the hip still feels unstable, then this position cannot be accepted.

If there is inadequate concentric reduction or there is not a safe zone of reduction then these should be achieved by an open reduction. The author's usual method of open reduction in these young children is the medial open reduction. This can be performed at as early as six weeks of age and enables the surgeon to identify the chief obstructions to reduction with a minimum of blood loss.

Management 6–12 months

This is a common time for presentation. Children of this age are examined by infant welfare nurses and

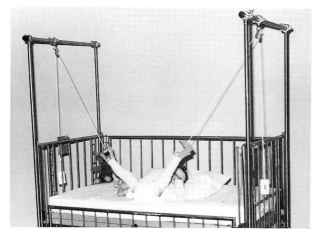

Figure 16.8 Abduction traction is used in some centres before an attempted reduction of the hip. It is important that abduction does not exceed 60°.

often present with various clicks or asymmetry of the hips before walking starts.

Examination starts by looking for asymmetry of the skin creases. Flexing the hip and knee to 90° may reveal a true shortening of the limb above the level of the knee. Palpation of the greater trochanter and anterior superior iliac spine may reveal some asymmetry of their relative positions when compared to the normal side (if there is a normal side!). Stability of the hip is tested by a Barlow or Ortolani test depending on the size of the child. A radiograph is taken, and if the ossific nucleus has not formed an ultrasound examination should also be performed.

Under a general anaesthetic, the hip is assessed for a concentric reduction in the safe zone. A hip spica is then applied with the hip in the position of maximum stability: this is usually 90° of flexion and 60° of abduction. If a closed reduction is unsatisfactory a medial open reduction should be performed.

Preoperative traction is used in some centres (*Figure 16.8*). The rational is that this may reduce the risk of avascular necrosis and increase the probability of a successful closed reduction of the hip. However, there is no evidence to confirm this contention.

The child treated by closed reduction generally has a hip spica for three months. The cast may have to be changed to accommodate growth. After three months the hip spica is removed and an abduction device is worn until any acetabular dysplasia has resolved.

Management 1–3 years

Presentation after walking has started produces a characteristic Trendelenburg limp. When a child stands with unilateral DDH the contralateral leg flexes at the knee to accommodate the shortening in the affected leg. When the dislocation is bilateral the symmetry of the Trendelenburg gait makes it more difficult to recognize. In the bilateral case the peroneal gap is increased.

Ortolani and Barlow tests are not usually positive at this age because the hip generally cannot be reduced on the examination couch. By this age anatomical blocks to reduction have developed, as described in the section on anatomy.

Preoperative traction is commonly used in the belief that it increases the ease of reduction and reduces the incidence of avascular necrosis. In the past it has been used up to three weeks preoperatively, although in many centres it is now used for much shorter periods. Usually the traction is Gallow's traction with 90° of hip flexion. If abduction is used, this should not exceed 60° as more than 60° carries a higher risk of avascular necrosis. Many centres have abandoned preoperative traction because they believe it is ineffective and unnecessary.

If the hip can be concentrically reduced in a reasonable safe zone, then **a closed reduction** is acceptable. Postoperatively the position of reduction can be checked using CT or MRI. The hip is kept in a hip spica for 12 weeks and then put into an abduction device such as a Denis Browne (DB) bar. In those children whose position of stability was with internal rotation of the femur, this position can be maintained in a broomstick cast (Batchelor cast). The abduction device is discarded when the acetabulum is sufficiently developed. Acetabular dysplasia is common and may require secondary procedures.

Medial open reduction is used extensively up to the age of one year when the chief bars to reduction are tightness of the psoas tendon and inferior capsule, both of which can be better released through this approach. Between 1–2 years of age its use is more controversial because a capsulorrhaphy of the lateral part of the capsule cannot be carried out through this approach and subluxation or redislocation are therefore more likely. Few centres use medial open reduction in children over two years of age.

Anterolateral reduction has been the standard method of open reduction for the congenitally dislocated hip in the past. Because it is a more extensive procedure involving blood loss it has not been popular for the young child under six months and in the past reduction was often delayed until the child was older and bigger. Many centres use this as the only method of open reduction, and all centres use it as the method of open reduction for children over three years of age. It still relies on an adequate concentric reduction of the hip to stimulate the acetabulum and improve acetabular development.

Anterolateral reduction combined with Salter osteotomy is used routinely in some centres in children over 18 months of age. It is a method of addressing the acetabular dysplasia and the reduction of the dislocated hip at the same time. The advantage is that there are very few secondary operations required for acetabular dysplasia; the disadvantage is that it makes the operation more involved and technically more difficult, and the Salter osteotomy may be unnecessary in about 40% of cases.

Anterolateral reduction and femoral osteotomy has been a popular method of dealing with DDH in the UK. A standard anterolateral reduction of the hip is performed and the hip is splinted in significant internal rotation to counter the effect of persistent femoral anteversion. Six weeks later derotation osteotomy is performed in the upper part of the femur through a separate incision. This is a combination of varus and external rotation distal to the osteotomy to counteract the persistent femoral anteversion and valgus. It relies on the reduction of the femoral head stimulating the acetabulum. Acetabular development after concentric reduction of the femoral head is most effective under the age of four years, but also occurs, though less effectively, in children up to eight years of age.

Management over 3 years

At this stage the child may have developed lumbar lordosis together with a short leg and an abnormal Trendelenburg gait. Sometimes DDH is a coincidental finding when a radiograph is obtained for other reasons.

In the past it has been suggested that a unilateral DDH in a child over seven years of age and a bilateral DDH in a child over four years of age should be left untreated. The rationale for this is that the child will function adequately, but they may develop increasing pain in their forties. A total hip replacement of an untreated dislocated hip is, however, technically very demanding and the results are not as good as for an osteoarthritic reduced hip. This has meant that the age limits given above have been extended, so that if a hip replacement is needed at a later stage it is technically easier and the results are better because the hip has been reduced.

Most units now manage these hips using open reduction and femoral shortening in the subtrochanteric region in combination with an acetabuloplasty. In the past the Colonna arthroplasty has been popular and good results have been described, but we do not use it in our institution. The hip capsule is detached from the margins of the acetabulum and then closed over the femoral head. An acetabulum is fashioned with reamers to accept the femoral head and a suture may be passed through the ilium to stabilize the femoral head within the new acetabulum.

Complications of treatment

The complications of treatment include:

- Redislocation or subluxation.
- Avascular necrosis.
- Acetabular dysplasia.

Early redislocation in the first six months postoperatively is generally due to inadequate reduction with misinterpretation of the radiographs so that the hip has not been concentrically reduced. Late redislocation is due to femoral anteversion or progressive acetabular dysplasia. The management of the redislocated hip that has previously been operated upon is difficult and should only be attempted at specialist centres. The essential parts of operative management are:

- Release of soft tissue to ensure a full concentric reduction.
- Femoral osteotomy to ensure normal upper femoral anatomy. This is sometimes combined with shortening particularly in the child over 3 years of age to reduce the tension needed to obtain reduction.
- Acetabuloplasty, which may be in the form of a Salter or Pemberton to obtain good acetabular cover.

Avascular necrosis is due to a reduction in the blood supply to the femoral head. It may be a temporary phenomenon or it may progress to cause distortion of the femoral head and growth plate arrest, giving rise to abnormalities of the shape of the femoral head and upper femur (*Figure 16.9*). It can be recognized in the early stages by signs described by Salter (*Table 16.3*). Some of these recover while others develop the late effects described by Kalamchi and McEwen (*Table 16.4*). In grade 1 there is mild avascularity. Grade 2 is thought to be due to occlusion of the posterior branches of the medial circumflex artery. In grade 4 the ischaemia is more severe and affects all the femoral head and growth plate. There is relative overgrowth of the trochanter. The abnormal position of the greater trochanter produces a short lever arm and the abductors cannot function normally. A Trendelenburg gait develops.

Acetabular dysplasia may persist and the acetabulum may not develop normally if there is a failure to

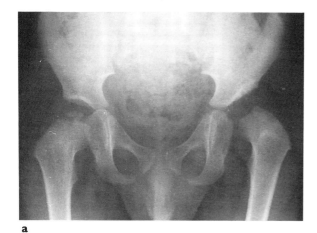

a

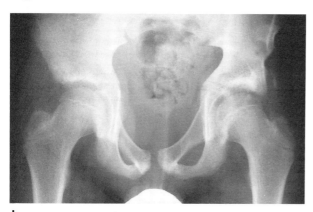

b

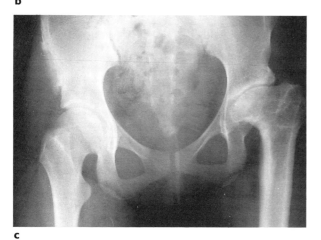

c

Figure 16.9 a This 2½-years-old boy developed avascular necrosis of both hips 12 months after a closed reduction of the left hip. **b** At 11 years of age, the boy has made a good radiological recovery from the avascular necrosis and a Salter osteotomy has been performed on the left hip for persistent acetabular dysplasia. **c** This 14-year-old girl, with grade 4 avascular change and a varus short neck and relative overgrowth of the trochanter, now has early osteoarthritic change. (Reproduced with permission from Brougham *et al.* (1988).)

Table 16.3 Salter signs for the early recognition of avascular necrosis (Salter *et al.*, 1969)

Mottling or fragmentation of the ossific nucleus
Delay in ossification of the ossific nucleus for at least 12 months
Areas of rarefaction, cyst formation or cupping of the metaphysis
Localised sclerosis of the growth plate
Abnormal growth arrest

Table 16.4 Kalamchi and McEwen classification of the late effects of avascular necrosis after treatment of developmental dysplasia of the hip (Kalamachi and McEwen, 1980)

Grade 1	Slight loss of epiphyseal height and slight coxa magna, but no significant sequelae
Grade 2	Growth plate arrest on the lateral part of the growth plate resulting in valgus orientation of the femoral head
Grade 3	Growth plate arrest of the central part resulting in a short femoral neck and relative overgrowth of the trochanter
Grade 4	Marked flattening of the femoral head, a short femoral neck tilted into varus, and overgrowth of the trochanter

obtain concentric reduction or in some cases if the reduction is late. The amount of acetabular development can be measured using the acetabular index. The acetabulum is dysplastic if the acetabular index is more than 25° over the age of four years. Acetabular dysplasia leads to an early onset of osteoarthritis and correction by acetabuloplasty can prevent this.

If there is acetabular dysplasia not improving on annual radiographs in a child over four years of age, then an innominate osteotomy is performed.

Operative procedures

Operative procedure for medial open reduction

The child is placed supine at the end of the operating table with the hips flexed and abducted. Bilateral medial open reduction can be undertaken under the same anaesthetic. The incision is centred over the adductor longus parallel to and 1 cm distal to the groin crease. The adductor longus tendon is divided close to its attachment to the pubis and through its bed the hip joint capsule is approached between pectineus and adductor brevis. It is also possible to approach the hip capsule through the interval between adductor brevis and adductor magnus. Branches of the medial circumflex vessels are identified as they pass between the psoas tendon and pectineus and protected by passing a loop around them. The psoas major tendon is cut at its attachment to the lesser trochanter. A T-shaped capsulotomy is performed using an incision parallel to the anterior margin of the acetabulum, followed by an axial incision extending from the mid-point to the attachment of the capsule to the neck of the femur. The transverse ligament of the acetabulum is divided through the capsulotomy and a good view of the acetabulum can be obtained by posterolateral displacement of the femoral head. The ligamentum teres is detached proximally and can then be used to pull the femoral head down into a concentrically-reduced position. The labrum of the acetabulum is usually squashed rather than inverted, but radial splits can be placed in the limbus if it is thought that this would improve the position of the labrum. In the reduced position the femoral head bulges through the opened capsule. The ligamentum teres is sutured to the capsule anteromedially for some temporary stability. A lateral capsulorrhaphy cannot be performed through this approach. The incision is closed and a double hip spica is applied. At six weeks the plaster can be removed, and generally the hips feel sufficiently stable for the child to be placed in an abduction splint. The splint is worn until the acetabulum has developed reasonably well.

Operative procedure for anterolateral open reduction

A straight oblique incision is made one finger-breadth below and parallel to the anterior one-third of the iliac crest and extending 2–4 cm anterior to the anterior superior iliac crest. This incision allows an anterior Smith Petersen approach to the hip. The lateral femoral cutaneous nerve of the thigh is identified and retracted medially. The interval between tensor fascia lata and sartorius is developed distally. The ascending branches of the lateral femoral circumflex vessel that cross this interval distally are identified and ligated. The interval is extended on to the iliac crest and the iliac apophysis is split. The abductors can now be elevated off the outer aspect of the ilium and retracted laterally. The sartorius is retracted medially. The two heads of rectus femoris are both divided and retracted medially. The capsule of the hip joint is then identified, and with the hip reduced any attachment of the capsule onto the lateral

aspect of the ilium is divided. The hip capsule is then opened using a T-shaped incision with one limb parallel to the edge of the acetabulum and the other running along the anterior aspect of the neck of the femur to its base.

The iliopsoas tendon is identified at its attachment onto the lesser trochanter and divided. The hip is inspected through the capsulotomy and any restriction to reduction identified. This requires division of the transverse acetabular ligament and sometimes excision of a bulky ligamentum teres. If inverted the labrum should be everted, although some authorities have removed the limbus in the past. The position of best stability can now be assessed and is usually one of flexion, abduction and slight internal rotation. If considerable internal rotation is necessary a femoral osteotomy may be required at a later stage. The capsule is repaired by double breasting the capsule. This should be carried out to remove redundant lax capsule rather than to force the femoral head into the acetabulum. The iliac apophysis is repaired and the child placed in a hip spica for up to 16 weeks with a change of cast as dictated by the growth of the child and the odour of the cast. The complete spica may be replaced by a broomstick cast at eight weeks.

If the reduction is being carried out in an older child, a femoral shortening may be undertaken at the same time. This ensures an easier reduction and relieves some of the pressure on the femoral head, which may reduce the incidence of significant avascular necrosis.

Operative procedure for Salter innominate osteotomy

The skin incision runs parallel to and just below the iliac crest from the junction of the posterior one-third and the middle-third to the anterior superior iliac spine and is then continued transversely to below the mid-point of the inguinal ligament. The interval between tensor fascia lata and sartorius is identified and followed proximally to the iliac crest. The iliac apophysis is split and the abductor muscles are peeled off the outer aspect of the ilium and retracted laterally. Sartorius is divided from its insertion onto the anterior inferior iliac spine. Iliacus is then elevated from the inner wall of the ilium and the ilium is cleared back to the greater sciatic notch. The psoas tendon is divided. With great care and avoiding the gluteal vessels, a Gigli saw is then passed into the greater sciatic notch. The pelvic osteotomy is performed transversely and superiorly to the acetabulum. The distal segment is then angulated forwards and laterally, and this manoeuvre can be helped by a 'figure four' position

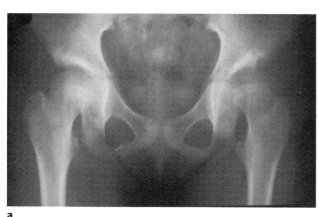
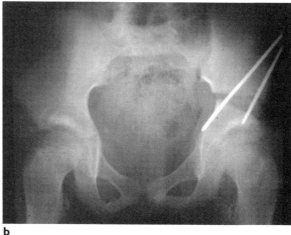

Figure 16.10 **a** This child has persistent acetabular dysplasia in the left hip after closed reduction of developmental dysplasia of hip. **b** A Salter osteotomy has been performed and stabilized with two wires.

of the hip. A wedge of bone is cut from the iliac crest and placed into the defect. Threaded Steinman pins are then passed from the iliac crest through the triangle of bone into the distal fragment into the posterior column behind the acetabulum. It is important that the orientation of these is correct to avoid any transgression into the acetabulum. A hip spica is applied after closing the skin wound. The wires should be removed after six weeks and the child can then mobilize (*Figure 16.10*).

Operative procedure for Pemberton acetabuloplasty

This is performed through a similar skin incision to that of the Salter innominate osteotomy. The abductors are reflected off the lateral wall of the ilium. A curved osteotomy is made in the bone above the acetabulum using osteotomes and the acetabulum is decreased in size by forward flexion of the osteotomized segment on the mobile triradiate cartilage. The opening is packed with bone graft. Internal fixation is not usually necessary.

Operative procedure for trochanteric surgery

For grade 3 and 4 avascular necrosis, the relevant overgrowth of the greater trochanter can be treated by epiphysiodesis or trochanteric advancement. Epiphysiodesis is only effective if carried out under the age of six years. In children over six years of age the greater trochanter is repositioned, pulling the trochanter laterally and distally. If the overgrowth of the trochanter is combined with a short varus neck,

the trochanter can be moved laterally, the femoral neck reorientated, and the femoral shaft moved laterally as described by Wagner. In this way the femoral neck is lengthened and the anatomy of the upper femur is restored.

THE ADOLESCENT WITH HIP DYSPLASIA

Acetabular Dysplasia

Acetabular dysplasia is an abnormality of development of the acetabulum. The shape may be abnormal with an enlarged, shallow saucer-like acetabulum lacking a well-defined lip rather than a cup-shaped acetabulum. The acetabulum may be directed laterally rather than anterolaterally and distally.

Aetiology

Acetabular dysplasia may be secondary to DDH or a primary problem without foregoing DDH, and this can present at any age. The acetabulum may be deficient in conditions in which there is muscle imbalance such as cerebral palsy, spina bifida or polio. If there is muscle imbalance there may be a deficiency in the posterior lip of the acetabulum. The acetabulum in Perthes disease may develop dysplasia with the deficiency of the acetabulum exaggerated by the large femoral head.

Clinical Features

Acetabular dysplasia may be a coincidental radiological finding or it may become evident during follow-up of DDH or another pre-existing condition. It may also present with pain in the groin after activity, which is assumed to be due to stretching of the capsule, or pain due to early osteoarthritic change.

Radiology

Traditionally a two-dimensional assessment has been made on the anteroposterior radiograph. The CE angle gives some idea of the amount of acetabular dysplasia. The upper femoral anatomy can also be assessed, looking at the relative overgrowth of the trochanter and the valgus or varus orientation of the femoral neck.

Three-dimensional reconstructions using CT or MRI have greatly improved understanding of the anatomy of the dysplastic hip. An appreciation of the orientation of the acetabulum and rim deficiencies helps in the planning of an appropriate acetabuloplasty, while the orientation of the upper femur in terms of anteversion and the neck–shaft angle aids in planning femoral surgery (*Figure 16.6*).

Management

Indications for treatment
Capsular pain and early osteoarthritic pain are treated surgically. Whether asymptomatic acetabular dysplasia should be improved to prevent the subsequent onset of osteoarthritis is always the subject of great discussion. We would advocate an acetabuloplasty if the CE angle is less than 10°. If there is distortion of the upper femoral anatomy then the acetabuloplasty should be combined with an intertrochanteric osteotomy.

Changing the shape of the acetabulum
Pemberton osteotomy is particularly used in children aged 2–6 years. This is combined with an open reduction of a dislocated hip if it is unlikely that follow-up is possible. This approach has been used in nomads and has also been very useful in the management of children with spina bifida for whom multiple operations should be avoided.

An ischioplasty has also been described if the deficiency lies mainly in the posterior wall. This is similar to a Pemberton osteotomy, but is a partial osteotomy of the posterior wall with a bone graft to give posterior cover.

Changing the direction of the acetabulum
The **Salter innominate osteotomy** can be performed in children up to ten years of age. The prerequisites for this osteotomy are listed in *Table 16.5*.

The **Sutherland osteotomy** is a double pelvic osteotomy. It consists of the Salter innominate osteotomy combined with division of the pubis close to the pubic symphysis. This is used for children in their early teenage years in whom there is insufficient mobility of the symphysis for a Salter osteotomy to be effective.

The **Steel or triple osteotomy** can be used in the adolescent and adult patient and provides much more manoeuvrability of the acetabulum. It includes an osteotomy through the ischium, through the superior pubic ramus and through the ilium (*Figure 16.11*). It is a major undertaking and problems have been described around the ischial component of the osteotomy with non-union and damage to the sciatic nerve. Various modifications of the basic technique have been described to reduce the risk of complications, to improve the exposure, and to increase the ability to reposition the acetabulum, such as the **Tonnis procedure**.

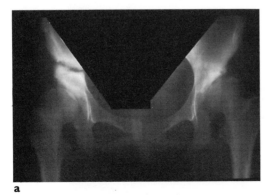
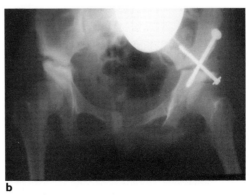

a   b

Figure 16.11   **a** This shows persistent acetabular dysplasia of the left hip. The right hip has previously been treated by a Salter osteotomy, which has failed to unite.   **b** The left hip has been treated by a triple osteotomy with good cover of the femoral head.

Table 16.5 The prerequisites for a Salter innominate osteotomy

Concentric hip
Femoral head containable with less than 25° of
    abduction
Undeformed femoral head and acetabulum
No osteoarthritis.

The **Dial osteotomy** (as described by Wagner) is a periacetabular osteotomy in which an osteotomy is made around the acetabulum and then the socket rotated into an improved position. This gives excellent manoeuvrability of the segment to improve cover and is inherently stable. Again it is a major undertaking and avascular necrosis of the acetabulum has been described. There is a prolonged recovery from this procedure with limping.

Salvage of the acetabulum

Acetabular salvage can be performed if the four prerequisites for redirectional osteotomy are absent. It is designed to provide better cover for the femoral head, but relies on the development of fibrocartilage between the covering bone and the femoral head rather then the redirection of acetabular cartilage. The **shelf procedure** consists of placing a piece of bone taken from the outer wing of the ilium at the anterolateral lip of the acetabulum to give better cover. This can be inherently stable by positioning underneath the reflected head of rectus femoris. A modification has recently been described by Staheli (1981) with bone grafting behind the shelf. The bone in the area usually hypertrophies to give good cover.

The **Chiari osteotomy** is a medial displacement osteotomy of the acetabulum to leave the ilium as cover for the femoral head (*Figure 16.12*). It has proved to be effective in cerebral palsy and in paralytic conditions, and the head can be higher than is acceptable for the shelf procedure. It is not commonly used for DDH.

The shelf procedure and Chiari osteotomy can be combined in various ways to provide increased cover, particularly for children with cerebral palsy.

Upper Femoral Dysplasia

If radiological studies indicate that the femoral head is better contained in a position of abduction and internal rotation a femoral osteotomy may be indicated (*Figure 16.13*).

Often the upper femoral growth plate has prematurely closed due to avascular necrosis, resulting in a relative overgrowth of the trochanter. A trochanteric advancement may be indicated to improve the limping of the Trendelenburg gait. It can also be combined with a valgus osteotomy of the femoral neck to effectively lengthen the femoral neck in cases of short femoral necks secondary to early growth plate closure as described by Wagner.

In managing adolescent dysplasia it is important that consideration is given to subsequent surgery as many of these patients develop osteoarthritis in later life. It is therefore important not to distort the upper femur so that a femoral component of a total hip replacement can be easily placed and that adequate bone stock is maintained around the acetabulum to

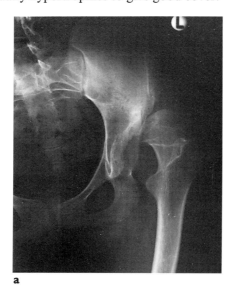
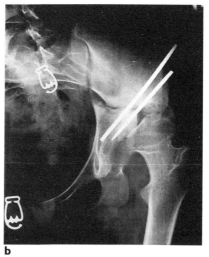

a   b

Figure 16.12 a Recurrent dislocation of the hip in cerebral palsy, **b** treated by a Chiari osteotomy.

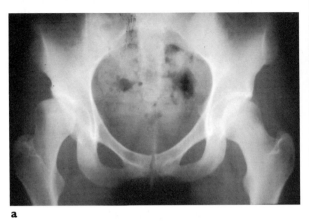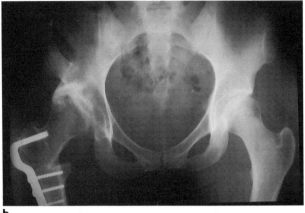

a   b

Figure 16.13 **a** Persistent acetabular dysplasia with recurrent subluxation of the right hip. **b** The persistent acetabular dysplasia has been treated by varus derotation osteotomy of the upper femur together with a shelf arthroplasty of the acetabulum (reproduced with permission from Williams PF, Cole WG. *Orthopaedic Management in Childhood.* Chapman & Hall, London).

provide improved seating for an acetabular component.

REFERENCES AND FURTHER READING

Blockey NJ. Derotation osteotomy in the management of congenital dislocation of the hip. *J Bone Joint Surg* 1984; **66B**: 485–490.

Brougham DI, Broughton NS, Cole WG, Menelaus MB. The predictability of acetabular development after closed reduction for congenital dislocation of the hip. *J Bone Joint Surg* 1988; **70B**: 733–736.

Coleman SS. *Congenital Dysplasia and Dislocation of the Hip.* CV Mosby, St Louis, 1978.

Ferguson AB. Primary open reduction of congenital dislocation of the hips using a median adductor approach. *J Bone Joint Surg* 1973; **55A**: 671–689.

Graf R. Classification of hip joint dysplasia by means of sonography. *Arch Orthop Trauma Surg* 1984; **102**: 248–255.

Harcke HT, Clarke NMP, Lee SM. Examination of the infant hip with real-time ultrasonography. *J Ultrasound Med* 1984; **3**: 131–137.

Kalamchi A, MacEwen GD. Avascular necrosis following treatment of congenital dislocation of the hip. *J Bone Joint Surg* 1980; **62A**: 876–888.

Kasser JR, Bowen JR, MacEwen GD. Varus derotation osteotomy in the treatment of persisting dysplasia in congenital dislocation of the hip. *J Bone Joint Surg* 1985; **67A**: 195–202.

Klisic P. Combined procedure of open reduction and shortening of the femur in treatment of congenital dislocation of the hip in older children. *Clin Orthop Rel Research* 1976; **119**: 60–69.

Love BRT, Stevens PM, Williams PF. A long term review of shelf arthroplasty. *J Bone Joint Surg* 1980; **62B**: 321–325.

Pemberton PA. Pericapsular osteotomy of the ilium for treatment of congenital subluxation and dislocation of the hip. *J Bone Joint Surg* 1965; **47A**: 65–86.

Reynolds DA. Chiari innominate osteotomy in adults: technique, indications and contra-indications. *J Bone Joint Surg* 1986; **68B**: 45–54.

Salter RB. Innominate osteotomy in the treatment of congenital dislocation and subluxation of the hip. *J Bone Joint Surg* 1961; **43B**: 518–539.

Salter RB, Kostuik J, Dallas S. Avascular necrosis of the femoral head as a complication of treatment for congenital dislocation of the hip in young children: a clinical and experimental investigation. *Can J Surg* 1969; **12**: 44–61.

Staheli LT. Slotted acetabular augmentation. *J Pediatr Orthop* 1981; **1**: 321–327.

Thomas IH, Dunin AJ, Cole WG, Menelaus MB. Avascular necrosis after open reduction for congenital dislocation of the hip: analysis of causative factors and natural history. *J Pediatr Orthop* 1989; **9**: 525–531.

Tonnis D. *Congenital Dysplasia and Dislocation of the Hip.* Springer, Berlin, 1986.

Weinstein SL, Ponseti IV. Congenital dislocation of the hip. Open reduction through a medial approach. *J Bone Joint Surg* 1979 **61A**: 119–124.

Chapter 17
Perthes Disease

Malcolm B Menelaus

Perthes disease is a condition characterized by avascular necrosis of a portion or of the whole of the femoral head; this is followed by revascularization. It is one of a group of conditions loosely grouped together under the title 'osteochondritis juvenilis.' These conditions are characterized by avascular changes with a specific age and sex incidence for each condition.

Incidence

Perthes disease is more common in boys than girls with a ratio of 4:1. It is bilateral in approximately 15% of cases. Bilateral involvement should always raise the question as to whether the condition represents epiphyseal dysplasia rather than Perthes disease. It is most common in children aged 4–10 years, though it may be seen as early as two years and as late as 15 years of age. The condition occurs in approximately 1 in 740 boys under the age of 15 years (though the incidence varies for different races and geographical regions). The condition is more common in lower socioeconomic groups.

Aetiology

The basic cause of Perthes disease remains uncertain. Whatever it is, it mediates its effect by interfering with the blood supply to the head of the femur. It is likely that several episodes of impaired circulation produce the condition. The blood supply to the femoral head in children aged approximately 4–8 years is almost exclusively from the lateral epiphyseal vessel. These vessels might be thrombosed or occluded by trauma, increased pressure due to an effusion or by some other insult.

Children of low birth weight and with a delayed bone age are more commonly affected by the condition. Occasionally, there is a history of recurrent hip irritability months or even years before the radiological appearance of Perthes disease.

Pathology

In the early stages, the synovial membrane is thickened and more vascular than normal. The pulvinar is swollen and thickened. This may be responsible for the lateral displacement of the femoral head that is sometimes seen in early radiographs (*Figure 17.1*). Microscopy reveals villi on the surface of the synovial membrane. The articular cartilage remains normal.

Bone death is followed by bone repair. Bone death is evident by the death of osteocytes and coagulation of the bone marrow. The trabecular pattern and mineral content at this stage remain unaltered and there is therefore no radiological change in density or trabecular pattern. Repair is accompanied by:

- Revascularization by granulation tissue leading to resorption of dead bone.
- Reossification with increased trabecular width and bulk as a result of new bone being laid down on the dead bone. This leads to a radiologically visible increase in bone density. Different areas are affected at different times.
- Resorption of dead bone. This is a slow process over a period of years. As the bone revascularizes some dead trabeculae may be absorbed, but most act as a framework for appositional bone growth. If dead trabeculae become completely ensheathed they present no free surface for absorption and are never absorbed. The early new bone is woven bone and is more mouldable or plastic.

Perthes disease affects varying portions of the head of the femur, and if only part of the femoral head is affected it is the anterior part. The physis may be involved and this may lead to premature fusion of part or whole of the growth plate with resultant broadening and shortening of the femoral neck (*Figure 17.2*).

In more severe forms of the condition the femoral head is not well covered by the acetabulum, either as a result of lateral extrusion of the femoral head with

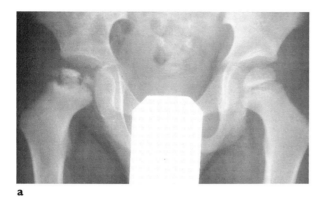
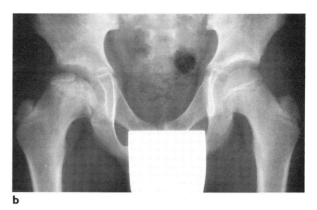

a   b

Figure 17.1   a Fragmentation and lateral displacement of the femoral head in Perthes disease at five years of age (bone age four and a half years); the head to teardrop distance is increased more than the superior joint space due to inflammatory change in the pulvinar.   **b** At seven years of age the displacement of the femoral head has corrected. There is a broader growth plate accounting for the larger head and acetabulum.

increased head to teardrop distance or a broadening of the neck and the head of the femur. There is increased vascularity of the metaphysis adjacent to the affected portion of the femoral head.

The acetabulum is affected in that if the head becomes enlarged so the acetabulum tends to become enlarged (particularly in those children who have the condition at a younger age) and its lateral margin becomes rounded.

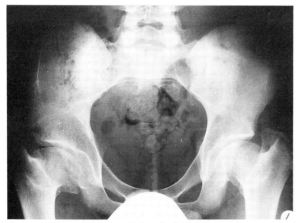

Figure 17.2   Bilateral healed Perthes disease in a male aged 19 years. There has been major involvement of both heads and of the growth plates resulting in coxa magna; note the 'sagging rope' curved line of sclerosis in the inter-trochanteric regions at the distal margin of the large femoral heads. There has been an early arrest of growth with resultant coxa breva, and the tip of the trochanters lie proximal to the articular surface of the femoral heads. There is congruity between the heads and acetabula.

Later in life (and seldom before the age of 30 years) the changes of osteoarthritis of the hip may supervene and are more likely in those patients in whom there is marked deformity of the femoral head and an incongruous relationship between the head and the acetabulum.

Clinical Features

Symptoms
The most common presentation is with a history of painless intermittent limp. The limp may become more persistent and pain may develop. Sometimes, the child is reluctant to walk on rising in the morning and may limp then and after prolonged activity.

The condition may be diagnosed as an incidental finding during a radiological investigation of the urinary tract. This raises the question as to whether the condition may be much more common than the incidence quoted above, and these asymptomatic cases may be responsible for some cases of 'idiopathic' osteoarthritis of the hip in adults.

Signs
Physical examination in the early stages generally reveals a limitation of all movements of the hip joint, flexion being the least affected. At a late stage the most characteristic findings are restriction of abduction in extension, adduction in flexion, and internal rotation; there is wasting of the thigh and buttock, and shortening of the limb. These changes are generally reversed with healing of the condition. The degree of limp generally parallels the degree to which hip motion is restricted. Some patients have a fixed abduction contracture of the hip while the disease is active.

Radiology

Radiographs

The radiological changes vary both in the amount of femoral head involved and the severity of these changes. The rate of radiological progression also varies. The more extensive the involvement of the femoral head, the more likely it is that permanent deformity of the femoral head will occur and that there will be growth plate involvement as described above. The clinical features may be similar regardless of the degree of involvement of the head, but consistent limitation of joint motion is more common in children with extensive involvement of the femoral head.

Initially radiographs may be normal. The earliest change is a concentric widening of the joint space. This is generally more marked medially in association with an increase in the head to teardrop distance. Sometimes there is a subchondral radiotranslucency, which occurs as a lucent line in the lateral radiograph. This demarcates the extent of involvement of the head of the femur (Salter and Thompson, 1984). The translucency may be so clearly defined as to suggest a fracture line (*Figure 17.3*).

As avascular necrosis occurs the head develops a relative increase in density in an irregular fashion. As revascularization occurs a true increase in density (relative to the opposite hip) occurs due to the laying down of appositional bone. When revascularization is complete the head eventually regains its normal density. If less than 50% of the head is involved, normal head height is maintained and there is usually little increase in the width of the femoral neck or tendency for the head to extend beyond the confines of the acetabulum. If more than 50% of the head is involved there may be a loss of epiphyseal height, increased width of the head and neck, and reduced

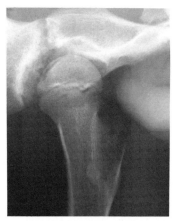

Figure 17.3 Salter sign. The length of the subchondral fracture line indicates the extent of the involvement of the underlying femoral head. Here the anterior one-third of the head is involved.

covering of the head with a loss of sphericity (*Figure 17.2*).

In addition to epiphyseal changes there are metaphyseal changes on the radiograph with irregular rarefaction of the metaphysis. This may be so severe as to suggest the development of metaphyseal cysts adjacent to the growth plate. The degree of this change (which is assumed to be due to increased vascularity) varies with the degree of involvement of the head and underlies the involved portion of the femoral head. If there is premature closure of the growth plate (which occurs in the more severe forms of the condition) then shortening and widening of the femoral neck occurs.

Isotope scan

A radioisotope bone scan using technetium-99m diphosphonate will demonstrate avascularity of the femoral head before any radiological features are evident (*Figure 17.4a*). Specialized pinhole images of

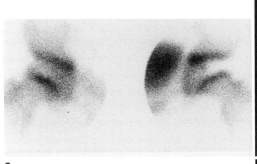
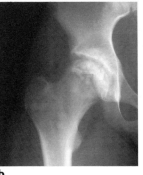
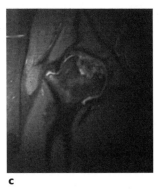

Figure 17.4 a Isotope scan showing left Perthes disease. Magnified pinhole image of both femoral heads revealing abscence of uptake on the left. **b** Radiograph of Perthes disease in an older child than that shown in Figure 17.4a. **c** Magnetic resonance image of same child as in Figure 17.4b. The area involved is well defined.

the hips are generally required. These magnify the region, improve resolution and permit assessment of the extent of any change within the femoral head. Perthes disease is readily distinguished from other hip diseases in which femoral head vascularity is intact. The investigation is useful for diagnosis and monitoring progress. Bone scanning is accurate with very few false positive or false negative studies. Bensahel *et al.* (1983) suggest a 97% sensitivity in differentiating Perthes disease from non-specific synovitis.

Magnetic resonance imaging

Magnetic resonance imaging (MRI) easily demonstrates the area involved, but its value in the management of these children is yet to be defined (*Figure 17.4c*).

Differential Diagnosis

The irritable hip or observation hip

This is the principal differential diagnosis in a small group of children who present before there is any radiological change. If there is persistent irritability a bone scan should be performed.

Multiple epiphyseal dysplasia

This is to be suspected in bilateral cases and a skeletal survey should be performed.

Tuberculosis of the hip

This remains the principal differential diagnosis in countries where joint tuberculosis is still common. In tuberculosis, there is narrowing rather than widening of the joint space and widespread osteoporosis.

Osteochondritis dissecans

Some patients with localized Perthes disease have radiological changes resembling and sometimes progressing to osteochondritis dissecans of the hip (*Figure 17.5*).

Other causes of avascular necrosis of the femoral head

Avascular necrosis may also occur in association with fractures of the femoral neck, corticosteroid therapy, infection, juvenile chronic arthritis, after radiotherapy or in renal disease. It may also occur in the adolescent with a haemoglobinopathy such as sickle cell disease and thalassaemia. Cretinism can also produce an appearance similar to bilateral avascular necrosis of the upper femoral epiphyses.

There are patients who present as teenagers with a condition that resembles Perthes disease. In these late-onset cases the condition commonly runs a

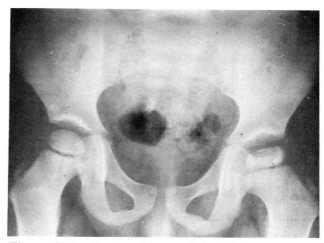

Figure 17.5 Perthes disease of the left hip in a boy with a chronological age of five years and a bone age of four years. The involved portion of the head is central. This very localized involvement without involvement of the full depth of the head down to the growth plate sometimes precedes the development of osteochondritis dissecans of the hip. According to the lateral column classification this is in Group A with no loss of lateral column height. The prognosis is excellent.

prolonged course, results in severe deformity of the femoral head, and unlike Perthes disease in the younger child, results in loss of articular cartilage from the femoral head.

Prognosis

Long-term studies of Perthes disease indicate that most children who have had the condition lead an active life through their later childhood and have no symptoms in early adult life. During this period there is commonly some persistent restriction of hip motion and there may be intermittent episodes of hip pain over the years requiring a short course of anti-inflammatory tablets.

At 30 years following the onset of the condition approximately one-third of the patients have no symptoms and few physical signs, one-third have discomfort and intermittent pain in the hip, and one-third have frank osteoarthritis of the hip requiring treatment (McAndrew and Weinstein, 1984). Those patients who at the conclusion of the pathological process do not have a spherical head (as measured by Moses rings on anteroposterior and lateral radiographs of the femoral head) or who have poorly covered heads are more likely to develop osteoarthritis. If the disease begins under the age of five years, a spherical head and a good long-term prognosis are more likely to ensue, although a poor radiological and clinical result is sometimes seen in those in whom the condition starts when they are under three years of age.

Clinical factors affecting prognosis

These include age, physical signs and sex. Children who present over the age of ten years have a poor prognosis with a few developing a loss of the radiological joint space due to changes in the articular cartilage. It is important to perform a bone age estimation on children with Perthes disease as the bone age is commonly retarded in relationship to the chronological age and the prognosis more closely relates to bone age.

Children who have persistent restriction of joint motion or recurrent episodes of hip stiffness, despite adequate treatment, also have a poor prognosis, and in general girls have a worse prognosis than boys.

Radiological factors affecting prognosis

Lateral pillar classification (Herring *et al.*, 1993): it has been found that the femoral head is more likely to undergo progressive flattening in those patients with more severe lateral pillar involvement. The three groups in the lateral pillar classification are - A, B, and C.

- In group A, there is no collapse of the lateral pillar and no significant radiolucency in the lateral pillar (*Figure 17.5*).
- In group B, the lateral pillar has maintained at least 50% of its height compared to the original height (*Figure 17.6*).
- In group C, there is a loss of lateral pillar height of over 50% of the original height (*Figure 17.7*).

It must be repeated that this, and all other prognostic factors, indicate a probability, but not a certainty with regard to outcome. Herring *et al.* (1993) suggest that progressive flattening with more severe lateral pillar involvement is more likely to occur in older patients and in those with prolonged reossification.

Uncovering of the femoral head at presentation: previous studies have indicated that the more the degree of uncovering at presentation the worse the clinical end-result (Dickens and Menelaus, 1978). More than about 3 mm of uncovering (in excess of that on the normal side) indicates a poor prognosis. The uncovering is measured as the horizontal distance between a vertical line through the outer lip of the acetabulum and a second vertical line through the lateral edge of the femoral capital growth plate. The measurements should be compared on the two sides. Others have expressed this measurement as a ratio: the percentage of the width of the femoral head

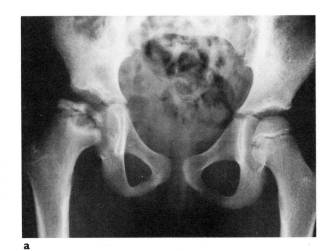

a

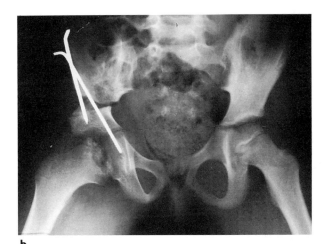

b

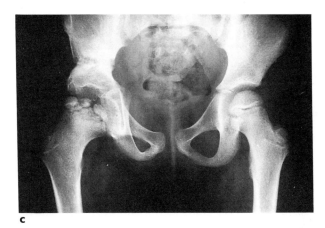

c

Figure 17.6 a Girl with a bone age of six years with less than 50% loss of lateral column height (Group B). **b** Immediately following innominate osteotomy. Note the lateral displacement of the inferior quadrant of the pelvis and the asymmetry of the obturator foramina, indicating forward rotation of the distal pelvis. **c** Appearance one year later. Note the improved containment of the femoral head.

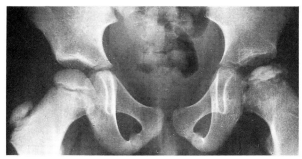

Figure 17.7 Perthes disease of the left hip in a boy with a chronological age of five years and a bone age of four and a half years. According to the lateral column classification he is in Group C (over 50% loss of lateral column height, though this is somewhat masked by some recent lateral ossification, which also indicates a poor prognosis). There is a large central area which has undergone avascular neurosis. There is a horizontal V-shaped defect at the junction of the growth plate and the lateral aspect of the neck. This is Gage sign and indicates a poor prognosis as does the broad band of metaphyseal rarefaction and uncovering of the head.

that is lateral to the Perkin line with the hip in neutral position compared to the percentage width on the opposite side.

Catterall assessment Catterall (1971) groups patients with Perthes disease into four groups depending on the amount of femoral head involvement as assessed in radiographs (*Table 17.1*). Those in which only the anterior 50% of the head is involved (groups I and II) have a good prognosis, while those in whom the greater part of the head is involved (groups III and IV) have a poorer prognosis in that there is more likely to be permanent deformation of the hip joint. Catterall has also drawn attention to various factors that worsen the prognosis whatever the radiological group. He described these as the 'head at risk' factors. They include:

- The radiological signs of lateral displacement of the head, calcification of the epiphysis lying lateral to the acetabulum, a radiolucent bite out of the

lateral edge of the epiphysis, growth plate and metaphysis known as Gage sign, a horizontal epiphyseal line, and gross metaphyseal change.
- Clinical factors such as progressive loss of motion, adduction contracture, flexion with abduction and the heavy child (*Figure 17.8*).

It may be difficult to determine the Catterall grouping for a period of up to eight months after presentation. Studies have shown difficulties in the assessment of the Catterall grades, with a significant amount of interobserver variability (Simmons *et al.*, 1990).

Salter sign (Salter and Thompson, 1984) drew attention to the fact that early radiographs may show a subchondral fracture, which is of prognostic value since the extent of involvement of the head is likely to be that portion of the head which underlies the fracture line (*Figure 17.3*). Salter also described a simple classification of Perthes disease into group A with less than 50% of the head involved and group B with more than 50% of the head involved. Group B heads tend to subluxate and the condition has a worse prognosis than group A Perthes disease.

Stage of the disease at the time of diagnosis and prognosis

Treatment is more likely to be successful in improving the prognosis if it commences early in the disease and before significant deformity has occurred.

Management

It should always be the aim to carry out management that interferes least with the patient's home and school lifestyle. Only those children who are likely to have arthritis later in life require vigorous treatment and less than 50% of patients with Perthes disease are likely to benefit from treatment. For the remainder, the prognosis cannot be improved by treatment. Clearly it is necessary to identify the child with a poor prognosis who is likely to benefit from treatment. Children who do not fall into this category may require treatment for phases of irrit-

Table 17.1 Catterall classification of Perthes disease

	Group I	Group II	Group III	Group IV
Percentage of head involved in disease process	Up to 25%	Up to 50%	Up to 75%	100%
Collapse of head	None	None or slight	Moderate	Severe
Sequestrum formation	None	Present	Present	Present
Metaphyseal change	Seldom and if present mild	Anterior	Extensive	Extensive

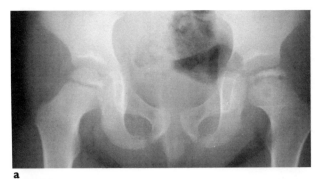

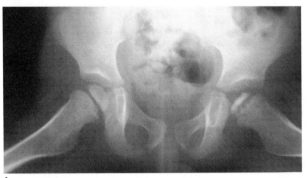

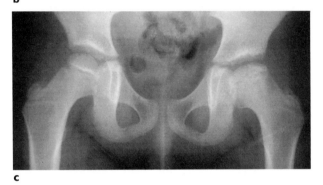

Figure 17.8 a,b A four-year-old boy (bone age three years) who has Perthes disease with a good prognosis. He has whole head involvement (Catterall group IV) and a metaphyseal cyst. **c** At eight years of age the boy has a spherical well-contained head. There is reconstitution of the head by bone with a normal trabecular pattern. There is loss of head height (distance from the growth plate to the joint space) and narrowing of the growth plate, both of which are common following whole head involvement.

ability (see below). The child with a poor prognosis typically presents with:

- A bone age of six years or more.
- Uncovering of the femoral head of more than 3 mm in excess of the uncovering on the unaffected side.
- Collapse of the lateral pillar of more than 50%.
- Catterall grading of III or IV (Catterall, 1971).

If the prognosis is good

Many children recover with an excellent clinical result when the condition has merely been treated symptomatically. Symptomatic treatment may involve periods of restricted activity if the child limps badly or complains of pain, but in general few restrictions are necessary and the child will moderate his activities according to his abilities. It may be necessary to take the child to and from school by car if he has been limping a lot and to avoid long trudges in the supermarket. Long-distance running and some regular sporting activities may have to be curtailed, but swimming is to be encouraged. The hip is observed clinically and radiologically at four monthly intervals. If despite periods of rest at home, the child limps badly and complains of pain, then he is admitted to hospital and the affected leg is suspended from a frame by two slings attached to springs. One sling supports the thigh and the other the calf. A period of ten days on slings and springs is usually adequate to convert an irritable hip into one with a painless range of motion, though that range is restricted when compared to normal.

If the prognosis is poor

If the prognosis is considered to be poor at the onset or if features suggesting a poor prognosis develop, then treatment designed to contain the femoral head within the acetabulum is instituted. Clearly this is only appropriate if the child has not presented too late for such treatment to be effective. It may be that examination under anaesthesia and arthrography are necessary to determine whether this is the case. If containment treatment cannot be carried out because of a late presentation and because an unacceptable degree of abduction of the leg is necessary to contain the head within the socket, the patient receives symptomatic treatment for the phases of irritability.

There is no evidence to suggest that any one method of containment gives superior results, nor does logic suggest that this should be the case. Prolonged conservative methods of containment have been used in the past such as the Birmingham splint. They are not usually used now because they disturb the child's life unnecessarily at an age when activity is desirable for normal physical and emotional development.

Conservative containment: many forms of orthoses and casts have been used to achieve containment by non-operative means. Broomstick casts are used for those children who have a poor prognosis yet lack the hip mobility, which is a necessary prerequisite for surgical containment. If the affected hip will not abduct sufficiently to allow the cast to be applied with the head properly covered, then a period on slings and springs may achieve this.

Some children exhibit the phenomenon of 'hinge abduction' (i.e. when the leg is abducted the lateral margin of the articular cartilage hinges on the lateral lip of the acetabulum instead of the head rotating normally within the acetabulum (*Figure 17.9*)). This can be demonstrated if the clinician holds the legs in full abduction while the radiographs are taken.

If the clinician finds that hinge abduction does not occur with the patient anaesthetized then there is a place for adductor and psoas tenotomy and then placing the hip in a broomstick cast in wide abduction for a period, before deciding whether to continue with non-operative containment or a form of operative containment. A broomstick cast may be used as a definitive form of management or a device such as the Scottish Rite brace can be employed (*Figure 17.9c*).

A difficulty in the use of conservative containment is the timing of treatment, whereas there is no end-point if the hip has been contained surgically because that containment will remain indefinitely. For conservative containment, the clinician must choose the time beyond which containment is not likely to improve the prognosis. It is generally considered appropriate to cease conservative containment when the hip is entering the reparative phase with the appearance of:

- Ossification in the epiphysis.
- The removal of all dense bone and a continuous line of bone along the surface of the femoral head.
- Some normal trabecular bone in the epiphysis.

In general, conservative containment is not used for a period shorter than 12 months and longer than 18 months.

Operative containment: the advantage of operative containment is that the child can generally resume a normal life without further interruptions for treatment; surgery therefore shortens the clinical course of the condition. Both innominate osteotomy (Salter, 1966) and femoral osteotomy are capable of giving similar results.

Innominate osteotomy (*Figure 17.6*) is capable of shortening the clinical course of the disease more than any other method of treatment. It is appropriate only if:

- Radiographs suggest that the condition is not longstanding and preferably when the symptoms have been present for less than six months.
- There is nearly a full range of movement of the hip. It is acceptable for the hip to lack 10° of movement in any direction, but no more than this.

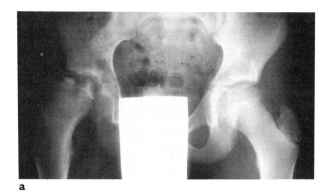

a

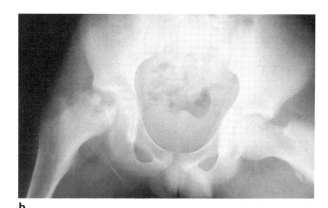

b

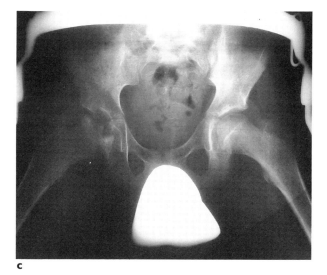

c

Figure 17.9 a This ten-year-old boy with late-onset Perthes disease presented with a gross increase in the head to teardrop distance accompanied by lateral displacement of the femoral head. **b** The range of abduction of the hip was approximately 15° only. The head impinges on the lateral lip of the acetabulum on abduction rather than rotating concentrically within the socket: this is 'hinge-abduction.' **c** Following adductor and psoas release, three months in a cast in abduction the head is concentric. This position was maintained in a Scottish Rite Brace (shown here) for a further three months.

- Radiographs in full abduction demonstrate that the femoral head can be covered by the acetabulum. An arthrogram to demonstrate that the cartilaginous head is spherical is not necessary if surgery is performed only on patients with early disease.

Innominate osteotomy carries the disadvantage of sometimes producing permanent restriction in motion at the hip joint, but this should not occur if it is performed on a mobile hip that has not had recurrent episodes of restricted movement.

Femoral osteotomy is appropriate for patients suitable for surgical containment but lacking the free range of motion necessary for innominate osteotomy (Evans et al., 1988). Some surgeons prefer femoral osteotomy to innominate osteotomy in all circumstances. The main aim of femoral osteotomy is to produce varus at the osteotomy site. This can be combined with derotation to reduce the degree of anteversion and extension. The alteration in the upper femoral anatomy is planned in order to better contain the femoral head within the acetabulum. The operation is less extensive and to some surgeons technically less demanding than a pelvic osteotomy. However the disadvantage of the procedure is that it results in shortening of the leg, a prominent trochanter, and in bilateral cases, an unsightly widening of the perineum. The amount of shortening and varus commonly lessens with the years, but this is not invariably the case. Femoral varus, derotation, extension osteotomy, as for Salter osteotomy, requires a second operative procedure to remove the internal fixation device.

Other surgical procedures: Chiari osteotomy and shelf arthroplasty have been performed by some to better contain the head. Cheilectomy (excision of the extruded anterolateral portion of the femoral head) does not have a good reputation and should be performed only after fusion of the growth plate.

In patients who have healed with a severely flattened head, the lateral portion of the head may impinge on the lateral lip of the acetabulum on abduction. This is commonly accompanied by pain, limp, shortening and limited abduction or fixed adduction. In these circumstances an abduction–extension femoral osteotomy is appropriate.

Removal of a loose body from the hip joint or drilling of a central avascular fragment of bone is very rarely indicated in those patients who have a form of Perthes disease similar to osteochondritis dissecans or in whom Perthes disease has preceded the development of osteochondritis dissecans.

Distal and lateral transfer of the greater trochanter is occasionally necessary in patients who have had premature closure of the proximal femoral growth plate with gross coxa breva and a high greater trochanter and have a Trendelenburg limp and fatigue pain.

REFERENCES AND FURTHER READING

Bensahel H, Bok B, Cavailloles F, Csukonyi Z. Bone scintigraphy in Perthes disease. *J Pediatr Orthop* 1983; **3**: 302–305.

Catterall A. The natural history of Perthes disease. *J Bone Joint Surg* 1971; **53B**: 37–53.

Catterall A. *Legg–Calvé–Perthes Disease*. Churchill Livingstone, Edinburgh, 1982.

Dickens DRV, Menelaus MB. The assessment of prognosis in Perthes disease. *J Bone Joint Surg* 1978; **60B**: 189–194.

Evans IK, Deluca PA, Gage JR. A comparative study of ambulation–abduction bracing and varus derotation osteotomy in the treatment of severe Legg–Calvé–Perthes disease in children over 6 years of age. *J Pediatr Orthop* 1988; **8**: 676–682.

Herring JA, Williams JJ, Neustadt MD, Early JS Evolution of femoral head deformity during the healing phase of Legg–Calvé–Perthes disease. *J Pediatr Orthop* 1993; **13**: 41–45.

McAndrew MP, Weinstein SL. A long-term follow-up of Legg–Calvé–Perthes disease. *J Bone Joint Surg* 1984; **66A**: 860–869.

Salter RB. Experimental and clinical aspects of Perthes disease. In: Proceedings of the Joint Meeting of the American Physicians Fellowship and the Israeli Orthopaedic Society. *J Bone Joint Surg* 1966; **48B**: 393–394.

Salter RB, Thompson GH. Legg–Calvé–Perthes disease. The prognostic significance of the subchondral fracture and a two-group classification of the femoral head involvement. *J Bone Joint Surg* 1984; **66A**: 479–489.

Simmons ED, Graham HK, Szalai JP. Interobserver variability in grading Perthes disease. *J Bone Joint Surg* 1990; **72B**: 202–204.

Stevens PM, Williams P, Menelaus M. Innominate osteotomy for Perthes disease. *J Pediatr Orthop* 1981; **1**: 47–54.

Chapter 18
Slipped Upper Femoral Epiphysis

Gary R Nattrass

Slipped upper femoral epiphysis (SUFE) is a disorder in which a dehiscence occurs through the growth plate of the immature hip. There is a progressive posterior and inferior displacement of the femoral head relative to the neck of the femur.

Incidence

The condition affects about three per 100,000 children and is more common in boys than girls (4:1). The condition usually occurs in boys between 12–14 years of age, but occurs earlier in girls at 11–13 years of age. There is familial association with a 7% risk to a second family member. It has previously been said to be bilateral in about 25% of cases, but recent work indicates that at maturity it can be seen that 60% have had involvement on both sides. The left side is more commonly affected than the right.

Aetiology

Most slips are idiopathic without any underlying cause. The boys may be overweight with delayed puberty, but this is not invariable. It has been postulated that these boys have an imbalance between growth hormone (which causes physeal hypertrophy and rapid growth) and the gonadal hormones (which stimulate physeal fusion). However, this has never been proven. In a few cases there may be an aetiological factor (*Table 18.1*). If there is an unusual presentation such as the child is not in the expected age group, or there is a history of medical problems, specific aetiologies should be considered. It is currently believed that endocrine screening laboratory tests are not indicated unless there is a clinical suspicion that there may be an underlying disorder.

Table 18.1 Aetiology of slipped upper femoral epiphysis

Weight	Adipogenital syndrome
Endocrine disorder	Hypothyroidism Hypogonadism Hypopituitarism Growth hormone therapy
Cranial disorder	Head injury Craniopharyngioma
Renal disorder	Renal osteodystrophy
Connective tissue disorder	Marfan syndrome, Down syndrome
Iatrogenic	Chemotherapy, radiation

Pathology

The abnormality of SUFE lies in the zone of hypertrophy of the growth plate. Disorganization of the chondrocyte columns occurs, with the normal longitudinal and transverse collagenous septa being replaced by an homogeneous matrix with scattered, irregularly-orientated fibrils. This is distinct from the pathology of a Salter I physeal fracture, which occurs between the zone of hypertrophy and zone of provisional calcification.

The direction of the slip results in the epiphysis lying posterior to the metaphysis, and then secondarily, the epiphysis slips inferiorly to the metaphysis. Approximately 70% are chronic slips and remodelling of the posterior femoral neck can be seen on the lateral radiograph. Most of the rest are acute-on-chronic, with evidence of remodelling on the posterior femoral neck with a sudden slip further than this. An acute slip with no remodelling is unusual.

Table 18.2   Classification of slipped upper femoral epiphysis

Chronological	
Acute	Less than three weeks of symptoms
Acute-on-chronic	An acute exacerbation with a background of symptoms lasting longer than three weeks
Chronic	Symptoms lasting longer than three weeks.

Extent of slip	
Pre-slip	No movement
Mild	Less than one-third slip
Moderate	One-third to one-half slip
Severe	Greater than one-half slip

Clinical Features

Symptoms

Presentation of SUFE is with either hip or knee pain or both. Commonly there is only knee pain and the unwary clinician may decide the knee is normal and not consider hip pathology. Some patients present after many months of mild pain whereas others present acutely with signs similar to those of a fracture after a mild injury. Classification of the slip is by the symptoms and the severity on radiographs (*Table 18.2*). The patients with acute slips have great difficulty in walking, whereas the children with chronic slips can usually walk without aids.

Signs

The patient lies on the examination couch with an external rotation deformity of the hip. There is restriction of flexion, abduction and internal rotation, and all these movements cause pain. In flexion the limb goes into abduction and external rotation. There may be a small amount of real leg length discrepancy.

Radiology

Plain radiographs (anteroposterior and frog leg lateral) must be obtained for any child suspected of having hip pathology. Most cases can be diagnosed from these two views (*Figure 18.1*). The severity of the slip is assessed by the amount of displacement. The angle of displacement can also be measured (*Figures 18.2, 18.3*). Fortunately the two correspond,

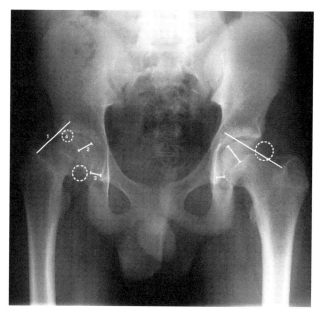

Figure 18.1   Findings of a slipped upper femoral epiphysis on the anteroposterior radiograph compared to the normal side. (1) The Klein or Trethowan line demonstrates the migration of the neck superior to the epiphysis. (2) The apparent height of the epiphysis is decreased as it has slipped posteriorly. (3) The joint space is relatively increased inferiorly. (4) The changes of remodelling of the neck reveal this to be a chronic slip.

ALSO:- SHENTONS LINE DISRUPTED
    :- AFFECTED SIDE IS OSTEOPENIC in CHRONIC
        CASES.

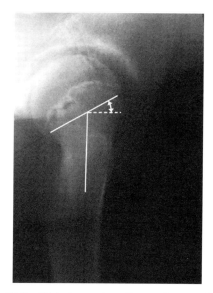

Figure 18.2   This lateral radiograph reveals posterior displacement of the epiphysis relative to the neck as well as the signs of remodelling in this chronic slip.

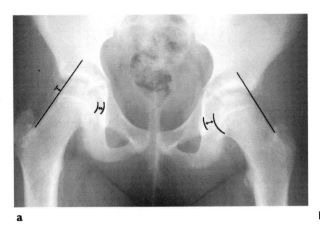 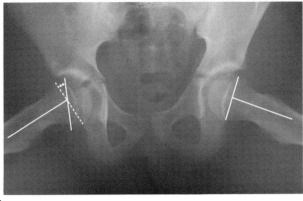

a   b

Figure 18.3 **a** Mild slips can be difficult to diagnose radiologically. Comparison with the opposite hip on this anteroposterior radiograph of the pelvis shows the abnormality in the Klein (or Trethowan) line as well as the increased joint space in this patient with a mild right slip. **b** Frog leg lateral view of the pelvis confirms the posterior displacement of the head relative to the neck.

so 30% displacement is usually about 30° of angulation. Severity measurements in degrees are mild (0–30°), moderate (30–50°) and severe (over 50°).

Acute and chronic slips can be differentiated by the presence of remodelling of the posterior femoral neck on the lateral radiograph. Some patients present in a pre-slip phase where there has been no movement, but there is pain, and in these cases there is often widening or irregularity of the growth plate on the radiograph. Computerized tomography (CT) can be useful to show the degree of slip, while ultrasound may be useful in quantifying the severity of the slip, defining a haemarthrosis and identifying remodelling indicating a chronic slip (*Table 18.3*).

Management

The goal of treatment is to prevent further displacement before physeal closure and to ensure that the treatment itself does not cause complications.

The child is kept non-weight bearing and admitted urgently to hospital.

In the child with mild or moderate chronic SUFE the hip is pinned *in situ*, while for the child with the severe chronic SUFE, reduction of the upper femoral epiphysis or an osteotomy to realign the upper femoral anatomy can be considered. In our institution all chronic cases are pinned *in situ*. An osteotomy is considered at a later stage for severe slips depending on the gait and degree of clinical deformity of the leg.

For the child with an acute or acute-on-chronic presentation with a mild or moderate deformity, *in situ* pinning is performed. Manipulation of these cases has been abandoned in most centres because of the unacceptable risk of avascular necrosis, but some centres use open reduction or osteotomy for the severe case. In our institution we aspirate the hip and then use gentle traction, aiming for a slow reduction over a few days, and then pin *in situ*. It is important not to manipulate the hip or use excessive traction because of the risk of avascular necrosis. The aim is to bring the epiphysis back to its position before the acute component of the slip. Overcorrection leads to stretching of the posterior retinacular

Table 18.3 Radiographic findings of slipped upper femoral epiphysis

Plain radiographs
Anteroposterior view of the pelvis
Migration of neck superiorly relative to epiphysis (Klein or Trethowan line)
Widening or irregularity of physis
Decreased apparent size of epiphysis
Widening of joint space

Frog leg lateral view
Posterior displacement or angulation of the epiphysis relative to the neck
Signs of remodelling indicating chronic slip

Computerized tomography
Posterior displacement of the epiphysis relative to the neck

Ultrasound
Presence or absence of effusion (acute or chronic)
Evidence of metaphyseal remodelling

vessels over the bump of remodelling on the posterior part of the femoral neck and may lead to avascular necrosis.

Traction

This is only used for acute slips as a gentle and slow method of reduction. Longitudinal traction of 2–3 kg is used over 2–4 days, together with 0.5 kg of internal rotation. Skeletal traction is used for the larger child over 55 kg and skin traction for smaller children.

In situ pinning

This is presently the 'gold standard' of treatment. Although many fixation devices have been used in the past (e.g. Knowles, Steinman, and Haigie pins), we now use a cannulated screw. Multiple pins have been used, but most centres would now advocate the use of a single well-placed screw across the physis. While there is a slight mechanical advantage to using two screws, there is a greatly increased chance of perforation into the joint and subsequent chondrolysis.

Some of the factors for successful *in situ* pinning are listed in Table 18.4. There is an increased incidence of avascular necrosis when a fracture table is used, presumably due to inadvertent reduction of the epiphysis when positioning the patient. We use a radiolucent table with a sandbag to partially turn the patient and place the guide wire percutaneously. A frog leg lateral image is obtained before advancing through the growth plate.

Table 18.4 Key points in the placement of the screw

Image intensifier
Radiolucent table
Anterior entry site on neck (*this is NOT a pinning of a fractured hip!*)
Do not cross physis until biplanar alignment is achieved
Ensure that the pin is into epiphysis and not into the joint by multiplanar radiographic evaluation

Perforation into the joint by the pin should be avoided. If the screw is left protruding through the head into the joint, there is direct articular cartilage damage and a higher incidence of chondrolysis. It has now been shown that a protruding screw or drill that is immediately removed from the joint is not associated with an increased incidence of chondrolysis. Using an anterior entry site and passing across the neck from anterior to posterior ensures that the centre of the epiphysis is pinned in its slipped position (*Figures 18.4, 18.5*). Breakage of the drill or screw can occur and the broken hardware should be removed if possible.

Postoperatively the patient is kept partially weight-bearing until the limb is comfortable and the quadriceps is strong. Activities can be increased as tolerated.

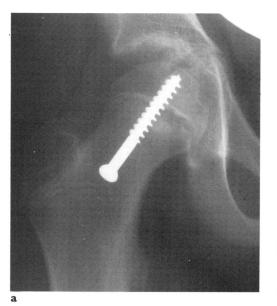
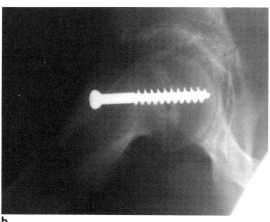

a   b

Figure 18.4 a Pin placement of the mild slip should be central in the plate and epiphysis. **b** In the lateral view the line of the screw is at right angles to the plate in both planes. The entry point is on the anterior part of the femoral neck.

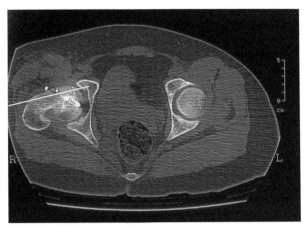

Figure 18.5 Computerized tomographic (CT) scan of a chronic severe slip with a marked posterior displacement of the epiphysis. It is essential to place the screw through an anterior entry site on the neck. If the screw is placed along the axis of the neck, as shown, the epiphysis is missed or poorly held. CT scans can be used to confirm the position when the plain radiographs are difficult to interpret.

Screw removal

The screw should be left in until there is definite radiographic evidence of physeal closure. This is at approximately one year after the pinning, but will vary between individuals. Removal of the hardware is desirable as many of these patients will eventually require further surgery on the hip. Removal of the screw before physeal closure can lead to further slipping. Follow-up radiographs should also ensure that the epiphysis does not grow off the implant as further slipping can occur. The use of a screw seems to have abolished this complication which occurred with some of the smooth pins used in the past.

Pin removal has been difficult in the past because of bony overgrowth. The cannulated screw has a large head, which helps in its removal and reverse cutting. We use an image intensifier so the incision can be as small as possible.

Prophylactic pinning

Some centres advocate prophylactic pinning of all contralateral hips because of the high incidence of bilateral slips. Other centres, fearful of the incidence of chondrolysis in the contralateral pinned hip, only pin for symptoms. We advocate contralateral prophylactic pinning in those who present young or have a metabolic aetiology, in nomads and if there may be poor compliance.

Other treatment options

Cast immobilization

This has been used in the past in an attempt to prevent further slipping until the physis closes. However, the treatment has to be continued for several months and poor results have been reported. It appears that it neither prevents further slipping nor prevents the operative complications of chondrolysis and avascular necrosis. It is not a practical option.

Manipulation

Although this has been carried out on many acute-on-chronic slips in the past, it has now been abandoned in most centres because of the high incidence of avascular necrosis.

Open epiphyseodesis

This achieves a quick fusion of the growth plate and is advocated by some, but good results have not been achieved by all. It has a possible role in the treatment of severe slips, but requires an experienced surgeon. There are high reported rates of avascular necrosis and chondrolysis.

Open reduction and epiphyseodesis

This has been advocated for severe slips in an attempt to reduce the late incidence of osteoarthritis due to anatomical malalignment. The epiphysis is further displaced through an open approach without stretching the posterior retinacular vessels. The remodelling on the posterior neck is removed and the neck is shortened. The epiphysis is reduced and fixed with pins. Although the incidence of avascular necrosis is low in the hands of experts, great skill is required to obtain a successful outcome. It should not be carried out if there is already partial fusion of the growth plate.

Primary osteotomy

Osteotomies have also been advocated as a primary treatment in an attempt to correct the deformity of the slip and later osteoarthritis. These have been described at the cervical level, but the incidence of avascular necrosis is unacceptably high, although the alignment is good. Basal cervical osteotomies such as the Sugioko, give good correction, but the incidence of complications is high. Trochanteric osteotomies have been described, but these are technically very demanding and no long-term results are available. Correction at the subtrochanteric level, such as the biplanar osteotomy of Southwick, is safe with a low risk of avascular necrosis. The rationale is to place the epiphysis within the acetabulum in its normal

Table 18.5 Royal Children's Hospital, Melbourne, protocol for managing slipped upper femoral epiphysis

Acute or acute-on-chronic	
Immediate admission.	
Mild	Percutaneous pin *in situ*
Moderate or severe	Aspiration of hip
	Gentle longitudinal and rotational traction
	Percutaneous pinning at 2–4 days
Chronic	
Percutaneous pinning *in situ* without preceding aspiration or traction	
Subtrochanteric osteotomy later for severe clinical deformity	

orientation. This often distorts the upper femoral anatomy to such an extent that it can be very difficult to place a femoral component in a subsequent total hip replacement.

Cheilectomy

In the moderate to severe slip, abduction may be restricted by the bump on the lateral aspect of the femoral neck. This may be removed by cheilectomy to improve abduction. Cheilectomy combined with an open epiphyseodesis has been described as a primary treatment – the Herndon–Heyman procedure. Although the results from one centre are good, this is not widely practised.

Our strategy for managing the severe slip is to pin it *in situ* then carry out an osteotomy at a later stage if necessary. This is an easy operation with few complications with the expectation of some remodelling. Alternative strategies involve a more difficult initial procedure with more complications except in expert hands. However, anatomy is restored to try to prevent premature osteoarthritis. Our strategy has been developed to keep our complication rate of avascular necrosis and chondrolysis as low as possible as these are terrible and virtually untreatable complications in young people. Some patients may end up with premature osteoarthritis as a result of this policy, but we believe that this can be dealt with at a later stage (*Table 18.5*).

Remodelling of the deformity

Approximately 70% of all slips will develop an acceptable functional range of motion. It has been thought that remodelling over the first one or two years causes this improvement, but it may be a product of stretching of the soft tissues.

The late deformity is of external rotation with a lack of flexion and abduction. Patients complain of

difficulty in activities such as sitting at the theatre or on public transport and in running. The indication for surgery is residual deformity after one year causing significant functional impairment. Osteotomy to rectify this can be performed at any level of the upper femur, but most would correct at the subtrochanteric level. The Southwick biplanar osteotomy corrects the extension and adduction deformity by a flexion and abduction osteotomy with correction of the external rotation deformity. Other upper femoral osteotomies such as the basi-cervical as described by Sugioko or Griffiths are technically more demanding and long-term results are not impressive.

Complications

Chondrolysis

Chondrolysis is a global loss of articular cartilage within the hip joint. It has been described in 10–20% of SUFEs and the incidence is greater in acute slips and after manipulation. It can occur where no treatment is given for the slip and rarely it can occur in a normal hip. It is probably an immunological reaction, and is more common with pin protrusion (*Figure 18.6*). It presents with pain, a decreased range of motion and radiographic findings of joint space narrowing.

Treatment consists of rest, maintenance of the maximal range of motion and oral anti-inflammatories. About 50% resolve satisfactorily, but the rest cause continuing pain and result in a degenerative arthritis and there maybe a fixed flexion deformity. Recently there has been some enthusiasm for distraction arthroplasty using external fixation devices (Orthofix or Ilizarov). These still allow flexion and extension while 'reconstituting' a joint space. While the short-term results are encouraging, the long-term

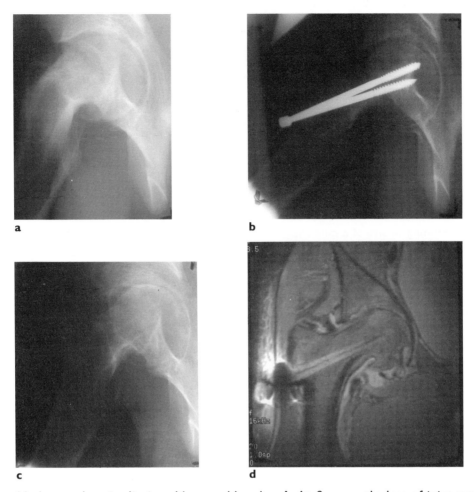

a   b

c   d

Figure 18.6 a Moderate chronic slip in a 16-year-old male. **b** At five months loss of joint space is evident. **c** At ten months the joint space narrowing has progressed when the screws were removed. **d** Magnetic resonance image nine months after screw removal shows complete loss of articular cartilage.

outcome is still unknown. Late treatment includes osteotomy to realign any deformity and arthrodesis of the joint, and eventually some need total hip replacement.

Avascular necrosis

The incidence of avascular necrosis is about 5% in the chronic slips, but this is higher after attempts at manipulation and if the pin placement has been in the posterosuperior quadrant. In acute-on-chronic cases the incidence is about 20% and even higher in those that are manipulated (*Figure 18.7*). The natural history is for increasing pain, restricted movement and degenerative change.

Treatment comprises rest, anti-inflammatory drugs and range of motion exercises, but the prognosis is poor. Surgical treatment is on an individual basis. If the head collapses there may be a risk of

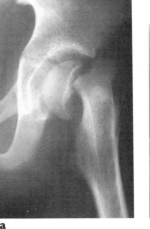 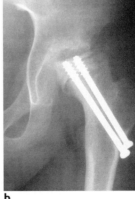

a   b

Figure 18.7 a Eight-year-old Down syndrome boy with an acute severe slip. **b** Radiographs nine months later demonstrate avascular necrosis.

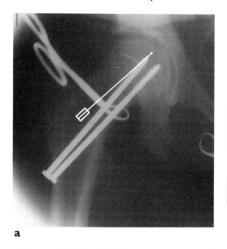 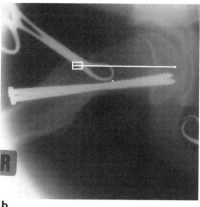 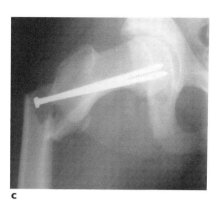

a   b   c

Figure 18.8 a,b Pinning *in situ* of a mild slip. The entry site is too low and lateral. The added line shows the preferred line of the screws. **c** Two weeks later this 11-year-old girl sustained a fracture, which was treated by a hip screw.

pin penetration, so the pins should be removed and placed in a better position if the physis is still open. Some may respond to realignment of any preserved articular cartilage by valgus osteotomy or a Sugioko osteotomy. Sometimes there may be subluxation of the femoral head and a shelf acetabuloplasty may provide better cover. Often the decision is between an arthrodesis and a total hip replacement.

Deformity

The common residual deformity is that of external rotation and extension. If the deformity is symptomatic it is treated by a biplanar osteotomy at the subtrochanteric level, but there is no evidence that this reduces the incidence of osteoarthritis.

Fracture

This is uncommon, but can occur when the placement of the pins has been started too low. Treatment is by open reduction and internal fixation (*Figure 18.8*).

Further slipping

Occasionally the femoral head can grow off the end of the pins and the epiphysis can slip further. It is uncommon but may occur if:

- The patient is young and the physis does not fuse with the placement of the pin.
- The fixation device is removed before fusion of the physis.
- The original placement of the pin was not into the epiphysis or was very eccentric in the epiphysis.

Osteoarthritis

Follow-up studies have revealed a high incidence of osteoarthritis in well-treated slips without any complications. The natural history of the malunited slip is of a slow deterioration and the development of degenerative change.

In addition many early-presenting cases of hip osteoarthritis have a 'bullet-shaped' head on the anteroposterior radiograph, indicating an earlier asymptomatic slip. Stulberg found that approximately 40% of a group of patients with idiopathic osteoarthritis had radiographic changes identical to those of a group of patients known to have had a SUFE. Some may be improved by osteotomy, but many require total hip replacement.

REFERENCES AND FURTHER READING

Aadalen RJ, Weiner DS, Hoyt W, Herndon CH. Acute slipped capital femoral epiphysis. *J Bone Joint Surg* 1974; **56A**: 1473–1487.

Aldegheri R, Trivella G, Saleh M. Articulated distraction of the hip. *Clin Orthop Rel Research* 1994; **301**: 94–101.

Boyer DW, Mickelson MR, Ponseti IV. Slipped capital femoral epiphysis: long-term follow-up study of one hundred and twenty-one patients. *J Bone Joint Surg* 1981; **63A**: 85–95.

Broughton NS, Todd RC, Dunn DM, Angel JC. Open reduction of the severely slipped upper femoral epiphysis. *J Bone Joint Surg* 1988; **70B**: 435–439.

Carey R, Moran P, Cole W. The place of threaded pin fixation in the treatment of slipped upper femoral epiphysis. *Clin Orthop Rel Research* 1987; **224**: 45–51.

Carney R, Weinstein S, Noble J. Long term follow-up of slipped capital femoral epiphysis. *J Bone Joint Surg* 1991; **73A**: 667–674.

Fish JB. Cuneiform osteotomy of the femoral neck in the treatment of slipped capital femoral epiphysis. *J Bone Joint Surg* 1984; **66A**: 1153–1168.

Hagglund G, Hansson LI, Ordeberg G, Sandstrom S. Bilaterality in slipped upper femoral epiphysis. *J Bone Joint Surg* 1988; **70B**: 179–181.

Heyman CH, Herndon CH, Bell DM. Treatment of slipped capital femoral epiphysis by epiphysiodesis and osteoplasty of the femoral neck. *J Bone Joint Surg* 1963; **45A**: 999–1012.

Kallio PE, Paterson DC, Foster BK, Lequesne GW. Classification in slipped capital femoral epiphysis. Sonographic assessment of stability and remodelling. *Clin Orthop Rel Research* 1993; **294**: 196–203.

Mickelson MR, Ponseti IV, Cooper RR, Maynard MA. The ultrastructure of the growth plate in slipped capital femoral epiphysis. *J Bone Joint Surg* 1977; **59A**: 1076–1081.

O'Brien ET, Fahey JJ. Remodeling of the femoral neck after in situ pinning for slipped capital femoral epiphysis. *J Bone Joint Surg* 1977; **59A**: 62–68.

Salvati EA, Robinson HJ, O'Dowd TJ. Southwick osteotomy for severe chronic slipped capital femoral epiphysis. *J Bone Joint Surg* 1980; **62A**: 561–570.

Sugioko Y. Transtrochanteric anterior rotational osteotomy of femoral head in the treatment of osteonecrosis affecting the hip. *Clin Orthop Rel Research* 1978; **130**: 191–201.

Weiner DS. Bone graft epiphysiodesis in the treatment of slipped capital femoral epiphysis. *Instructional Course Lectures* 1989; **38**: 263–272.

Wells D, King J, Roe T, Kaufman F. Review of slipped capital femoral epiphysis associated with endocrine disease. *J Pediatr Orthop* 1993; **13**: 610–614.

Chapter 19
The Knee

Nigel S Broughton

CONGENITAL RECURVATUM OF THE KNEE

This is recognized at birth with hyperextension of the knee. The knee is mobile, but flexion is limited. It can be treated by malleable splints to hold the knee in increasing degrees of flexion, and as the condition improves a Pavlik harness can be used to maintain this flexed posture. The prognosis is good.

CONGENITAL DISLOCATION OF THE KNEE

This is a rare condition with an incidence of two per 100,000 live births. Approximately 35% of cases are bilateral. It is more common in girls in a ratio of 2:1. In 45% of cases there is an associated developmental dysplasia of the hip (DDH) and 30% of cases have talipes equinovarus. It is a feature of Larsen syndrome, a condition of ligamentous laxity, when it is usually bilateral and associated with bilateral hip dislocation. It is also seen in Down syndrome and arthrogryposis.

Pathology

The child is born with a hyperextension deformity of the knee. The appearance is similar to congenital recurvatum of the knee, but in congenital dislocation of the knee the tibia is dislocated anteriorly to the femur and the quadriceps are tight (*Figure 19.1*). There may also be a valgus deformity and lateral displacement of the tibia. The patella is high and the anterior capsule is tight. The cruciates are usually absent and because of the forward displacement of the tibia on the femur the hamstrings act as extensors.

Management

The knee is usually too stiff to allow splintage in a corrected position and an open reduction is usually required at the age of 3–6 months. Surgical correction consists of quadriceps lengthening and capsular release to reduce the tibia on to the femur; the knee is then splinted in a flexed position. The condition is difficult to treat successfully and patients often have knee problems as they mature due to ligamentous instability.

PATELLAR DISLOCATION

Congenital Patellar Dislocation

Congenital dislocation of the patella is rare. The presentation is of a newborn with a fixed flexion deformity of the knee and lateral rotation of the tibia. It is commonly bilateral, often familial, and occurs in Down syndrome, arthrogryposis and other

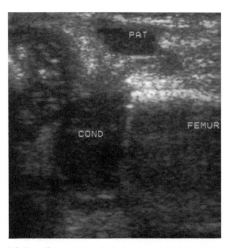

Figure 19.1 Congenital dislocation of the knee. The ultrasound demonstrates the forward displacement of the tibia on the femur.

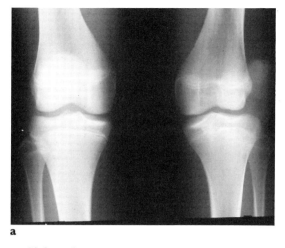
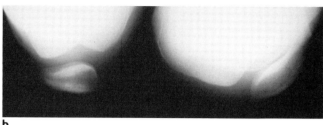

Figure 19.2 a Congenital dislocation of the patella. The anteroposterior view shows lateral displacement of the patella. **b** Skyline view confirms lateral displacement of the patella.

syndromes. It is often difficult to palpate the patella in its dislocated position high and lateral to the lateral femoral condyle, and diagnosis is often delayed until the child starts walking (*Figure 19.2*). Radiography is unrewarding in the early stages because the patella does not have an ossific nucleus until the child is aged three years, but ultrasound demonstrates the abnormality.

Management

Treatment is by surgery when the condition is diagnosed, with a large lateral release, medial plication, a Roux–Goldthwaite and a tenodesis using semitendinosus. Sometimes in an older chid the tight hamstrings may have to be addressed. Problems in later life are common despite adequate early surgery because of the flat retropatellar surface and the flat femoral trochlea.

Habitual Patellar Dislocation

Habitual patellar dislocation or subluxation can occur in flexion or in extension. It occurs every time the knee is moved and can be demonstrated clearly by a careful examination (*Figure 19.3*). It is always in a lateral direction in a knee that has not had previous surgery, but can occasionally be seen in a medial direction after overenthusiastic surgery. When the dislocation occurs in flexion, if the patella is held in the midline, flexion is restricted to about 30°; if the patella is allowed to dislocate full flexion can be obtained.

Aetiology

Aetiological factors include:

- Contracture of the vastus lateralis, which is sometimes due to neonatal intramuscular injections into the thigh.

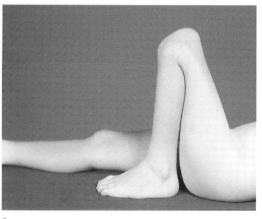
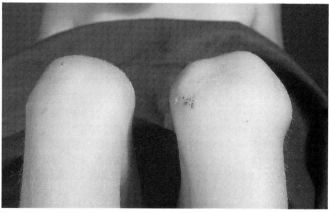

Figure 19.3a,b   Habitual dislocation of the patella in flexion.

- Ligamentous laxity syndromes. This condition is relatively common in children with Down syndrome who have a combination of tight lateral structures and lax medial structures.
- Patella alta in which the patella is usually high in habitual dislocation in extension, and the patella escapes from the lateral femoral condyle on extension.

Management

This is a difficult condition to treat and recurrence is common. Arthroscopic closed lateral release is unlikely to be effective. An open procedure is usually required. The proximal realignment consists of a large lateral release with a complete detachment of the vastus lateralis; if full flexion is still not possible then rectus femoris should be lengthened. The distal realignment consists of 'medialization' of the attachment of the patellar tendon onto the tibia. If the growth plate has fused the whole of the tibial tubercle can be shifted medially, but in the younger child the lateral half of the patellar tendon is detached, threaded under the rest of the patellar tendon and reattached onto the periosteum of the tibia more medially to avoid damaging the upper tibial growth plate (Roux–Goldthwaite). In more difficult cases semitendinosus tenodesis may be used, and in some the patella alta may have to be addressed by distal transfer of the patellar tendon and a V–Y quadricepsplasty.

Acute Patellar Dislocation

Clinical Features

History
Following a twisting fall, the quadriceps contracts and pulls the patella over the lateral femoral condyle. The knee is stuck in flexion. The pain is poorly localized as the medial retinaculum is torn and painful. Usually the patient feels a large lump (the patella) on the lateral aspect of the knee, but sometimes there is confusion because the undue prominence of the medial femoral condyle can raise the suggestion that this is a medial dislocation of the patella. However, medial dislocation of the patella does not occur in a knee that has had no previous operations. Often the patella spontaneously reduces and the differentiation from a torn anterior cruciate or a displacing torn meniscus can be difficult.

Examination
If the child presents with the patella dislocated the diagnosis is straightforward. If reduction has already taken place, the knee is swollen with a haemarthrosis and there is tenderness over the torn medial retinaculum.

Management

If the patella is still dislocated, it should be immediately reduced under sedation by medial pressure on the patella as the knee is extended. Radiographs are then taken. These often show the haemarthrosis, but their main purpose is to identify any osteochondral fracture (from the retropatellar surface or the lateral femoral condyle) or an avulsion fracture from the medial aspect of the patella.

Indications for surgery after an acute patellar dislocation are for an osteochondral loose fragment and an avulsion fracture of the medial aspect of the patella.

Arthroscopy is performed if a loose body is seen on the radiograph and is removed or reattached according to its size. An open approach is performed if reattachment of an avulsed fragment from the medial side of the patella is necessary and in the rare circumstances where the patella cannot be reduced closed. Enthusiasts have widened the indications for arthroscopy after all acute patellar dislocations:

- To speed up rehabilitation by washing out the haemarthrosis.
- To remove chondral fragments that do not show up on plain radiographs.
- To perform lateral release and medial plication as up to 50% of acute dislocations will recur.

In those patients who do not require operative intervention, the knee is aspirated to relieve pain and supported in a bandage and splint for comfort and to keep the knee extended. Quadriceps exercises are commenced when possible and the splint is discarded when the knee is comfortable and the quadriceps strong. In the long term vastus medialis is strengthened in an attempt to prevent recurrent dislocations.

Recurrent Acute Patellar Dislocation

Clinical Features

Approximately 50% of acute dislocations recur. The condition is often bilateral and more common in girls (2:1), and there is a familial association.

On examination, if the knee is flexed past 30° with a thumb on the medial side of the patella pushing laterally, the patient often stops the test by grasping the examiner's hand. This is a positive apprehension test.

Aetiology

Aetiological factors include:

- Ligamentous laxity. Often there is generalized ligamentous laxity and the patella is freely mobile.
- Muscle abnormality with a weak or poorly developed vastus medialis. There may be tight bands in the lateral retinaculum or a short vastus lateralis.
- Abnormal Q angle. The Q angle is defined as the angle of deviation between a line along the quadriceps and a line along the patellar tendon (*Figure 19.4a*). It should not be more than 20°. Lateral

rotation of the tibia and genu valgum can contribute to an abnormal Q angle.
- Abnormal shape to the patellofemoral articulation. The patella may be high riding (patella alta), the retropatellar surface may be flat and the lateral femoral condyle may be deficient, giving rise to a flat femoral trochlea groove.

Radiology

An anteroposterior view, a lateral view, a notch view and a skyline view should be performed. This allows the identification of any loose body, patella alta and the relationship of the patella to the femoral trochlea. If the lateral view is taken at 30° flexion the superior pole of the patella should not be higher than a line extended from the central part of the distal femoral growth plate (Blumensaat line) (*Figure 19.4b*). Insall and Salvati described the determination

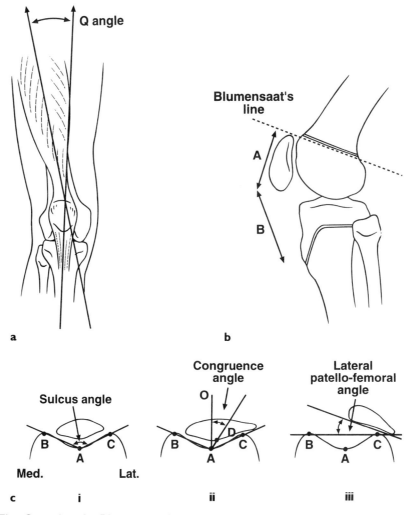

Figure 19.4 a The Q angle. **b** Blumensaat line. **c** Radiological measurements on the skyline view. In the measurement of congruence angle, the line OA bisects the angle BAC.

of patella alta on the lateral view by measuring the greatest dimension of the patella and comparing it to the distance between the inferior pole of the patella and the site of attachment of the patellar tendon to the tibial tuberosity. Patella alta is defined when the patellar tendon length is more than 20% greater than the patella size.

Various skyline views have been described. We use the Laurin technique where the patient lies supine with the knees flexed to 30°. The plate is held by the patient and the beam is placed over the patient's feet to shoot proximally. This gives a good view of the patellofemoral articulation.

The sulcus angle describes the depth of the femoral trochlea. The congruence angle measures the amount of lateral subluxation and is said to be abnormal if more than 16°. The lateral patellofemoral angle is a measurement of lateral tilt and is abnormal if zero or less (*Figure 19.4c*). Although various other angles have been constructed from skyline views we have not found any of these to be useful in deciding whether to operate on these children.

Management

The urge to operate on all children who present with an acute dislocation of the patella must be resisted. Generally we offer surgery to children who have sustained more than two dislocations in one year. Many children grow out of the tendency to dislocate and can avoid the need for surgery with vastus medialis strengthening. However, recurrent dislocators run the risk of causing osteochondral damage, producing loose bodies in the joint, and leading to osteoarthritis in later life.

Arthroscopic closed lateral release allows a careful appraisal of any intraarticular pathology, can be carried out through minimal incisions and is associated with a relatively quick recovery. Its success rate is in the order of 70%, but it is less reliable when the Q angle is high, if there is excessive ligamentous laxity and if there is demonstrable habitual subluxation. In these circumstances or where an arthroscopic lateral release has failed, an open approach should be performed.

Proximal realignment
A lateral release, plication of the medial retinaculum, and advancement or lateralization of the vastus medialis onto the anterior surface of the patella is performed. A semitendinosus tenodesis can also be carried out by detaching the tendon proximally, leaving it attached distally and passing it through a drill hole in the patella to prevent any lateral displacement. There is also a sling procedure in which a strip of the medial retinaculum is detached distally, passed under the quadriceps and then around the muscle, and then sutured back onto itself, but this is now rarely used.

Distal realignment
Various techniques have been described, although they all aim to move the vector of the pull through the patellar tendon more medially and reduce the Q angle. If the upper tibial growth plate is open, the tibial tubercle cannot be moved because of the risk of partial growth plate arrest and the unsightly complication of recurvatum. In these circumstances the patellar tendon should be split and the lateral half passed under the rest of the tendon and attached via the periosteum to the tibia in a more medial position (Roux–Goldthwaite technique). If the growth plate has fused the tibial tubercle should be moved laterally. Distal advancement and a more posterior positioning of the tibial attachment by placing the transposed tubercle into a slot (Hauser technique) are now contraindicated because of the risk of patellofemoral osteoarthritis. The most popular transposition now is medial angulation of a long tapering cut of the tubercle and fixation with one or two screws in the manner of the Elmslie technique. This achieves the objective of keeping the level of attachment at the same place on an anteroposterior and lateral radiograph in the expectation of not increasing the risk of osteoarthritis (*Figure 19.5*).

ANTERIOR KNEE PAIN

Anterior knee pain is a descriptive term that could be used for any specific disorder causing pain around the front of the knee. Generally, it is now used to describe pain arising from the patellofemoral articulation. Many names have been used to describe the syndrome in the past, including patellar pain syndrome, excess lateral patellar pressure, and chondromalacia patellae. However, children with the clinical picture of painful patellofemoral articulation often do not have the pathology of chondromalacia on the retropatellar surface, and the changes of chondromalacia patellae may be seen where there are no specific symptoms from it. Anterior knee pain seems to be as good a term as any to describe this common clinical condition.

Anterior knee pain is common in adolescents and can be a cause of great concern in communities where sporting endeavour at school is important. It is usually bilateral and affects girls more than boys. When the incidence has been carefully sought, up to 20% of adolescents may report some symptoms. It

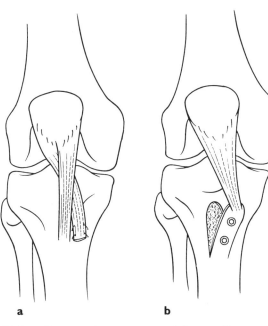

a　　　　　　　b　　　　　　　b

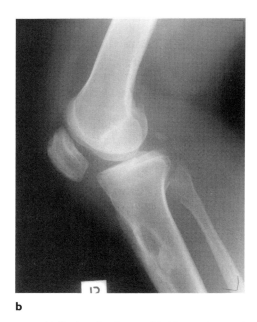

Figure 19.5　a Moving the insertion of the patellar tendon more medially by the Roux–Goldthwaite technique.
b The Elmslie technique used when the growth plate has fused.　**c** Patella baja and early osteoarthritis after using the Hauser technique for medialization of the insertion of the patellar tendon.

may be used as an excuse to retire from exercise and can put considerable stress on family dynamics. Sometimes there is a clear psychological element.

Clinical Features

History

The child complains of pain around the front of the knee either during or after exercise. Night pain is unusual, but the pain is worse on climbing stairs or hills. There are often descriptions of clicking or grating as the knee is flexed. Pseudolocking can occur after sitting in one position for a long time. Sitting in the back seat of a car for a prolonged period may produce the description of the 'knees locking up' and having to be 'clicked free' when the child gets out of the car.

Examination

The knee usually looks normal, although rarely there may be an effusion. There is tenderness around the patella and on the retropatellar surface. Movement of the patella on the underlying trochlea may produce pain and crepitus. There is no tenderness over the medial or lateral joint lines. There may be crepitus of the patellofemoral articulation on flexing the knee. The patella may track abnormally with lateral tracking or subluxation on flexion.

Radiology

Radiographs should be taken of the knee, and lateral subluxation may be seen in the skyline views taken at 30° and 60° flexion. Generally the radiographs exclude other abnormality such as osteochondritis dissecans and are not helpful in directing the management of the anterior knee pain.

Aetiology

Occasionally symptoms may be referred back to an injury with direct force applied to the patella, indicating a traumatic basis. Excessive pressure on the lateral facet of the patella may underlie the development of symptoms. There may be incongruence of the patellofemoral articulation and lateral subluxation of the patella. There may be an abnormal Q angle and weakness of the vastus medialis. Goodfellow charted out the contact areas of the patellofemoral joint using an ink staining method and abnormalities in the contact areas can produce high stresses through a small area and degeneration of the underlying articular cartilage. Abnormalities of the molecular structure of the articular cartilage proteoglycans may also be a factor in the development of chondromalacia. The condition is more common in children who play a lot of sport and it behaves as an overuse syndrome.

Pathology

The pathology of anterior knee pain is variable. Chondromalacia of the patella may be present. Once the collagen layers on the outer layers of the articular surface are disrupted the cartilage over-hydrates as a result of the osmotic effect of the proteoglycan molecules. There is softening and splitting of the cartilage and then fibrillation.

Management

Non-operative

Reassurance that anterior knee pain is a common phenomenon and that the child will grow out of it is very important. Often the parent feels guilty that the child is going to 'ruin his knees' as he plays. It is unlikely that the avoidance of sport influences its natural history, but reducing the amount of sport reduces the amount of pain the child experiences. It is useful to refer to the condition as an immaturity of the retropatellar surface, which is therefore unable to withstand the increased stress and strain as the rest of the child grows, when discussing it with the parents.

If specific treatment is indicated and the pain persists despite playing less sport, exercises to improve the function of the vastus medialis have a theoretical basis and are often successful. Various knee braces have been described to stabilize the patella. Some of these are effective because they reduce the child's activity. Some children with associated flat feet are helped by a medial arch support. However, the response is unpredictable and just as effective with a simple cheap medial arch support as with an expensive custom-moulded insole.

Operative

Rarely are the symptoms severe enough to require surgery.

Arthroscopy can be indicated for various reasons. It is useful if other conditions are suspected and may reassure the surgeon and parent that there is no significant pathology. Inspection of the retropatellar surface may reveal areas of fibrillation. Although there is a placebo effect in some children, it should only be performed for specific indications. Arthroscopic shaving of areas of fibrillation may be helpful in some children. However, the cartilage does not regenerate normally and there is concern about the long-term damage that may result from this procedure. Arthroscopic closed lateral release may be performed if there is lateral subluxation or a lateral tilt of the patella. These procedures are often successful for a short time, but the condition may recur and the long-term prognosis is unclear.

Realignment procedures have been tried to overcome the excessive lateral pressure on the patella. These are similar to those already described for the dislocating patella. Indications for their use in anterior knee pain are less clear and there is concern about the development of osteoarthritic change in the patellofemoral joint in the long term.

Differential Diagnosis

Plica syndrome

Some children present with pain that involves more of the anteromedial aspect of the knee. They may have a palpable band to the medial side of the patella that can be rolled and flicked to produce pain by side to side movement of the examining finger. Their symptoms may be more suggestive of clicking and catching as a tight band flicks over the medial femoral condyle on knee flexion and extension. Differentiation from chondromalacia patellae can be very difficult.

These children often respond to a reduction in sport and strengthening the vastus medialis. At arthroscopy the medial synovial shelf is inflamed or sometimes split or damaged. Some respond to arthroscopic excision or division of the medial synovial shelf. Recurrence can occur. However, this operation has a poor reputation because a normal shelf may be removed when no other cause for the pain can be found, with no subsequent improvement in the pain. However, for the right indications it can be successful.

Bipartite patella

The patella forms from the coalescence of two or three ossification centres and sometimes this coalescence is incomplete. The anteroposterior radiograph may show a separate fragment of the patella at its superolateral aspect. The border between it and the rest of the patella is usually sclerotic and looks quite unlike a fracture, which the less experienced may diagnose. It occurs in one or two per 100 children and rarely gives symptoms. When it occurs in a child with anterior knee pain, the usual non-operative treatment should be used and it usually settles producing no persistent symptoms. If the child comes to surgery on the basis of persistent significant symptoms, arthroscopy may reveal fibrillation on the fragment or a loose fragment, and excision of the bipartite fragment may be successful.

Osteochondritis

The osteochondritic syndromes of the patella should be differentiated from anterior knee pain, i.e. (Osgood–Schlatter disease, Larsen–Johannson disease and Menelaus–Batten syndrome (see Chapter 13). Osteochondritis dissecans is considered in the next section.

Meniscal tear

Meniscal pathology in the young child is exceptionally rare, except the discoid lateral meniscus discussed below. A torn meniscus may present in the child approaching skeletal maturity with a history of a significant injury or twisting fall. A locked knee in children under ten years of age may mimic the adult torn meniscus, but the child usually has pseudolocking, which resolves with a non-operative approach.

Slipped upper femoral epiphysis

Never forget that the child with a slipped upper femoral epiphysis may present with knee pain only, but has an external rotation deformity on the couch and when walking. The hip should always be examined and an anteroposterior and lateral radiograph of the hip obtained if there is any pain or restriction of movement (see Chapter 18).

Osteochondritis Dissecans

Osteochondritis dissecans is a small area of avascular bone on an articular surface (*Figure 19.6*). There is often a well-defined demarcation between the avascular and normal bone, and sometimes the avascular area with its overlying articular cartilage can become partially loose and then detach itself to form a loose body. This is reflected in its name dissecans, meaning 'to cut out from.'

Ostechondritis dissecans most frequently presents on the lateral aspect of the medial femoral condyle. It can also present on the lateral femoral condyle, the patella and in other joints, such as the hip, elbow and ankle (see Chapter 13). It is not common with an incidence of four per 1000 in males. It is more common in boys (3:1), is bilateral in about 25%, and there is sometimes a family history. It usually presents between 10–20 years of age.

Aetiology

The aetiology is unknown, but most believe it is due to trauma, either a single event or repetitive microtrauma in a susceptible area and in a susceptible patient. Other theories include an ischaemic event or abnormalities of ossification.

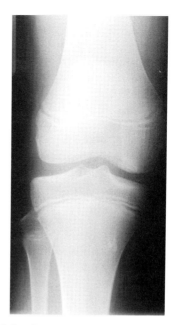

Figure 19.6   Osteochondritis dissecans in the classic position on the lateral part of the medial femoral condyle. The fragment is not displaced, but there is a clear line of demarcation surrounding the area.

Clinical Features

Patients present with intermittent ache, swelling and catching of the joint. They often describe a 'giving way' sensation, not on twisting but when walking in a straight line when increased stress is placed on the joint, such as when preparing to jump.

On examination there is often quadriceps wasting and a small effusion. If the knee is flexed to a right angle and the tibia is then internally rotated, there is often pain as the knee is extended, which can be relieved by external rotation; this is Wilson's sign.

Radiology

Plain radiography defines the lesion. A tunnel view of the intercondylar notch is required to show up the area most commonly affected on the lateral aspect of the medial femoral condyle. In the skeletally immature in whom the growth plates are still open the appearance is often of fragmentation of a subchondral area. In the skeletally mature the area affected is demarcated by a lucent and sclerotic line and detachment to form a loose body is more common. However, the radiological appearance is variable at any age. It should not be confused with the ragged epiphysis in which the border of the lateral femoral epiphysis is sclerotic and irregular. This is a variant of normal, is commonly seen in children aged 2–8 years and has no significant sequelae.

Arthrography may be useful to determine whether the articular surface is intact. If the fragment is loose dye leaks into the space between the fragment and the normal bone.

Computerized tomography (CT) may be useful for deciding whether the fragment is loose and injection of dye is then unnecessary.

Bone scanning may show whether the lesion is healing. If there is no activity around the fragment there is unlikely to be any further healing.

Magnetic resonance imaging (MRI) may have a yet unproven role.

Management

Non-operative

If the lesion is intact a period of observation is recommended with avoidance of sport. Radiological follow-up over the next year usually demonstrates healing of the lesion. This is particularly appropriate in the skeletally immature and if the area is fragmented but not detached.

Operative

If the symptoms persist or are unacceptable or the fragment appears to be detached arthroscopy is indicated. The appearance of the lesion can be graded according to Guhl classification (*Table 19.1*). If the articular surface is intact, the lesion may heal spontaneously. The lesion may be drilled with extension of the drilling into the adjacent normal bone. The intention is for the normal bone to extend into and encourage healing of the abnormal section. The drilling may be carried out arthroscopically through the articular surface or with image intensifier control through the medial femoral condyle into the abnormal bone so the articular surface is not breached. There is great debate about what is the correct management. If there are signs of early separation the lesion may be drilled, but internal fixation is probably more successful.

If the fragment is partially detached the fragment should be held firm by internal fixation to encourage healing of the fracture. Various methods of fixation

Table 19.1 Guhl arthroscopic classification of osteochondritis dissecans (Guhl, 1982)

1	Articular cartilage intact
2	Signs of early separation
3	Fragment partially detached
4	Crater on articular surface with loose bodies (salvageable and unsalvageable)

have been described, some of which allow removal of the internal fixation after healing. We often use Herbert screws in these circumstances as the differential pitch allows compression of the fragment onto the normal bone and the head can be buried inside the fragment. These can sometimes be placed arthroscopically.

If the fragment is detached and loose it has to be decided whether it can be reattached. If the fragment has not been detached for long and fits well into its crater, it should be internally fixed. If the fragment is small and does not involve much weight-bearing area it is removed and the crater smoothed with a shaver and then drilled to encourage the development of fibrocartilage. Reattachment of a large fragment should be carried out open and may require considerable skill to shape appropriately and fill the crater.

DISCOID LATERAL MENISCUS

The cartilages form *in utero* from a mesenchymal mass separating the femur and tibia. In the normal child the central section is absorbed to produce the characteristic semilunar or C-shaped meniscus. The resorption fails to take place in the discoid lateral meniscus and leaves the meniscus as a D-shape. This condition affects 1–2 per 100 children and is often bilateral. The condition rarely affects the medial meniscus. There are two types.

- The Wrisberg ligament type is not complete, but attaches to the posterior part of the knee only through the Wrisberg (lateral meniscofemoral) ligament. The posterior part of the cartilage is hypermobile.
- The complete type has normal attachments and is much less symptomatic than the Wrisberg ligament type.

Clinical Features

The condition may become apparent in someone as young as four years of age or it may be undetected even in old age. Most cause problems, which implies the meniscus has an inherent propensity to tear. The child presents with a palpable clunk in the knee as the knee is flexed or extended past about 110°.

A plain radiograph may show an increased joint space in the lateral compartment, and MRI demonstrates the abnormality.

Management

Operative correction should be delayed until skeletal maturity if possible. In the past the meniscus has often been removed completely through an open approach. However, arthroscopic removal of the complete type to leave a rim of normal meniscus is preferable. The Wrisberg ligament type should be removed completely and this should be achievable with the arthroscope.

POPLITEAL CYST

Juvenile popliteal cysts are not infrequent. They occur more commonly in boys (2:1) and are usually unilateral. They usually present in children aged 5–8 years as a painless mass behind the knee. Sometimes they cause great parental concern because they fear a malignancy, particularly if seen by an inexperienced clinician. On examination the mass is fluctuant and transilluminable and the rest of the knee is normal. They may present at a later age in patients with juvenile chronic arthritis or pigmented villonodular synovitis of the knee.

Most popliteal cysts are bursal originating from the gastrocnemius–semimembranosus bursa, but some are herniations from the knee joint. About two-thirds communicate with the knee joint.

Although contrast radiography, ultrasound and CT scans demonstrate the lesion well, they are unnecessary in the diagnosis and management.

Management

Reassurance that the lesion is benign is essential. The vast majority resolve spontaneously and there are few indications for surgery. Aspiration is unnecessary. The desire for surgery should be fiercely resisted because it is not necessary and recurrence has been reported in 40% after surgery.

BLOUNT DISEASE AND TIBIA VARA

Tibia vara is common in children. It is usually physiological and improves with growth (see Chapter 14). In some children there is a progressive varus deformity with an abnormality of the medial part of the upper tibial growth plate. This is rare in caucasian communities but common in blacks, particularly in the West Indies. The cause is probably excessive pressure on the posteromedial part of the growth plate, but there is debate as to whether the infantile form is secondary to severe physiological bowing or a separate condition (*Figure 19.7*).

Clinical Features

Blount disease may present in the infant, when it is usually bilateral, or at a later stage in the 8–14-year-old, when it is commonly unilateral. The child may be overweight. The deformity is progressive.

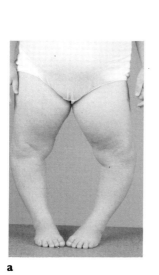 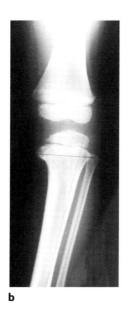 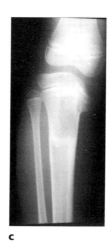 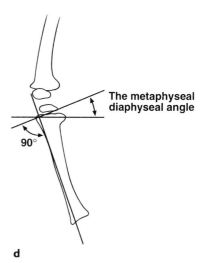

The metaphyseal diaphyseal angle

90°

a **b** **c** **d**

Figure 19.7 a The clinical appearance of Blount disease. **b** The radiological appearance in early Blount disease. **c** The radiological appearance in a later case of Blount disease. **d** Radiological measurement of the metaphyseal–diaphyseal angle.

Table 19.2 Langenskoild (1989) classification of Blount disease

Stage	Age (years)	Radiological features
I	2–3	Irregularity of the growth plate, medial beaking
II	2–4	Saucer-shaped defect in medial metaphysis at its junction with growth plate. Wedging of upper tibial epiphysis
III	4–6	Deepening of 'saucer' into a 'step'. Irregularity of medial epiphysis
IV	5–10	Growth plate inclined distally at medial side. Irregularity of medial epiphysis
V	9–11	The epiphysis is split in two, with the medial aspect inclined distally; this gives the appearance of a double epiphyseal plate
VI	10–13	The medial growth plate ossifies, but the lateral part remains

Radiology

There is an abnormality of the posteromedial part of the upper tibial growth plate, with beaking of the medial metaphysis. There is fragmentation around the growth plate and in the adolescent form, wedging of the medial part of the upper tibial epiphysis. The metaphyseal–diaphyseal angle is measured in an attempt to differentiate severe physiological genu varum, which is likely to resolve, and Blount disease, which is likely to be progressive. Although there is no clear cut-off point metaphyseal–diaphyseal angles of more than 11° are likely to be progressive.

Langenskoild (1989) has described six grades based on the age of the child and the severity of the radiological appearance (*Table 19.2. Figure 19.8*).

Management

In the first two years of life the child is observed. Treatment is decided according to the severity of the deformity. Some use orthotics in the young child while weight-bearing, but we have no experience in their use. If progression is likely, surgery is advised.

If the physiological seven degrees of valgus orientation of the knee can be restored, resolution is usual for stages I and II and possible for stages III and IV. Stages V and VI indicate irreversible changes, so progressive angular deformity will occur if the tibia is only realigned.

Various methods of corrective osteotomy have been described. A closing lateral wedge is the simplest, but an upside down dome (smiley dome) just below the attachment of the patellar tendon produces less shortening. Fixation may be by crossed K wires or a plate or ring fixators for the older child with complex deformity. A fibular osteotomy must always be performed and a decompression of the anterior compartment to prevent the development of a compartment syndrome.

For stage V and VI the tibial osteotomy should be combined with a total epiphyseodesis of the affected limb to prevent further progression. There are also techniques to elevate the medial aspect of the metaphysis and straighten the upper tibial articular surface (*Figure 19.8b*). Consideration should also be given to epiphyseodesis of the other limb to achieve limb length equalization at skeletal maturity.

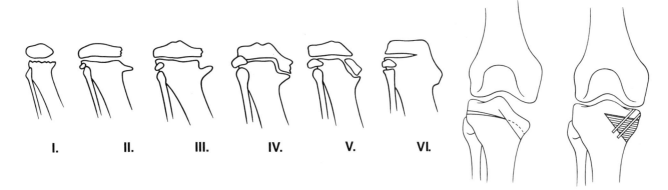

I.   II.   III.   IV.   V.   VI.

Figure 19.8 a The grades of severity of Blount disease. **b** Osteotomy technique for correction of stage V and VI Blount disease.

REFERENCES AND FURTHER READING

Aichroth P. Osteochondritis dissecans of the knee: a clinical survey. *J Bone Joint Surg* 1971; **53B**: 440–447.

Bentley G. Articular cartilage changes in chondromalacia patellae. *J Bone Joint Surg* 1985; **67B**: 769–774.

Bergman N, Williams PF. Habitual dislocation of the patella in flexion. *J Bone Joint Surg* 1988; **70B**: 415–419.

Curtis BH, Fisher RL. Congenital hyperextension with anterior subluxation of the knee. *J Bone Joint Surg* 1969; **51A**: 255–258.

Dickhaut SC, DeLee JC. The discoid lateral meniscus syndrome. *J Bone Joint Surg* 1982; **64A**: 1068–1073.

Dinham JM. Popliteal cysts in children. *J Bone Joint Surg* 1975; **57B**: 69–71.

Dowd GSE, Bentley G. Radiographic assessment in patellar instability and chondromalacia patellae. *J Bone Joint Surg* 1986; **68B**: 297–300.

Green JP, Waugh W. Congenital lateral dislocation of the patella. *J Bone Joint Surg* 1968; **50B**: 285–289.

Goodfellow JW, Hungerford DS, Zindel M. Patello-femoral mechanics and pathology I. Functional anatomy of the patello-femoral joint. *J Bone Joint Surg* 1976; **58B**: 287–299.

Guhl J. Arthroscopic treatment of osteochondritis dissecans. *Clin Orthop Rel Research* 1982; **167**: 65–74.

Hampson WGJ, Hill P. Late results of transfer of the tibial tubercle for recurrent dislocation of the patella. *J Bone Joint Surg* 1975; **57B**: 209–213.

Langenskoild A. Tibia vara. A critical review. *Clin Orthop Rel Research* 1989; **246**: 195–207.

Outerbridge RE. The aetiology of chondromalacia patellae. *J Bone Joint Surg* 1961; **43B**: 752–757.

Chapter 20
The Foot

D Robert V Dickens

CONGENITAL TALIPES EQUINOVARUS

The management of congenital talipes equinovarus (CTEV) is one of the most challenging problems in paediatric orthopaedics. The condition can range from a very severe fixed deformity for which surgical intervention is almost inevitable (*Figure 20.1*), to mild fixed deformity for which one would expect resolution with serial casting. Prediction of the end result at presentation is extremely difficult. This same variability makes a comparison of results almost impossible.

Aetiology

The aetiology of CTEV is unknown, but there have been numerous theories. At the five-week stage of gestation, the growing limb bud is in a position of equinovarus and an arrest of normal development from this stage may be the cause. Other theories include abnormal tendon and ligamentous insertions and neurological abnormalities, particularly lower motor neurone lesions. A high proportion of type I fibres have been described in the affected muscles (Handelsman and Badalamente, 1981). Intrauterine

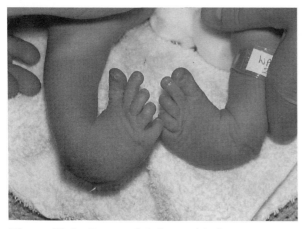

Figure 20.1   Severe club feet at birth.

posture may cause some moulding of foot posture, but does not cause the calf wasting seen in severe CTEV.

Incidence

There is a racial variation in the incidence of CTEV. The incidence in Caucasians is approximately one per 1000 live births compared with 0.5 per 1000 in the Oriental races and about five per 1000 in the Polynesian races.

The sex incidence is one of males predominating by a ratio of 2:1, and 50% are bilateral. The inheritance pattern suggests a polygenic inheritance.

Pathology

The basic pathology of CTEV is an abnormality of the articulation of the talus with the navicular and the calcaneum. The navicular is placed medially on the talus and can even be in contact with the medial malleolus. The body of the talus is directed laterally within the ankle mortice, but the neck of the talus is angulated medially. The talocalcaneal relationship is also abnormal; the calcaneum is in a varus position with the distal end of the calcaneum displaced medially. The forefoot is in an adducted and supinated position as a consequence of this displacement of the tarsal bones. (This anatomical situation is well recognized when performing posteromedial release procedures for CTEV.) The calcaneocuboid joint is abnormal with medial displacement of the cuboid on the calcaneum, the degree of displacement being a good indication of the severity of the condition.

Associated with these bone and joint deformities are contractures of the capsules and ligaments of the ankle and subtalar joints. There is also a contracture of the ligaments and capsule of the talonavicular joint and the calcaneonavicular spring ligament. The tendons of tibialis posterior, flexor hallucis longus and flexor digitorum longus are contracted. Sometimes there is a contracture of the plantar structures, which produces a cavus deformity.

Clinical Features

The condition is easily recognized at birth as a fixed deformity of equinus, varus and forefoot adduction. This is in contrast to positional congenital talipes equinovarus, which can be fully corrected or even overcorrected. The degree of deformity at birth should be accurately recorded and there have been various attempts to grade severity using clinical and radiographic criteria.

The clinical deformity is varus of the hind foot with adduction and supination of the forefoot; the foot is in equinus. The relationship of the navicular to the medial malleolus can be palpated. The crease on the medial aspect of the foot indicates a significant deformity. Calf atrophy is noted in a number of patients at birth.

CTEV may be associated with other disorders. The most common are spina bifida and arthrogryposis,

and less commonly conditions such as diastrophic dwarfism. The prognosis for these teratogenic talipes is much worse than for idiopathic CTEV.

Radiology

Radiological investigation of CTEV is an important parameter in assessing the severity of the condition and the results of treatment. The radiographic techniques are well described by Simon (1977). The radiographs required are a weight-bearing or simulated weight-bearing anteroposterior (AP) film and a forced dorsiflexion lateral film.

- On the AP film the angle between the longitudinal axis of the talus and the axis of the calcaneum describes the talocalcaneal angle, which has a normal range of 20–40°. If this angle is less than 20° the hind foot is in varus (*Figure 20.2*).
- On the lateral dorsiflexion film the talocalcaneal angle should be 25–50° and if it is less than 25°

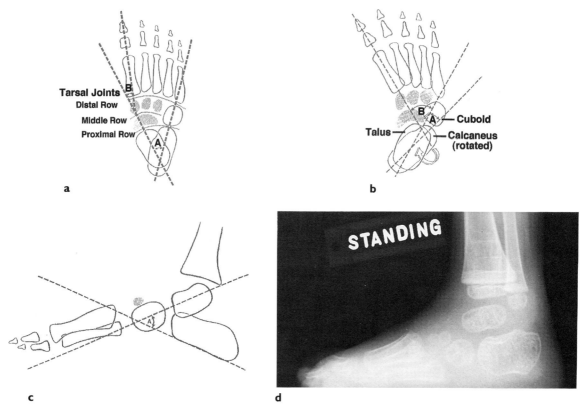

a

b

c

d

Figure 20.2 **a** Anteroposterior radiograph of the normal foot showing a talocalcaneal angle (A) of 20–30°. The angle between the axis of the talus and the first metatarsal (B) is small. **b** In a club foot the talocalcaneal angle is less than 20° (A). The angle between the talus and the first metatarsal is increased (B). **c** Normal lateral view of the foot shows a talocalcaneal angle of 20–50°. **d** Lateral radiograph of a club foot showing that the talus and calcaneum are parallel.

indicates parallelism and therefore inadequate reduction (see *Figure 20.2*).

Management

It is important to recognize the relative strengths of the involved structures. The strongest are the ligaments, the next strongest is bone, and the structure least able to withstand pressure is the articular surface. Forced stretching of the ligaments can have adverse effects on the articular cartilage causing stiffness and recurrent deformity.

Clinicians have used a variety of methods of treatment to correct the deformity. The options available are serial casting, splints (e.g. Denis Browne) and strapping (*Figure 20.3*). The use of maternal manipulation, physiotherapy and other modalities is not recommended.

The most appropriate method is that which the surgeon finds most suitable in his practice. Each form of treatment is equally effective in experienced hands.

Conservative treatment is appropriate for all patients presenting with CTEV, even if it is unlikely to correct the deformity. At least it produces a stretching effect on the skin, which may be a critical factor in the success of later surgical treatment.

Serial casting
Gentle manipulation of the deformity into a corrected position is followed by the application of the plaster cast. When applying the cast it is important that the baby is relaxed. Feeding as the cast is applied or immediately before is recommended. The cast is applied below the knee initially and pressure has to be exerted to avoid a spurious correction. Gentle moulding of the cast, first to correct the forefoot deformity of adduction and supination, and subse-

quently to correct the equinus, will result in serial correction of the deformity. In correcting the equinus it is important that the pressure is placed in the region of the cuboid to avoid a boating deformity of the foot. Having obtained the maximum correction available by gentle manipulation and application of a below-knee cast, the cast is then extended to an above-knee position so that an external rotation corrective force can be applied.

This form of treatment requires repeated change of casts weekly or two-weekly initially, and gradual correction of the deformity. At 3–4 months a decision is then made as to whether surgery is required. Using serial casting 40–60% will be corrected.

The Denis Browne splint is an equally effective method of correction, but requires meticulous attention to detail when applying the splints.

Strapping
Strapping can be just as effective as casts or Denis Browne splints. One inch zinc oxide tape is applied to skin prepared with tincture of iodine. One length is applied to the medial aspect of the heel, led under the heel and applied to the lateral aspect of the lower leg, to correct the varus heel. Another length is applied to the dorsum of the forefoot, led around the medial aspect onto the plantar aspect of the forefoot and then up to the lateral aspect of the lower leg. With the knee flexed to 90° the tape is applied around the knee to the medial aspect of the knee so that forced extension of the knee produces dorsiflexion at the ankle. A bandage over the tape protects it and the strapping is changed weekly. The tape can be soaked off in warm water before the child comes to the clinic.

Splinting
If correction has been achieved by conservative measures, the foot position must be maintained and

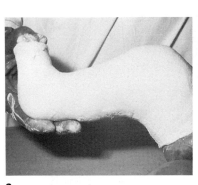 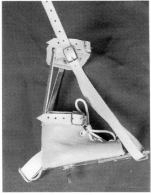 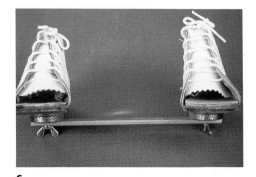

a   b   c

Figure 20.3 a Plaster cast for club foot (reproduced with permission from Williams PF, Cole WG. *Orthopaedic Management in Childhood*. Chapman & Hall, London). **b** Unilateral splint to correct equinus varus and adductus. **c** Denis Browne splints.

held to allow adaptive changes to produce a stable situation. Initially the splints should be worn day and night and the calcaneus splint is appropriate. For bilateral cases the use of the Denis Browne splint may be more convenient. Splintage is continued until the child starts to stand holding on to furniture. Splintage can be then continued at night up to the age of 18 months to two years.

The requirement of any splint is that it holds the correction of abduction and external rotation and also provides a degree of dorsiflexion at the ankle.

Surgery

Surgery should be undertaken if conservative treatment has failed to fully correct the deformity. The timing of such surgery is debatable. In general, surgical procedures are easier after the child is over three months of age and preferably closer to six months. In the past authors have suggested later periods for such surgery, for example Turco (1979) advocates 1–2 years. After five years soft-tissue releases are unlikely to be successful because the repositioning of the foot into a reduced position is usually not maintained as the capacity for bony remodelling is reduced.

The exact form of surgery should be tailored to the individual case. Generally we advocate the use of a posteromedial release for CTEV because the most important pathology is at the talonavicular joint. However, we recognize that other centres report good results following an early posterior release (8–12 weeks) followed by a late posteromedial release (at 12 months) in those cases with residual deformity.

The Cincinnati incision, popularized by Crawford *et al.* (1982), is an excellent way of exposing the anatomical structures medially, posteriorly and laterally (*Figure 20.4*), the only slight deficiency being the difficulty in getting adequate exposure of the tendo Achillis for lengthening.

The standard operative procedure for CTEV is a posterior and medial release of the contracted structures. The neurovascular bundle is identified and protected by vascular loops. Posteriorly the tendo Achillis is divided in a Z-lengthening procedure and the capsules of the ankle and subtalar joint are released. The ankle joint is released from the tip of the lateral malleolus to the tip of the medial malleolus, but ligaments anterior to this are preserved. More dorsiflexion can be obtained by dividing the syndesmosis between the tibia and fibula posteriorly.

On the medial side the tibialis posterior is lengthened. The ligaments between the talus and navicular together with the talonavicular capsule are released. The plantar calcaneonavicular ligament or spring ligament is released and the sheaths of the tendon of flexor digitorum and tibialis posterior are released. The capsule of the subtalar joint is released on the medial aspect together with the talocalcaneal interosseous ligaments. A decision is then made whether the tendon of the flexor digitorum longus requires lengthening, and depends on the degree of clawing of the toes. The flexor digitorum longus and flexor hallucis longus may be lengthened or divided. It may also be necessary to release the calcaneocuboid joint capsule through the lateral arm of the Cincinnati incision to effect a full correction. Uncommonly it is noted that there is a cavus deformity during primary club foot surgery and if this is regarded as significant a plantar release may be performed through the medial incision.

Once the release is complete a pin is placed in the talus to use as a gear stick to redirect the talus. The

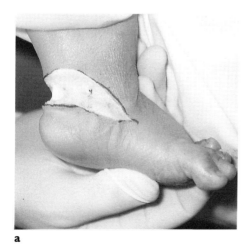

a

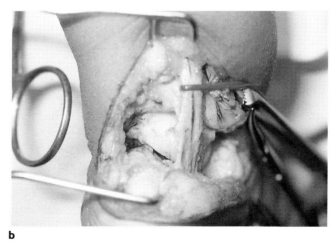

b

Figure 20.4 a The Cincinnati incision for posteromedial release of club foot. **b** View of the posterior ankle showing the intact neurovascular bundle protected by a loop and opened ankle and subtalar joints.

abnormal lateral rotation of the talus can now be appreciated. If the release is adequate the anterior aspect of the talus can be rotated medially and the navicular pushed laterally to reduce the talonavicular joint. A second wire is driven through the talus into the navicular and out through the forefoot to emerge between the first and second metatarsals. The gear stick wire is removed. A wire is then passed from the sole of the foot up through the calcaneum into the talus to immobilize the talocalcaneal correction in the appropriate position. Having repaired the lengthened tendons, the wound is closed in two layers. The foot is then placed into a relaxed position and immobilized using an above-knee plaster slab over wool and a crepe bandage.

Ten days postoperatively a new plaster is applied under general anaesthetic. The pins are removed either at this stage or after six weeks, depending on the preference of the surgeon. The plaster is applied with the foot in a slightly overcorrected position, and is maintained for a minimum of eight weeks and usually for 12 weeks.

Complications

Pressure sores can result from inappropriate or excessive corrective forces being used during the application of plasters or splintage. A rocker bottom foot can be caused by applying the dorsiflexion force too far forward on the sole of the foot. Excessive force at manipulation can cause damage to the articular surface of the talus resulting in a flat-topped talus. Physeal damage with partial growth plate arrest may occur and physeal separation has been reported.

Skin necrosis
Closure of the skin after surgery without undue tension is important. Skin necrosis can result in excessive scarring and therefore recurrence. Scar excision and closure of the wound with some form of vascularized pedicle graft may then be necessary.

Scars sometimes hypertrophy and cause rubbing in shoes, and may become attached to bony structures such as the medial malleolus and cause a significant problem.

Overcorrection
Valgus posture of the foot can be caused by over-zealous soft-tissue release combined with overcorrection in the postoperative cast (*Figure 20.5a*). It can be treated by subtalar fusion by the Grice technique. Calcaneus may be due to overlengthening of the tendo Achillis or excessive dorsiflexion positioning of the foot after surgical correction. This is more difficult to treat and may require a transfer of tibialis anterior to the calcaneum (Wijesinha and Menelaus, 1989).

Recurrence
Recurrence of CTEV can occur after successful correction by conservative methods or after surgical intervention (*Figure 20.5b*). In the child under four years of age, it is an indication for a repeat postero-

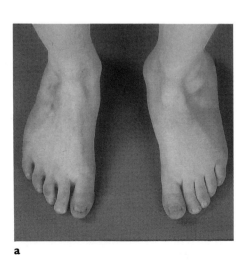

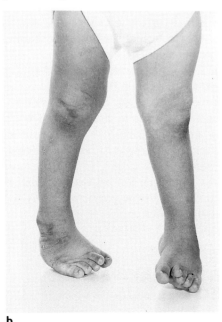

a

b

Figure 20.5 **a** Overcorrection: a complication of posteromedial release of club foot. **b** Recurrence after posteromedial release of club foot.

medial release, which may be combined with procedures to correct any muscle imbalance such as a tibialis anterior transfer (either a split tendon transfer or a full transfer).

In a child aged 5–6 years the soft-tissue procedures should be combined with minor bony procedures to effect a correction. The Dillwyn Evans procedure is a method of equalizing the medial and lateral columns. It combines a soft-tissue medial release and medial column lengthening with a lateral column shortening by bony excision. The classic description is by excision and fusion of the calcaneocuboid joint. This can be modified to shorten the lateral column by decancellation of the cuboid or the distal end of the calcaneum. If the deformity seems to be further forward in the forefoot, metatarsal osteotomies can be used. For the severe recurrence, hind foot procedures such as calcaneal shift or astragalectomy are occasionally necessary.

Triple arthrodesis gives good correction of all the elements of a recurrent clubfoot. Its use should be withheld until the foot has fully grown because it shortens the foot and stops further growth. In the mature foot it is the treatment of choice for most recurrent club feet. It is performed with an excision technique from the lateral side.

Following surgery on a club foot the child may sometimes still walk with an intoe gait. This is usually due to recurrence of the deformity, but may be due to internal tibial torsion. Most severe club feet have a compensatory external tibial torsion, which can be demonstrated by palpation of the lateral malleolus at a level behind the medial malleolus. If there is internal tibial torsion and the radiographs show appropriate correction of the foot, a rotational tibial osteotomy can be very successful.

The use of the Ilizarov apparatus to correct CTEV is now being used more frequently. Under the age of eight years soft-tissue correction can be considered, and the Ilizarov frame used to hold the corrected position or to gradually improve the position. However, for a very fixed deformity, even under this age, osteotomies may be necessary. In the older age group the Ilizarov technique can be used with osteotomies and immediate or slow correction obtained through the osteotomy sites.

CONGENITAL TALIPES CALCANEOVALGUS

This should not be confused with CTEV, but is often given the broad term of talipes. At birth, the foot is noted to be dorsiflexed and in valgus. The deformity

may be so severe that the dorsum of the foot lies along the lateral border of the lower limb. It is thought to be a packaging defect due to intrauterine position. It is frequently associated with developmental dysplasia of the hip (DDH) and a careful examination of the hips is mandatory.

The deformity is quite benign and corrects within the first year of life. The mother is often instructed in gentle manipulation to correct the deformity and this may accelerate the spontaneous resolution. This condition has none of the disabling implications of CTEV and does not require splintage.

METATARSUS ADDUCTUS

This condition is discussed in Chapter 14.

CONGENITAL VERTICAL TALUS

Congenital vertical talus is rare. It frequently presents with other deformities such as arthrogryposis multiplex congenita, myelomeningocoele and trisomy 18, and sometimes with DDH. Other names for this condition have been congenital flat foot and congenital rocker bottom flat foot, and some prefer the term congenital convex pes valgus (*Figure 20.6*).

Aetiology

The aetiology of congenital vertical talus is unknown. It is thought that intrauterine muscle imbalance or arrested development of the foot might be causes.

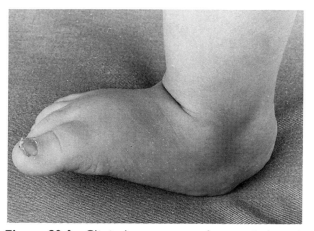

Figure 20.6   Clinical appearance of congenital vertical talus with a rocker bottom foot.

Pathology

The talus is in a vertical position. There is lateral displacement of the calcaneum and hypoplasia of the sustentaculum tali, which allows the talus to fall off and lie to the medial side of the calcaneus. The talonavicular joint is dislocated, with the navicular lying on the dorsum and neck of the talus. The calcaneus is in an equinus position, producing a characteristic rocker bottom foot. There is also an associated but lesser degree of displacement of the calcaneocuboid joint with lateral displacement of the cuboid on the calcaneus, producing abductus of the forefoot. The soft tissues are contracted, particularly the ligaments associated with the talonavicular joint. The tendons on the dorsum of the foot are also contracted including tibialis anterior, extensor digitorum longus, extensor hallucis longus and peroneus tertius, and to the lateral side peroneus brevis and longus. Posteriorly the tendo Achillis is also tight, creating the equinus position of the calcaneus.

Clinical Features

The condition is a rigid deformity, which cannot be corrected by manipulation to create a longitudinal arch. It is immediately apparent at birth: the forefoot is dorsiflexed and abducted and the heel is in valgus and equinus. The head of the talus is easily palpable on the medial border of the foot, creating a rocker bottom deformity.

Radiology

The talus is in a vertical position compared to the calcaneum. The talonavicular joint is dislocated, with the navicular lying anterior to the long axis of the talus. The calcaneus is in equinus.

Differential Diagnosis

Vertical talus is also seen in other circumstances. The most common is a mobile deformity associated with ligamentous laxity, which is easily correctable. In talipes calcaneovalgus, the talus may have a more vertical position than normal. It is the lack of rigidity that distinguishes these two conditions from true congenital vertical talus.

Management

Serial casting
Serial casting has limited value, but may stretch some of the soft tissues to allow easier closure at surgery. It is used in the first 6–12 weeks.

Surgery
Surgical correction is appropriate at the age of about 12 weeks. The Cincinnati incision is used to obtain access to the medial, lateral and posterior components of the deformity. Through this incision the tendo Achillis, extensor hallucis longus, extensor digitorum longus and tibialis anterior are lengthened. Peroneus brevis may also require lengthening. The capsules of the talonavicular and subtalar joints are then divided medially, laterally and posteriorly. The navicular is then reduced on to the head of the talus and held in place with a K wire. The talocalcaneal articulation is then orientated and K wires passed up from the plantar aspect. A bone graft may be placed into the subtalar joint to obtain fusion. A further K wire may be passed through the calcaneocuboid joint to hold the reduction. This is radical surgery, but necessary to obtain a full correction. The wounds are then closed and the foot placed into a plaster slab. This is changed at three weeks, and the wires are removed. Plaster is maintained for 12 weeks after surgery. A mounded ankle–foot orthosis is then used to hold the position until walking starts.

Severe or late-presenting case
Management is very difficult. Excision of the navicular has been advocated by some for the severe or late-presenting case, but our results have been poor. Waiting for skeletal maturity and then performing an excisional triple arthrodesis is probably preferable for the late-presenting case.

PES PLANUS

Flat feet are common and usually physiological (*Figure 20.7a*). They are discussed in Chapter 14. A useful classification of flat feet is given in Table 20.1.

Flat Feet Associated With Ligamentous Laxity

Some patients such as those with Marfan or Down syndromes have marked ligamentous laxity associated with pes planus. Weight-bearing films demonstrate the talus to be in a more vertical position than normal. This condition can be associated with a mild contracture of the tendo Achillis. The management is mainly conservative, but in those with a progressive deformity there may be an indication for a Grice subtalar fusion at about seven years of age.

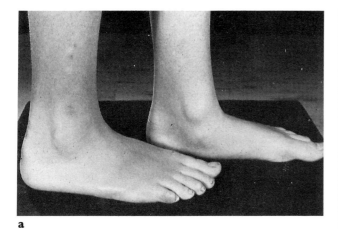
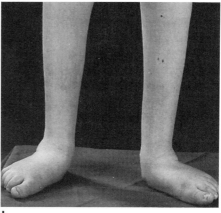

a   b

Figure 20.7 **a** Physiological flat feet. **b** Paralytic flat foot due to spina bifida.

Table 20.1 Classification of flat feet

Physiological (see Chapter 14)

Non-physiological
Congenital
   Congenital talipes calcaneovalgus
   Congenital vertical talus
Painless
   Flat foot associated with ligamentous laxity
   Flat foot associated with tightness of tendo
     Achillis
   Paralytic flat foot (cerebral palsy, spina bifida)
Painful or peroneal spasmodic flat foot
   Tarsal coalition
   Subtalar irritability (idiopathic, septic arthritis,
     osteoid osteoma, juvenile chronic arthritis,
     traumatic subtalar degenerative changes)

Paralytic Flat Feet

A paralytic flat foot is common in association with a variety of neuromuscular disorders such as cerebral palsy and spina bifida (*Figure 20.7b*). Management of this is along conservative lines with the use of orthotics to prevent excessive shoe wear or pressure effects on the foot. At maturity there may be a place for an inlay triple arthrodesis.

Peroneal Spasmodic Flat Foot

Children of 10–14 years of age may present with a rigid painful valgus foot. The subtalar joint is rigid and any attempt to bring the foot into inversion aggravates the pain and causes the peroneal muscles to go into spasm. This is described as a peroneal spasmodic flat foot. The cause of this clinical syndrome is a tarsal coalition or an irritable subtalar joint as listed in *Table 20.1*.

Flat Feet associated with tight tendo Achillis

Pes planus in association with a tight tendo Achillis is common. Many are variations of the normal physiological flat feet and should be treated along similar conservative lines. Occasionally there may be a place for a heel raise if symptoms are a problem. However, usually no surgical intervention is indicated. Very rarely, if the foot becomes progressively deformed, there is a place for elongation of the tendo Achillis combined with the use of insoles to maintain a medial arch to the foot.

Tarsal Coalition

Tarsal coalition is a well-recognized cause of painful flat foot associated with peroneal spasm. The commonest bony bridge accounting for about two-thirds of the cases is a calcaneonavicular coalition. The next commonest coalition is talocalcaneal, which occurs in approximately one-third of cases. The talocalcaneal bar is usually on the medial aspect of the middle facet. Presumably there is overgrowth of the bar producing a valgus deformity of the heel. Rare coalitions also occur between the calcaneum and the cuboid and the navicular and the cuboid.

Aetiology

The aetiology of this condition is thought to be a congenital cartilaginous bar between the two bones. Initially a pseudoarthrosis or synchondrosis develops which then becomes a fixed bony bar. There is a recognized familial association and the incidence has been variously estimated to be around 1%. Some cases are asymptomatic. It is common for the condition to be bilateral, particularly calcaneonavicular bars.

Clinical Features

Tarsal coalition usually presents at the age of 10–11 years. It is thought that this is because the midtarsal joint loses mobility as the abnormal connection ossifies. Pain in the calcaneonavicular bar is characteristically lateral, whereas the pain of talocalcaneal coalitions is more commonly felt under the medial malleolus. The symptoms are frequently more obvious when the patient has been active and may be difficult to detect if the patient is examined early in the day.

The clinical features are those of a child who has an antalgic gait associated with visible peroneal spasm and a flat foot. The posture of the foot is usually one of valgus of the hind foot and attempts to invert the foot result in increased peroneal spasm associated with discomfort.

The natural history of tarsal coalition is unclear. It is not uncommon to find relatives with the condition who are entirely symptom free. However, many of those who present with pain have evidence of degenerative changes in the hind foot joints and these inevitably progress.

Radiology

Plain films of the foot may not show the coalition. The calcaneonavicular bar is best seen on an oblique film of the hind foot. This demonstrates the relationship between the anterior end of the calcaneum with the lateral aspect of the navicular. Sometimes there is not a complete bony bar, but a connection resembling a fibrous union between the bones (*Figure 20.8a*). Talocalcaneal bars are difficult to diagnose on plain films and various axial views of the calcaneus have been described to demonstrate them. We no longer rely on plain films to diagnose talocalcaneal bars, but use CT scans, which demonstrate the bar well in the frontal plane (*Figure 20.8b*).

Management

The treatment of tarsal coalition depends on the severity of the symptoms. For mild cases there may be a place for no intervention or the use of a supportive insole. For the established symptomatic case attempts at overcoming the symptoms with manipulation under anaesthesia and immobilization in a below-knee plaster cast have not been successful, The vast majority of painful cases need surgical intervention.

Calcaneonavicular bar

An oblique incision (as described by Ollier) is made, starting below the lateral malleolus and extending across to the talonavicular joint. The dorsal branch of the superficial peroneal nerve is avoided and the common extensor muscle origin is exposed. The muscle is elevated to reveal the bar. A wide excision of bone is required, and a rectangle of bone is removed to leave a gap of about 1 cm. It is essential

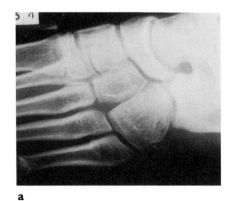
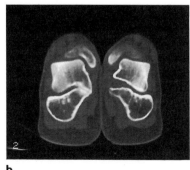

a   b

Figure 20.8 **a** Radiological appearance of a calcaneonavicular bar. **b** Computerized tomographic appearance of talocalcaneal bar in the left foot. The right foot shows the appearance following surgical excision of a similar bar.

to be able to see across the soft tissues on the medial side of the foot through the bed of the excised bar.

The defect is filled with soft tissue to prevent recurrence. Some use a fat graft from the buttock, but we prefer the substance of the extensor brevis muscle. The muscle belly is attached to a suture and pulled into the defect. The suture is then passed out onto the medial side of the foot and tied over a button or gauze swab. The foot is immobilized in a crepe bandage with a backslab for two weeks and then mobilized.

If presentation has been delayed to the age of 14–15 years there are often degenerative changes in the midtarsal joint. Bar excision is unlikely to be successful in these patients and an inlay triple arthrodesis is the preferred treatment.

Talocalcaneal bar

Painful talocalcaneal bars are unlikely to be improved by non-operative means. Bar excision has now been accepted as having a worthwhile success rate, but the chances of a good result are greater if the bar is small, if there is no degenerative change and if there is no significant valgus deformity of the hindfoot (Wilde *et al.*, 1994).

Using the medial limb of a Cincinnati incision, the subtalar joint is exposed. Normal articulation is identified anteriorly and posteriorly. The posterior aspect is approached through the sheath of flexor hallucis, which lies along the line of the posterior articulation. Having defined the bridge, it is removed using dental burrs; a good light source such as the fibreoptic light probe is helpful. Having excised the bar and created a situation where the articulation is evident and the talus is able to move freely on the calcaneum, the defect is then filled with a fat graft

from either the buttock or from the sole of the foot. The foot is treated with immobilization using a backslab for three weeks and then mobilized.

If bar excision is unlikely to produce a satisfactory result an arthrodesis of the subtalar joint can be considered, or alternatively, an inlay triple arthrodesis.

PES CAVUS

Pes cavus refers to a high arch of the foot. It can also be thought of as an equinus deformity of the forefoot on the hindfoot or a plantaris deformity. It can be divided into a pure cavus deformity and a cavovarus deformity.

- In a pure cavus deformity the plantaris is the same on the medial and lateral aspects of the forefoot so there is no consequent varus or valgus deformity on weight-bearing.
- In the cavovarus foot there is an associated varus of the hindfoot. This may be a fixed deformity. However, in some the varus only occurs on weight-bearing as a consequence of an asymmetrical plantaris. When the first ray is more plantarflexed than the lateral rays (otherwise known as a pronation deformity), the heel is forced into varus on weight-bearing because of the forefoot deformity. When not weight-bearing the heel can be corrected to neutral or into valgus (*Figure 20.9*).

Most of the idiopathic cases of pes cavus are simple cavus and most of the neurological cases are cavovarus, some due to fixed varus and some a consequence of the fixed pronation of the forefoot.

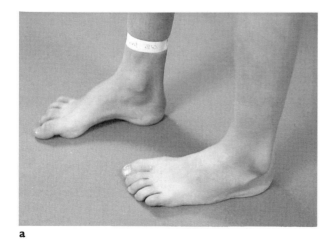
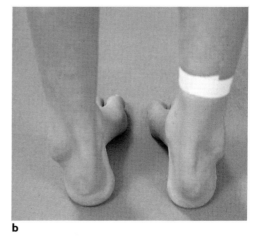

Figure 20.9 a Pes cavus due to peroneal muscular atrophy demonstrating the high arch and clawing of the toes. **b** Demonstrating the varus inclination of the heel secondary to a fixed pronation deformity of the forefoot.

Table 20.2 Classification of pes cavus

Idiopathic

Residual to congenital talipes equinovarus

Neuromuscular
    Muscle (e.g. Duchenne muscular dystrophy,
        compartment syndrome)
    Peripheral nerves (e.g. peroneal muscular
        atrophy)
    Spinal cord (e.g. spinal dysraphism, polio)
    Central (e.g. cerebral palsy, Friedreich ataxia)

Aetiology

A useful classification of the causes of pes cavus is given in Table 20.2.

Clinical Features

Idiopathic pes cavus usually presents in adolescence or adult life as a result of pressure effects on the deformed foot. Calluses under the prominent metatarsal heads become painful, and if there are associated claw toes, tender callosities may develop over the dorsum of the interphalangeal joints. Not uncommonly there is a family history of pes cavus.

Pes cavus of neuromuscular origin usually presents at a younger age. The parent may be concerned about the appearance of the foot or difficulty with shoe fitting. The presentation may be due to excessive uneven shoe wear, which may be over the lateral aspect of the forefoot in the cavovarus foot. The child may complain of recurrent 'giving way' into inversion of the ankle, either due to the deformity or due to the underlying neurological cause. There may be pain over the prominent metatarsal heads, particularly if there is restricted dorsiflexion of the ankle joint. Clawing of the toes can produce pressure sores on the dorsum of these digits. If there is a loss of sensation the condition may present with neuropathic ulcers over the prominent base of the fifth metatarsal.

The physical sign of pes cavus is a high arch deformity associated with a tight plantar fascia. There may be varus of the hind foot as described above. The Coleman block test should be performed to ascertain whether the varus is fixed or a consequence of a pronation deformity of the forefoot. A block is placed obliquely under the child's foot to support the heel and lateral aspect of the foot to the head of the fifth metatarsal (see *Figure 1.9*). If the varus is due to pronation of the forefoot the heel corrects to neutral when weight-bearing in this fashion. If the heel varus is unaltered by this manoeuvre, it is fixed. There may be an equinus deformity of the ankle and clawing of the toes.

A full neurological examination is essential in all these children. Any muscle wasting should be noted and the tendon reflexes and muscle strengths should be tested. Particular note is made of any spasticity or weakness in the peroneal muscles.

The investigation of the cavus deformity is aimed at diagnosing the cause of the deformity. Only when the aetiology has been ascertained can one decide on the prognosis and appropriate treatment. The commonest causes of the cavovarus foot are hereditary motor and sensory neuropathy and spinal dysraphism, and less commonly, cerebral palsy. Before any investigations are undertaken, it is therefore important to obtain a full family history, to look at the back for any markers of spinal dysraphism, and to perform a full neurological examination.

Examination by a paediatric neurologist is often very helpful. Nerve conduction studies, serum creatine phosphokinase and biopsies are performed as indicated. At least one plain radiograph of the spine and probably magnetic resonance imaging (MRI) should be undertaken to detect any spinal dysraphism.

Management

In the idiopathic group for whom the deformity is usually simple cavus a non-operative approach is appropriate. A moulded insole can relieve pain from prominent metatarsal heads and an extra-depth shoe can prevent rubbing on claw toes. If conservative measures fail a plantar release can be combined with a Dwyer calcaneal osteotomy to improve the posture of the foot. In the adult a midtarsal osteotomy may be necessary. An excisional wedge osteotomy can result in a very short foot. The V-shaped osteotomy as described by Japas can prevent this shortening. Others advocate a large excisional triple arthrodesis to correct the deformity. The operative options for the neuromuscular cavovarus foot are discussed in Chapter 10.

HALLUX VALGUS

Decisions about the timing and the surgical approach for hallux valgus are difficult, but fortunately presentation in children is not common. The condition presents more often in females and there is often a family history.

Aetiology

The condition is probably not due to inappropriate footwear. The aetiology would appear to be a variation in anatomical development with a genetic predisposition. Shoes, however, cause symptoms because of the pressure of the shoe over the bony prominences.

Pathology

The first metatarsal is deviated medially and there is an increase in the angle formed by the axes of the first and second metatarsals (called metatarsus primus varus). The hallux is deviated laterally causing a prominence of the first metatarsal head and there may be an overlying bursa (*Figure 20.10*).

Clinical Features

The usual presentation is a child over ten years of age with a prominence of the first metatarsal rubbing on shoes. Often the parents are concerned about the appearance and hope for successful treatment before it gets as bad as mother's or grandmother's.

The physical signs are the prominent bunion. There is metatarsus primus varus, apparent as a palpable deficiency between the metatarsal heads when the patient is weight-bearing. The great toe is laterally deviated, and in the more severe case may overlap the second toe and be rotated so that the toe nail is directed medially and may produce pain and infection. The overall appearance of the forefoot is broad, often with a bunionette over the fifth metatarsal head. When the hallux valgus is over 25°, the natural history is of increasing deformity and symp-

toms. The symptoms can be aggravated as the patient starts wearing more fashionable shoes. With increasing valgus deviation of the great toe the metatarsophalangeal joint becomes incongruent and arthritic.

Management

The treatment of adolescent hallux valgus is difficult. The results of surgery are not always satisfactory, so non-operative management in the form of shoe modification is recommended wherever possible. This reduces symptoms, but there is no evidence that orthotics or spacers between the hallux and second toe can slow down the progression of the deformity. Many patients ultimately request surgical correction because of the unsightly appearance and increasing symptoms.

The patient's expectations of surgery are frequently to create a foot with a perfect appearance, preferably without a scar, with normal mobility and no discomfort and for it to remain permanently corrected. These expectations are frequently not met and it is essential to be quite frank in discussing the difficulties of surgery.

The optimum age for surgery is between 12–15 years of age. The principles of surgical treatment are to correct the metatarsus primus varus by proximal or distal osteotomy, correct the valgus by medial capsular reefing and correction of the muscle imbalance, which may include tenotomy or transfer of the adductor hallucis and lengthening of extensor hallucis longus.

Distal osteotomies with soft-tissue procedures to the first metatarsal joint are popular. If there is significant metatarsus primus varus an osteotomy through the base of the first metatarsal combined with a soft tissue correction of the first metatarsophalangeal joint is usually preferred. Some authors describe the use of a pure soft tissue correction in children (McBride), but we have found few indications for this. If there is significant degenerative change in the first metatarsophalangeal joint treatment is along the lines suggested for hallux rigidus.

Distal first metatarsal osteotomy

Through a dorsomedial approach the capsule of the first metatarsophalangeal joint is exposed. A Y-shaped incision with its base pointing proximal is made. Various methods of dividing the neck of the metatarsal to obtain lateral displacement have been described. The oblique incision of Wilson can produce shortening of the hallux; however, if the degree of obliquity is reduced and the direction of the cut is rotated to prevent dorsal displacement of

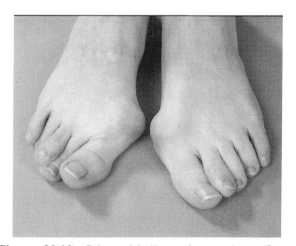

Figure 20.10 Bilateral hallux valgus and significant bunions.

the metatarsal head (as described by Helal *et al.* 1974) the position is stable and the results are good. The Chevron technique is stable and can significantly reduce any metatarsus primus varus, but occasionally the distal fragment becomes avascular. Closure of the capsule converts the Y into a V so correcting the hallux valgus. The feet are immobilized for six weeks. Some use a below-knee walking cast, but plaster slippers are adequate, and some surgeons use only reinforced bandages, particularly with the Chevron technique.

Simmonds–Menelaus operation

If the intermetatarsal angle is large a simple distal first metatarsal osteotomy is unlikely to give satisfactory results. The Simmonds–Menelaus operation is one method of obtaining a proximal bony correction of the first metatarsal and a distal soft tissue correction of the valgus deformity.

An incision is made between the first and second metatarsals to gain access to the adductor hallucis and the base of the first metatarsal. A second incision is made on the medial side over the first metatarsophalangeal joint. The capsule of the joint is elevated as a flap, the bony prominence excised, and the medial capsule advanced to correct the hallux valgus deformity. Through the first incision, adductor hallucis is detached from its insertion onto the base of the proximal phalanx, passed through a drill hole in the neck of the first metatarsal, and attached to the capsule. A simple division of adductor hallucis seems to be equally effective. The base of the first metatarsal is exposed and an osteotomy is performed. The excised exostosis is used as a graft in an opening wedge osteotomy to hold the first metatarsal deviated laterally. These patients are then immobilized in plaster for a period of six weeks, being able to walk on the plaster after about two weeks.

HALLUX RIGIDUS

Hallux rigidus occasionally occurs in children. It is more common in females and can be bilateral. It has been reported to be associated with an overlong first metatarsal, and a few cases are due to osteochondritis dissecans of the first metatarsal head.

Characteristically children presenting with hallux rigidus are in the adolescent age group and complain of pain in the great toe associated with restricted mobility. Movement is particularly restricted in dorsiflexion.

In the initial stages the symptoms and signs may be associated with relatively normal radiological appearances, but with time typical degenerative changes develop with sclerosis of the epiphysis of the proximal phalanx.

Management

Treatment of hallux rigidus in the adolescent is with metatarsal insoles designed to relieve weight under the metatarsal head. Frequently this is unsuccessful and often surgical intervention is required. Dorsal closing-wedge osteotomies of the base of the proximal phalanx or the neck of the first metatarsal have been described in an attempt to overcome the loss of dorsiflexion. If the degenerative changes are advanced, the condition is treated by arthrodesis with screw fixation in an appropriate position.

HEEL BUMPS

Bilateral heel bumps or calcaneal exostoses are common in adolescent boys and girls. The prominence is on the posterolateral aspect of the heel at the insertion of the tendo Achillis. They seem to be more troublesome in cooler climates and where hard backed shoes are worn. They present because of discomfort over the bump, rubbing on shoes and sometimes blistering. There is frequently overlying callus formation accentuating the prominence and sometimes a subcutaneous bursa forms.

The natural history is of resolution at skeletal maturity and therefore it is advisable wherever possible to pursue a non-operative approach. Care in choosing shoes is necessary and if trainers or sports shoes can be worn routinely there seems to be few symptoms.

If the symptoms are unacceptable, the prominence can be excised. The skin incision is lateral rather than posterior where it would rub on shoes. The bony bump is excised with an osteotome from the lateral side down to the insertion of the tendo Achillis.

CURLY TOES

Curly toes are common. They are usually present at birth, frequently run in families, and are often bilateral. They involve the third to fifth toes. The natural history is usually of continuing deformity, but some resolve as the child grows.

Clinical Features

The condition is usually not noticed by the parents until the child starts walking. The child is asymptomatic, but the parents are concerned about the

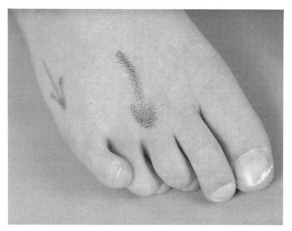

Figure 20.11 Curly third and fourth toes and an overriding fifth toe.

is no longer used. It is technically difficult and produces toes that are stiff in extension, often with a rotational abnormality.

Although many of these children present before the age of two years it is wise to delay surgical correction until after the age of four. It is easier to operate on a bigger toe and some may improve during the wait. It is ideal to have completed treatment before the child starts school, but the operation can be performed at any age up to about 12 years. After 12 years of age the deformity may become more rigid and less amenable to simple tenotomy.

Not infrequently the correction of one toe will reveal that the adjacent lateral toe also requires surgical intervention.

deformity and the natural history of the condition. There is frequently a family history of relatives who have had toe surgery. On occasions the child may indicate some discomfort, particularly if there is rotation of the toe so that the nail is weight-bearing. Rarely there may be pressure on the dorsum of the toe with foot wear or the prominent toe may catch when socks are put on.

A typical appearance is of a flexed third toe, deviated medially to underride the second toe and push it dorsally. The fourth and fifth toes curl in a similar way to the third toe, but usually not so much (*Figure 20.11*). The deformity increases with dorsiflexion of the ankle as the flexor tendons tighten. In normal people the fifth toe has a tendency to be slightly curled.

Management

There is little evidence that strapping the toes improves the chance of spontaneous resolution (Sweetnam, 1958).

Surgical treatment is advised if:

- There are symptoms.
- There is significant deformity.
- There is underriding of the toes under the adjacent medial toes.

Open flexor tenotomy is performed through the volar aspect of the toe between the skin creases overlying the proximal phalanx. All three flexor tendons are identified and divided. The most important part of the operation is to close the incision in such a way that it does not cause contractures across the skin creases. This simple procedure produces satisfactory results in the majority of patients. Transfer of the flexors into the extensor hood (Girdlestone transfer)

OVERRIDING FIFTH TOE

Overriding fifth toe may present at birth or may develop during childhood. It is usually bilateral. The fifth toe is hyperextended at the metatarsophalangeal joint with flexion at the interphalangeal joints. It is deviated medially to lie on top of the fourth toe. Often the toe is hypoplastic and there may be a rotational component so that the nail faces laterally. In many patients if this is left untreated the toe tends to flatten out and it is not uncommon to see adults with this deformity without symptoms.

The pathological anatomy is of contracture of the skin on the dorsum of the toe with shortening of the common extensor and the capsule of the metatarsophalangeal joint.

Patients present because there is concern about the appearance of the toe and the implications for the future. Very occasionally they present with pressure problems over the toe or catching of the toe when placing socks on the child.

Management

Conservative measures are not successful and surgical correction is necessary. There are many different approaches, but any surgical procedure must include a complete division of the extensor tendon with a wide capsular division including the collateral ligaments. In this way the toe can be brought down into its reduced position and also derotated. Correction of the skin contracture is best performed by a double racquet handle incision to move the toe into its corrected position as described by Butler (Cockin, 1968). The V–Y procedure often contracts and recurrence is common.

REFERENCES AND FURTHER READING

Carroll NC, Gross RH. Operative management of clubfoot. *Orthopedics* 1990; **13**: 1285–1296.

Catterall A. A method of assessment of the clubfoot deformity. *Clin Orthop Rel Research* 1991; **264**: 48–53.

Cockin J. Butler's operation for overriding 5th toe. *J Bone Joint Surg* 1968; **60B**: 78–81.

Coleman SS. *Complex Foot Deformities in Children*. Lea and Febiger, Philadelphia, 1983.

Crawford AH, Marxsen JL, Osterfeld DL. The Cincinnati incision: A comprehensive approach for surgical procedures for the foot and ankle in children. *J Bone Joint Surg* 1982; **64A**: 1355–1358.

Drennan JC. *The Child's Foot and Ankle*. Raven Press, New York, 1992.

Fraser RK, Menelaus MB, Williams PF, Cole WG. The Miller procedure for mobile flat feet. *J Bone Joint Surg* 1995; **77B**: 396–399.

Graham GP, Dent CM. The Dillwyn–Evans operation for relapsed club foot: long term results. *J Bone Joint Surg* 1992: **74B**: 445–448.

Handelsman JE, Badalamente MA. Neuromuscular studies in clubfoot. *J Pediatr Orthop* 1981; **1**: 23–32.

Helal B, Gupta SK, Gojaseni P. Surgery for adolescent hallux valgus. *Acta Orthop Scand* 1974; **45**: 271–290.

Hutchins PM, Foster BK, Paterson DC, Cole EA. Long-term results of early surgical release in club feet. *J Bone Joint Surg* 1985; **67B**: 791–799.

Menelaus MB, Ross ERS. Open flexor tenotomy for hammer toes and curly toes in childhood. *J Bone Joint Surg* 1984; **66B**: 770–771.

Simmons FA, Menelaus MB. Hallux valgus in adolescence. *J Bone Joint Surg* 1960; **42B**: 761–768.

Simon G. Analytical radiographs of club feet. *J Bone Joint Surg* 1977; **59B**: 485–489.

Sweetnam DR. Congenital curly toes. An investigation into the value of treatment. *Lancet* 1958; **2**: 398–400.

Turco VJ. Resistant congenital club foot. One stage posteromedial release with internal fixation. *J Bone Joint Surg* 1979; **61A**: 805–814.

Wijesinha SS, Menelaus MB. Operation for calcaneus deformity after surgery for club foot. *J Bone Joint Surg* 1989; **71B**: 234–236.

Wilde PH, Torode IP, Dickens DR, Cole WG. Resection for symptomatic talocalcaneal coalition. *J Bone Joint Surg* 1994; **76B**: 797–801.

Williams PF. Club foot. *Curr Orthop* 1987; **1**: 404–411.

Chapter 21
The Spine

D Robert V Dickens

SCOLIOSIS

The term 'scoliosis' simply describes a lateral curvature of the spine. Scoliosis has been recognized as a condition for many years and was first written about by Hippocrates. It can be classified into structural and non-structural:

- Non-structural scoliosis can occur in the presence of leg length discrepancy, muscle spasm from any cause, or as a voluntary act. There is no rotational element to the deformity as seen in structural scoliosis. When examining a child with a spinal curvature it is important to exclude non-structural scoliosis before considering the diagnosis of a true structural curve.
- Structural scoliosis has a three-dimensional component to the deformity including a rotational element, which produces a prominence of the ribs or loin musculature depending on the level of the curve particularly on forward flexion. It is fixed and is associated in most cases with a lordosis. On occasions it may be associated with a kyphosis. True structural scoliosis can be classified into a number of major groups as shown in Table 21.1.

Idiopathic scoliosis is the commonest form of scoliosis, accounting for about 70% of cases. Early- and late-onset scoliosis appear to be of a similar nature, although the long-term studies indicate that patients with early-onset scoliosis develop more severe curves.

Infantile Idiopathic Scoliosis

Infantile idiopathic scoliosis usually presents in the early months of life when the parent notices an asymmetry of the chest wall. The condition is a true scoliosis with rotation producing rib prominence. It is more common in boys, is more commonly a left-sided curve and is frequently associated with plagiocephaly. The condition is not common and the

Table 21.1 Structural scoliosis

Idiopathic scoliosis
Infantile
Adolescent
    Early onset
    Late onset

Congenital scoliosis
Failure of segmentation
Failure of formation

Neuromuscular scoliosis
Neuropathic
    Upper motor neurone
    Lower motor neurone
Myopathic

Scoliosis in other conditions
Neurofibromatosis
Marfan syndrome
Other conditions

natural history in the vast majority of patients is for spontaneous resolution, usually by the age of 2–3 years.

A small proportion of these children, however, develop progressive scoliosis. This can be suspected by observation and by measuring the progression of the rib–vertebral angle of Mehta on the spinal radiograph (*Figure 21.1*).

Adolescent Idiopathic Scoliosis

Adolescent idiopathic scoliosis affects approximately 4% of the population, with a male to female ratio of 1:1 (*Figure 21.2*). The male to female ratio of those requiring treatment, however, approaches 1:8. School screening studies suggest that for curves

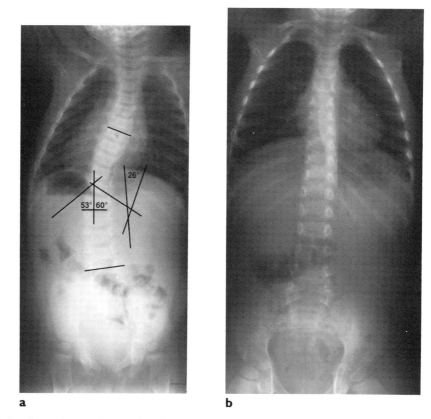

Figure 21.1 a Infantile idiopathic scoliosis. At 18 months the Cobb angle is 26° and the rib–vertebral angle of Mehta is 53° and 60°. **b** There has been complete resolution of the infantile idiopathic scoliosis without treatment at the age of three years.

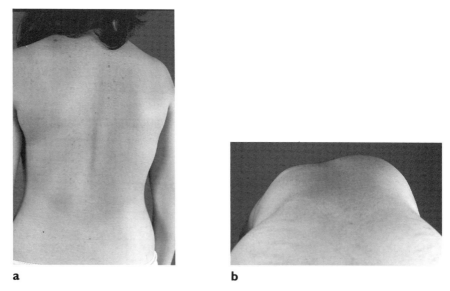

Figure 21.2 a Adolescent idiopathic scoliosis. The curve is convex to the right. This means that the convexity of the curve or the outer part of the curve is on the right side of the body, whereas the concavity or the inside of the curve is on the left side of the body. **b** The rib hump of adolescent idiopathic scoliosis becomes prominent on forward flexion because of the rotational abnormality of the vertebrae.

greater than 10°, the male to female ratio is 1:3.6 and for curves above 20°, 1:6.5. The proportion of children detected on a screening programme who require intervention is quite low (of the order of 1 in 10).

Adolescent idiopathic scoliosis has been recognized for many years as having a three-dimensional component to the deformity, but it is only in recent times that this three-dimensional characteristic of the curve has been recognized as important in the management of the condition. The majority of idiopathic curves are lordotic.

Aetiology

Little is known about the aetiology of idiopathic scoliosis. Sometimes there may be a subtle neurological cause, and using magnetic resonance imaging (MRI) it has become apparent that some of the previously labelled idiopathic curves may be associated with a spinal cord anomaly or Chiari malformation (*Figure 21.3*).

 Atypical features that indicate the need for investigation with an MRI to look for a cord anomaly include a left-sided curve, pain or stiffness, males and evidence of decompensation. Subtle neurological signs (e.g. absent superficial abdominal reflexes) should always be sought.

Clinical Features

History
The late-onset group usually present at 10–11 years of age. There is often a history of progression, the mother having become aware of it and then noticing an increase in the prominence of the rib hump with time. There is frequently a positive family history.

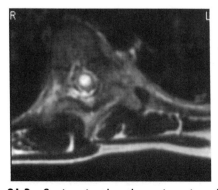

Figure 21.3 Syrinx in the thoracic spine. Dye has been used to enhance the central fluid-filled syrinx, which shows up white.

The history must include information on the antepartum and postpartum state of the child and any other medical condition that may have produced a neurological anomaly.

Examination
Examination of a child with scoliosis includes a full general and neurological examination for any features suggesting an aetiology. Inspection of the general body shape is important to exclude either short stature or Marfan syndrome. Skin abnormalities may suggest neurofibromatosis.

General body shape is inspected for shoulder height asymmetry, loin creases or waistline asymmetry, and rib or loin prominence. Leg length inequality gives rise to pelvic obliquity and a non-structural scoliosis, which can be corrected by blocks to equalize the leg lengths.

A forward flexion test is performed to observe the spinal alignment and at the same time to determine whether there is any rotational component to the curve producing a prominence on the convex side of the curve (see *Figure 21.2*).

Mobility of the curve is assessed by observing the spine in flexion, extension, lateral flexion and rotation, and by stressing the spine to determine the flexibility of the curve, either by forced lateral flexion or suspension.

Natural history
The natural history of idiopathic scoliosis is far better understood since the introduction of school screening. The likelihood of progression relates to age, and the earlier the onset of scoliosis the more likely there is to be significant progression. Late-onset scoliosis with minor curves developing close to skeletal maturity are unlikely to progress.

The natural history in the adult has also been extensively investigated. The Iowa Study (Weinstein *et al.*, 1981) suggests that in the skeletally mature, a thoracic curve of less than 30° will not progress, but curves greater than 50° tend to progress at a rate of up to 1° per year. In the lumbar spine, curves less than 30° in the skeletally mature are usually stable, but curves greater than this tend to progress.

In determining the likelihood of progression, it is necessary to estimate the skeletal maturity of the patient. Skeletal age is determined by a radiograph of the left hand and wrist, which is compared to the standards described by Greulich and Pyle charts. The spinal radiograph shows the iliac crests so that the development or progression of capping of the iliac apophyses can be assessed (Risser sign). In girls the onset of menarche is about two years before skeletal maturity.

The parents should be encouraged to keep growth charts at regular intervals, and using a combination of all information, one can estimate the period when growth ceases. It is during the period of rapid growth that scoliosis may progress significantly.

Radiology

Radiography

The most important assessment in the diagnosis of scoliosis and in determining its severity and progression is the plain radiograph. These films must be taken in a standard fashion so that serial radiographs can be compared. The patient is erect with a constant tube to cassette distance, with standard positioning of the patient in a relaxed position. 90 cm cassette films are preferable as they allow visualization of the full length of the spine. Appropriate radiation protection measures must be observed. The standard is to perform a posteroanterior (PA) rather than an anteroposterior (AP) film to reduce radiation to the breast tissue in the adolescent girls. A standing lateral film is also performed.

Supine forced lateral flexion films or suspension films, which are frequently used for patients with paralytic curves, are only indicated as a preliminary to surgical intervention. The aim is to determine the flexibility of the curve and the appropriate level for fusion. They should not be performed routinely in all scoliosis patients.

The follow-up of scoliosis requires serial radiographs and the effects of excessive radiation must be considered. For this reason, it is usually adequate to obtain six-monthly PA erect films to assess progression.

Bone scan

Bone scanning has a limited place in the investigation of scoliosis patients, predominantly in those presenting with painful scoliosis. Technetium is the isotope that is usually used because it indicates an increase in blood flow in areas where there is pathological activity. Tumour, infection and stress fractures can be excluded by a normal bone scan.

Computerized tomography

Computerized tomography (CT) of the spine has a limited place in patients with scoliosis. It is good for outlining bony architecture to define, for example, the nidus in an osteoid osteoma (see *Figure 7.6*) and the bony spur in diastematomyelia, but has little application in investigating the neurological structures in the spinal canal.

Magnetic resonance imaging

An MRI scan has become the investigation of choice for determining whether there is any intraneural or intraspinal pathology that may influence spinal cord function. The investigation is essential in patients with atypical curves and in those with neurological signs.

Management

Observation

The severity of the scoliosis is measured by the Cobb angle. On a standing PA film a line is drawn across the upper end-plate of the vertebrae with the greatest tilt and the lower end-plate of the vertebrae with the greatest tilt in the opposite direction. The angle created is the Cobb angle, which measures the severity of the curve (as drawn on *Figure 21.1*). Skeletal maturity is assessed by Risser sign and bone age.

Many children with adolescent idiopathic scoliosis present with relatively minor curves that have been detected on a school screening programme. If the curve is less than 20° it is appropriate to observe with a review film 6-monthly. If the curves remain at these minor levels no further intervention is necessary except in the rare circumstance where the cosmetic appearance appears to be worse than the radiological measurements.

Bracing

Over the years many forms of plaster cast and bracing have been attempted to control the progression of scoliosis. It is only very recently that a controlled study has indicated that bracing is more effective than no treatment at all.

Current bracing uses the Milwaukee brace (CTLSO, cervical thoracic lumbar sacral orthosis) or variants of it, and an underarm Boston-type of orthosis (TLSO, thoraco-lumbar sacral orthosis) (*Figure 21.4*).

It is essential that the decision to start a bracing programme involves not just the parent and doctor, but the patient as well. It must be recognized that this treatment is being imposed on a child at a delicate developmental stage, both physically and psychologically, and great empathy is required in this discussion process. It is essential that the expectation of the results of bracing should be explained. Bracing is used to control the curve, but is not expected to correct the curve. Surgical intervention can be avoided in the majority of cases, but at the end of the bracing programme curve severity is usually unchanged from the start of the programme. Although exercises do not have any place in prevent-

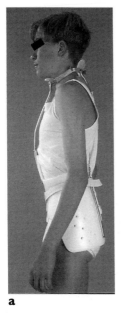 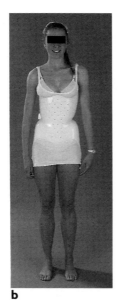

a   b

Figure 21.4 **a** The Milwaukee brace for adolescent idiopathic scoliosis (reproduced with permission from Williams PF, Cole WG. *Orthopaedic Management in Childhood*. Chapman & Hall, London). **b** The Boston underarm brace for adolescent idiopathic scoliosis.

ing the progression of scoliosis, it is important to encourage the patient to participate in activities while on the bracing programme.

The indications for bracing are curves in skeletally-immature children of:

- Greater than 30° but less than 45°.
- Greater than 20° with radiological progression.

A Milwaukee brace is used if the apex of the curve is above T8. Below T8, the Boston brace is preferred because it is more acceptable for the child. A skilled orthotist is imperative. The bracing programme should encourage the patient to wear the brace 23 hours a day until radiological and clinical skeletal maturity. Geographical considerations may influence these guidelines, for example the availability of the patient for review and the climate in which the patient wears the brace.

Bracing is used, but is not as effective, for patients with congenital scoliosis, Marfan syndrome, neurofibromatosis and paralytic disorders. In the latter category, it is used as a temporizing procedure aimed at reducing the rate of progression until the patient is old enough to contemplate surgery.

Patients in braces are seen three-monthly by the orthotist and have radiographs six-monthly to review progress and skeletal maturity.

Surgery

Curves greater than 40–45° with proven progression in skeletally-immature children, or curves greater than 50° in mature individuals are indications for surgical intervention. The likelihood of surgical intervention is much higher for early-onset scoliosis.

The ideal age for fusion is over 10–12 years of age as most of the skeletal growth has then occurred and there is unlikely to be any significant adverse effect on torso height.

Preoperative tests include radiographs with a lateral flexion film, general tests of the patient's health, respiratory function and cardiac assessment, and any other special investigations including MRIs that may be deemed necessary.

In the planning of surgery it is usual to fuse from neutral vertebrae to neutral vertebrae. In the lumbar area the concept of the stable vertebrae is important, this being determined by a vertical line drawn up from the mid-point at right angles to the sacrum. The vertebrae that are bisected by this line are said to be the stable vertebrae.

It is preferable not to fuse low into the lumbar spine as the lower the fusion extends the greater the incidence of long-term back pain. Below L3 this becomes a serious consideration and one should avoid going beyond this level if possible. The decision to fuse in front or behind is important. In general terms posterior fusions are appropriate for most curves, but in the thoracolumbar region in the presence of hyperlordosis, an anterior fusion of the Dwyer type is preferred.

In double structural scoliosis a decision has to be made as to whether one or both curves should be fused. If the lower curve is greater than the upper curve, and if the lower curve is less flexible than the upper curve, the lower curve should be fused and the upper curve can be left. If the thoracic curve is greater than the lumbar curve and is less flexible, generally the thoracic curve only should be fused (King *et al.*, 1983).

Anterior releases are performed for major curves with poor flexibility. A curve of 70° which on lateral flexion only corrects to 50° is probably best treated by anterior release before posterior instrumentation and fusion.

The junction between one scoliosis in which there is a lordotic component and the next level of the spine may result in a kyphotic component at that junctional level. In normal circumstances instrumentation should include the junctional kyphosis in the fusion. This may involve a reversal of instrumentation to bring the spine into balance in both coronal and sagittal planes.

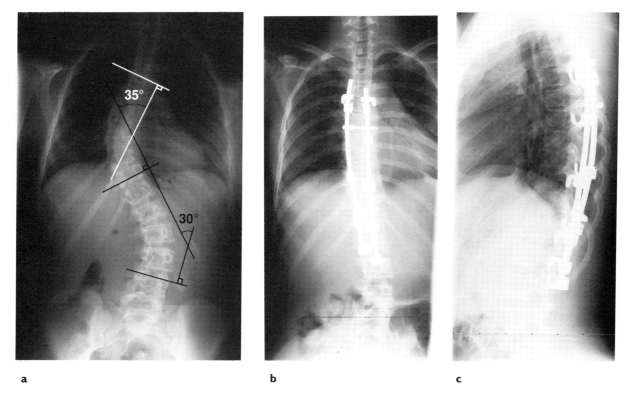

Figure 21.5 **a** Double structural curve in an adolescent with both Cobb angles marked. **b** Posterior instrumentation with Cotrel–Dubousset system including cross linkage. **c** The instrumentaion is contoured to preserve the thoracic kyphosis and lumbar lordosis.

Preoperative traction is rarely indicated and has been shown to be of little influence on the degree of correction in the vast majority of cases. For curves greater than 70° with poor flexibility, an anterior release may be performed and then the patient placed on halofemoral traction followed by posterior instrumentation and fusion performed as a staged procedure two weeks later. This is mainly reserved for the skeletally- mature patient with limited flexibility.

Internal fixation with fusion of the scoliotic spine has eliminated the previous necessity for prolonged bed rest. Posterior instrumentation originally used the Harrington system and corrected the coronal plane abnormality on the plain film, but failed to address the lordotic or kyphotic deformity and also the rotational component. The Luque system was developed to improve the correction of these other abnormalities and has been popular in the management of neuromuscular curves. The technique involves the use of multiple intralaminar wires. The Cotrel–Dubousset was the first posterior system to fully address the rotational component and has markedly improved the correction of the rotational element and the rib hump, which is often the most disfiguring part of the deformity (*Figure 21.5*). Other systems that now incorporate this rotational correc-

tion and rigid fixation allow rapid mobilization and discharge from hospital at 5–10 days without the need for any external bracing.

Popular anterior systems include the Zielke systems and its various modifications.

Congenital Scoliosis

Congenital scoliosis is not common, and the condition can vary from a mild non-progressive deformity to a rapidly progressing and severe curvature that compromises the spinal cord.

Aetiology

There are two types of congenital scoliosis.

- Failure of the natural segmentation of the individual vertebral component leads to asymmetrical fusion of adjacent vertebrae.
- Failure of formation in which only a part of the vertebra is formed (e.g. a hemivertebra).

In many of the patients it is common to see a combination of both a failure of formation and a failure of segmentation as the basis for the deformity

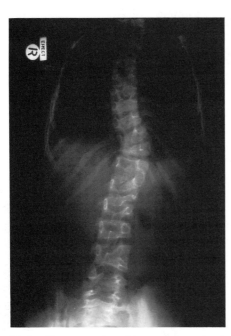

Figure 21.6 Congenital scoliosis with a combination of failure of formation on the right side and failure of segmentation on the left side.

(*Figure 21.6*). Failures of segmentation may be lateral, anterior or posterior, and produce the corresponding deformity. Similarly failures of formation may be lateral, producing scoliosis, or anterior, resulting in a kyphotic deformity. If there is a failure of formation that is mirrored by an adjacent vertebra there may be no consequence to the overall alignment of the spine. If the hemivertebra is incarcerated and not segmented the growth potential may be so small that a significant curvature does not develop. Failure of formation anteriorly and laterally results in a posterior and lateral hemivertebra with a very severe kyphotic deformity, progressive scoliosis, and early neurological problems.

The most significant curves are those with unilateral failure of segmentation. Others that are likely to progress are double convex hemivertebrae and single free convex hemivertebrae. Incarcerated hemivertebrae are less likely to be progressive.

Clinical Features

Congenital scoliosis may be recognized early in life or later, when increasing deformity becomes apparent. It is associated with other congenital abnormalities in the neuraxis (e.g. diastematomyelia), cardiac system, renal system, gastrointestinal system (e.g. tracheo-oesophageal fistula) and limbs (e.g. congenital absence of the radius and hypoplasia of the thumb). The natural history of congenital scoliosis depends on the type of lesion and its potential for acceleration or growth arrest determined by its position. Many minor congenital abnormalities are unrecognized and do not require treatment.

Management

Conservative
It is unlikely that any bracing programme has a major influence on the rate of progression. Bracing may act as a delaying procedure until the patient is at a more appropriate age for spinal fusion.

Surgery
Before surgical instrumentation an MRI is mandatory to look for cord involvement. The operative management depends on the aetiology, the age of the patient, and the rate of progression. As the unilateral unsegmented bar produces such a rapidly progressive curve, the patient should have a very early short-segment fusion on the convexity and anteriorly. This fusion *in situ* should be carried out before the curve becomes significant. Instrumentation is only used in the older age group if possible and if there is flexibility of the curve on lateral flexion studies.

For the rigid severe curves, there may be a place for hemivertebrae excision or osteotomy of the spine combined with a period in traction and then instrumentation posteriorly. In the younger age group it is essential to fuse both anteriorly and posteriorly to avoid the crankshaft phenomenon.

Neuromuscular Scoliosis

Although spinal deformities are common in many neuromuscular disorders, those most frequently presenting for correction are cerebral palsy, spina bifida and Duchenne muscular dystrophy. In some countries poliomyelitis remains an important cause of neuromuscular scoliosis.

Cerebral Palsy

Scoliosis presents mainly in the spastic quadriplegic patient, often as a long C-shaped curve. There is usually pelvic obliquity and hip subluxation or dislocation (*Figure 21.7*). These children have multiple problems including epilepsy, poor nutritional status, and poor swallowing with reflux and the risk of aspiration. Communication is often poor, but sensation is intact. Discomfort from a poor sitting balance and the associated pelvic obliquity may result in a miserable child, but one who has difficulty communicating his or her unhappiness.

Occasionally a child with less severe involvement may present with a mild curve that can be managed in a similar manner to that for idiopathic curves.

Management

Conservative

Orthoses for spinal deformity in cerebral palsy are only occasionally used. An orthosis may be useful for a moderate to mild curve in a child with a less severe involvement who is ambulant. There is occasionally a role for bracing in children who are floppy and have seating difficulties.

Seating modifications may simply involve the use of thigh pads and chest pads, but may progress to extremely elaborate custom-moulded seats. These do not alter the natural history of the curve, so repeated modifications may be necessary.

Surgery

The indication for surgery is an increasing deformity leading to loss of function. Most of these children are non-walkers and loss of function refers to difficulties with seating. Many of these children are institutionalized and if they cannot be seated, their outings are curtailed and their life is markedly constrained.

Planning of any operation must involve the parents because often a decision is philosophical as much as medical.

In patients with a thoracolumbar or lumbar curve associated with a significant pelvic obliquity, it is necessary to extend the instrumentation to the pelvis. The dictum is to fuse long rather than short in cerebral palsy. These spines usually contain good quality bone with intact posterior elements enabling good fixation. However, failure of fusion will lead to instrumentation breakage and recurrence of deformity.

For severe curves an anterior release of the thoracolumbar and lumbar segments may be necessary followed by posterior instrumentation using Luque rods with fixation into the pelvis (using the Galveston method). Recovery from anaesthesia and the immediate postoperative period are often the most stressful times for these children. Performing an anterior and posterior procedure at one sitting has definite advantages for selected cases.

Spina Bifida

Deformities of the spine are common in children with spina bifida. These deformities are related to muscle imbalance and deficiencies of the posterior elements

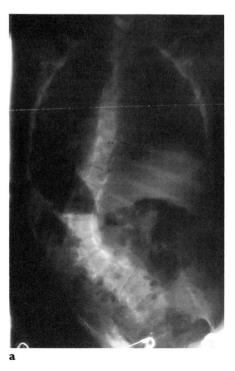
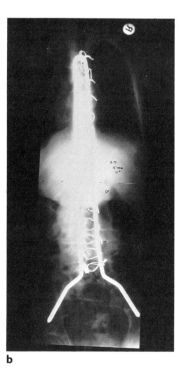

a   b

Figure 21.7   a The radiological appearance of scoliosis in cerebral palsy with a long C-shaped curve and pelvic obliquity. **b** Posterior instrumentation of scoliosis in cerebral palsy showing the Luque technique with Galveston fixation into the pelvis.

of the spine. Occasionally they are associated with bony anomalies and cord anomalies such as a syrinx or tethering. Commonly the deformities are severe and involve the thoracolumbar and lumbar spine with associated pelvic obliquity and dislocations of the hip.

In many patients with spina bifida, sensation is diminished or absent around the buttocks and thighs and therefore scoliosis producing significant pelvic obliquity can result in pressure areas that progress to skin breakdown and severe ulceration. Preservation of some mobility of the lumbosacral junction is important as these children often have good arm function and use manual wheelchairs requiring some mobility of the trunk for transfers and wheelchair propulsion.

These children often have a cerebrospinal fluid shunt, which can be put under traction by the correction of severe curves and malfunction. Rapid changes in fluid balance during surgical procedures can lead to difficulties with shunt management.

Management

Orthoses
Braces occasionally have a role in treating spinal deformities in spina bifida. However, the sensory deficiencies around the pelvis demand great care using a brace and rigorous inspection of the skin. Furthermore, orthoses do not prevent progression of the deformity.

Surgery
Many of these children have a long life, so it is necessary to obtain a solid reliable fusion. The lack of posterior elements and deficiencies in the transverse processes means that posterior fixation is unreliable, and generally an anterior and posterior fusion is performed.

An anterior release and fusion improves the correction in these children. Often it is not possible to provide corrective forces to the deficient posterior elements and a period of halofemoral traction may be used as an adjunct to an anterior release.

Instrumentation varies according to the pathology. We commonly use a combination of Luque sublaminar wiring in the thoracic spine where the posterior elements are usually intact and pedicle screws in the lumbar region (*Figure 21.8*). If fixation to the pelvis is necessary the Galveston technique can be used. However, the pelvis is often deficient and a more secure method is to use a sacral bar drilled through both iliac wings and the body of the sacrum. This technique requires a modified rod system.

Duchenne Muscular Dystrophy

Muscle weakness in Duchenne muscular dystrophy results in a wheelchair existence from about 11 years of age and it is at this stage that spinal deformities appear (see Chapter 10). Progression of the curve can be rapid so frequent assessment and early intervention are important. The characteristic curve pattern in Duchenne muscular dystrophy is a thoracolumbar or lumbar curve with associated pelvic obliquity. These boys have intact sensation, a normal intellect and good communication skills, so frequently complain of discomfort in seating when the pelvic obliquity becomes a problem.

Management

Conservative
Orthotic devices at best only slow the rate of progression of the curve and have a limited role. Orthotic devices may also reduce respiratory function. Seating modifications have had little success in slowing curve progression.

Surgery
The aim of surgery is to prevent progression and maintain seating ability and comfort. While spinal balance is maintained, the indications for surgery are few, but in most cases pelvic obliquity and a loss of balance require surgery. Respiratory function is assessed before surgery. Generally if lung function is more than 30% of normal levels, surgical intervention is possible without the need for postoperative intensive care or tracheostomy. Decisions about the surgical management of these children can only be undertaken after a frank and open discussion with the family and the patient outlining the aims of surgery and the risks involved. In these patients the spine has intact posterior elements, but the bone is porotic and fixation is difficult. The soft tissues in these patients are fibrotic and woody in character, and there is often significant blood loss during surgery.

The life expectancy of these patients is limited and usually a posterior instrumentation and fusion is all that is necessary to stabilize the spine during their remaining years of life. Segmental instrumentation using Luque wires and rods down into the pelvis is the preferred method of treatment. The rods should be contoured to maintain normal sagittal alignment and cross-linking ensures rigidity and promotes fusion. Simple stripping of the posterior elements with facet joint excision and grafting using local bone is sufficient for satisfactory fusion. Postoperatively

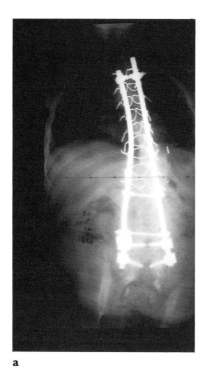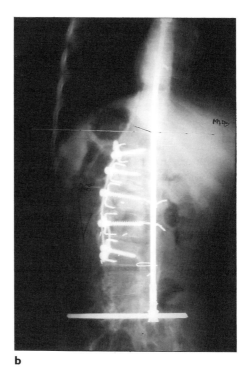

a   b

Figure 21.8 **a** Scoliosis in spina bifida. This shows a fixation method with thoracic sublaminar wiring and lumbar pedicle screws. Cross linkage has also been used. **b** Scoliosis in spina bifida. This shows anterior instrumentation with the Dwyer technique and posterior instrumentation with a sacral bar and some sublaminar wiring.

early mobilization maintains muscle function and improves respiratory rehabilitation.

Neurofibromatosis

Between 20–40% of patients with neurofibromatosis develop spinal deformities (see Chapter 5). Some are the typical idiopathic scolioses one expects to see in the general population; others are a short sharply-angled curve with kyphosis.

Characteristic radiological appearances are:

- Scalloping of the vertebrae, which is due to either dysplasia of the bone or dural ectasia.
- Wide neural foramina as a result of enlargement of the peripheral nerves.
- Ribboning of the ribs.
- The characteristic spinal deformity of a sharp short segment kyphoscoliosis.

Many patients with scoliosis associated with neurofibromatosis have cervical spine involvement, the severest form being cervical kyphosis.

The idiopathic type can be treated along standard lines, but presentation is often at an earlier age and the prognosis is worse than in normal children. The acute angular short segment kyphoscoliosis will pro-

gress. Fusion, usually anterior and posterior, is necessary. As these fusions are often carried out on young children posterior fusion alone allows curve progression due to anterior growth (the crankshaft phenomenon).

Marfan Syndrome

Scoliosis is present in about 50% of children with Marfan syndrome. It looks similar to that of adolescent idiopathic scoliosis, but most reported series show that bracing is ineffective treatment.

Surgical correction must address the frontal and sagittal components of the deformity in performing spinal fusion. Failure to recognize a junctional kyphosis in a double curve and to fuse beyond it allows progression of the curve and the need for re-fusion or fusion extension.

Osteogenesis Imperfecta

Children with mild osteogenesis imperfecta may develop mild to moderate curves and can be managed with orthoses in the usual manner. The curves that are most difficult to treat are those that occur in severe osteogenesis imperfecta; however, they do not usually produce pelvic obliquity and sitting problems and therefore do not always require intervention.

Instrumentation is difficult due to deformity of the bony elements and marked osteopenia. The posterior elements are usually the least involved component of the spine in terms of bone weakness.

SCHEUERMANN KYPHOSIS

Clinical Features

Patients typically present with a round shoulder deformity between 12–16 years of age. The deformity is usually painless. There is often great parental concern and the child's only concern is to avoid any painful treatment. Some patients dislike the appearance and avoid swimming as a result. On examination there is a fixed deformity, which does not correct on extension of the spine. The deformity is particularly apparent on forward flexion with a more angular component than the normal kyphosis (*Figure 21.9*).

Radiology

The radiological features of Scheuermann disease are kyphosis associated with irregular vertebral endplates, narrowing of the vertebral discs, wedging of the vertebral bodies and a kyphosis greater than the normal range (20–45°).

Management

The management depends on the age of the patient and the severity of the deformity. In the initial stages in a young patient where the spine remains fully correctable, hyperextension exercises are advocated, but it is unclear whether these influence the natural history of the disease. If the curve continues to progress, the use of a Milwaukee brace or an underarm orthosis aimed at creating a hyperextension three-point fixation over the apex of the kyphosis is effective in controlling progression and also in correcting deformity. Bracing is indicated for curves greater than normal, (i.e. over 45° but less than 60–65°). The individual undergoing bracing must be skeletally immature.

Surgery

Surgery for Scheuermann disease is a contentious issue and there are those who would suggest that the natural history of this condition is benign and there-

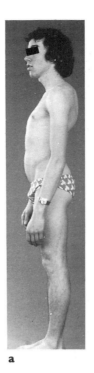
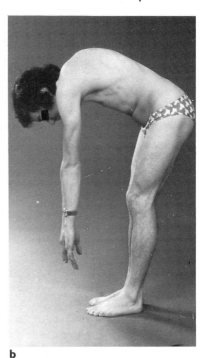

a   b

Figure 21.9 a Characteristic thoracic kyphosis of Scheuermann disease. **b** The kyphosis is accentuated on forward flexion.

fore there are limited, if any, indications for surgical correction. Indications for surgery are therefore based on concern about the cosmetic appearance of the spine, occasionally pain, and very uncommonly, neurological involvement, which can be associated with a significant kyphosis.

The operation of choice depends on the age of the patient and severity of the curve. If the curve is greater than 70° or if the patient is skeletally mature and the curve is greater than 60°, anterior release should be carried out before posterior instrumentation and correction. The implants of choice are Cotrel–Dubousset instrumentation or modifications. A claw is used at least two levels above the apex of the kyphosis and the rod–push effect is used to obtain correction. The lower attachment of the rod is stabilized using a combination of hooks and pedicle screws. The extent of the fusion is always difficult to assess, but it is essential to fuse all vertebral components within the kyphotic curve and extend beyond the end vertebra below wherever possible.

LORDOSIS

Lordosis is a natural component of the curvature of the spine in the cervical and lumbar region. Abnormal lordosis can be classified into postural and structural. Abnormal cervical lordosis is seen post-laminectomy. Thoracic lordosis is usually due to congenital abnormality. In the lumbosacral area, lordosis may be congenital or postlaminectomy or be associated with a neuromuscular scoliosis. Lordosis can also be secondary to fixed flexion deformity in the hip, proximal hamstring release and ventricular-peritoneal shunting for spina bifida. Proximal hamstring release has largely been abandoned now because of its tendency to produce this deformity. Lordosis caused by deformities around the hip is best treated by correcting the hip deformity.

Postural Lumbar Lordosis

This is a common presentation in girls between 8–10 years of age. There is parental concern about the accentuation of the lumbar lordosis with prominent buttocks posteriorly and abdomen anteriorly. On examination, there is no fixed deformity and full correction on forward flexion (*Figure 21.10*). Not infrequently there is an associated ligamentous laxity.

The natural history is for resolution with time and the only treatment required is to encourage the parents to allow the child to participate in normal activities.

SPONDYLOLYSIS/ SPONDYLOLISTHESIS

Radiological spondylolysis with or without spondylolisthesis is a common finding with an incidence of about 5%. In the adolescent or child, symptomatic spondylolysis is uncommon.

The classification of spondylolysis and spondylolisthesis as recommended by the International Society for the Study of the Lumbar Spine is outlined in Table 21.2 (Wiltse *et al.*, 1976).

The dysplastic form of spondylolisthesis is usually associated with congenital aplasia of the facet joints, often with spina bifida occulta. As the vertebrae slip forward there is attentuation of the pars interarticularis region.

The isthmic form of spondylolisthesis is graded into three types:

- Type A where there is a stress fracture.
- Type B where there is an attenuation of the pars followed by disruption of the isthmus.
- Type C, which is an acute fracture of the pars region (*Figure 21.11*).

The degenerative form usually occurs in people over 50 years of age, is more common in women and at the L4–5 level.

Traumatic spondylolisthesis refers to forward subluxation of a vertebra due to a fracture other than in

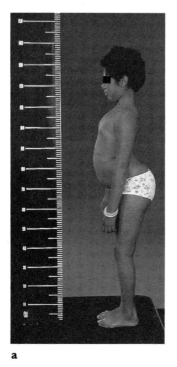
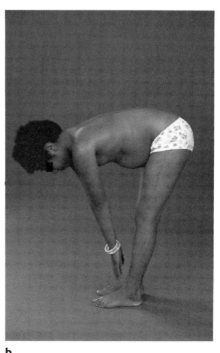

a   b

Figure 21.10 a Gross postural lumbar lordosis on standing. **b** The lumbar lordosis corrects completely on forward flexion.

Table 21.2 Classification of spondylolisthesis

Dysplastic
Isthmic
Degenerative
Traumatic
Pathological

the pars interarticularis. It is rare and usually associated with major traumatic episodes.

Pathological spondylolysis and spondylolisthesis is usually associated with abnormalities of the posterior elements, either generalized such as osteogenesis imperfecta, or localized such as tumours or rheumatoid arthritis.

Degenerative, traumatic and pathological spondylolisthesis is rare in childhood.

Clinical Features

Spondylolysis is most common at L5–S1 and has not been demonstrated in the newborn skeleton. The normal age at presentation is from around five years onwards. There is a familial tendency, particularly in the isthmic and dysplastic types, and the aetiology is thought to be traumatic. The condition is far more common in individuals who stress the lumbosacral junction (e.g. gymnasts, karate exponents). In the acute fracture of the isthmus there is frequently a history of active sport involvement, such as fast bowling in cricket.

The clinical presentation of spondylolysis and spondylolisthesis is varied and is often entirely asymptomatic in children and adolescents. Low back pain and deformity of the spine may be pre-

senting features (*Figure 21.12*), usually in the form of an accentuated lumbar lordosis. Hamstring tightness can result in an abnormal gait, and in those that are displaced, a palpable step at the level of the lesion. Neurological deficits can be demonstrated in some cases.

The natural history of spondylolysis and spondylolisthesis in the child with growth potential, particuarly at the time of adolescent growth spurt, is for increasing displacement. In the adult these displacements are usually stable and there is very slow progress or no progression at all. The likelihood of progression depends significantly on the age, the type of lesion, the percentage of slip and the degree of degenerative change in the disc.

Radiology

Standard AP and lateral radiographs frequently reveal the defect in the pars interarticularis region and demonstrate the degree of displacement. The significant radiographic features are the percentage slip and the sagittal rotation, which is a measure of kyphosis at the lumbosacral level (see *Figure 21.11*).

The defect can be seen more easily on oblique films or by a CT scan using a reversed gantry. In the presence of back pain where there is sclerosis in the pars, a bone scan can demonstrate bilateral stress fractures. An MRI is very helpful in diagnosing the state of the discs at the L5–S1 and more significantly at the L4–5 level.

Management

The treatment of spondylolysis and spondylolisthesis in children and adolescents depends on the symp-

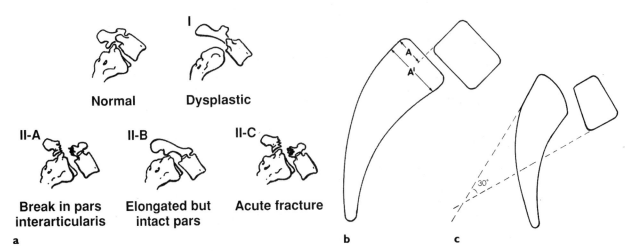

Figure 21.11 **a** Classification of spondylolisthesis commonly seen in children. **b** The measurement of anterior displacement in spondylolisthesis (A/A′ in %). **c** Measurement of sagittal rotation in spondylolisthesis.

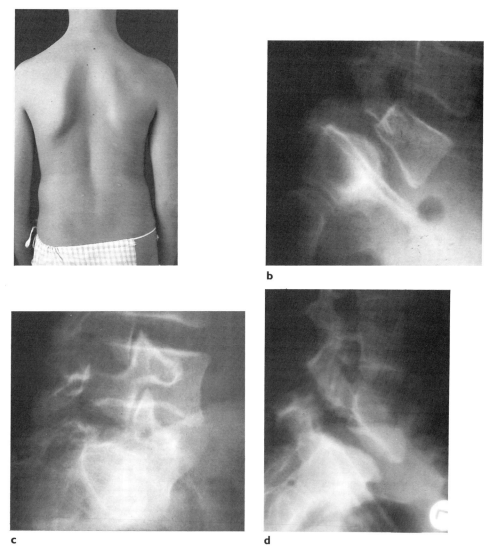

Figure 21.12 **a** Clinical photograph of spondylolisthesis. Note the bilateral loin creases. **b** There is anterior displacement of L5 on S1 of more than 50% in this case of spondylolisthesis. **c** The oblique view of the lumbar spine shows the characteristic Scottie dog shape with a normal neck. In spondylolisthesis with a defect in the pars this view shows a defect in the neck of the Scottie dog. **d** Lateral view of spondylolisthesis showing a bilateral defect in the pars interarticularis.

toms and likelihood of progression. Children who have minor discomfort or back pain and a slip of less than 50% are best treated by conservative measures in the form of rest, exercises and possibly bracing. In the unusual presentation of an acute fracture of the pars interarticularis, particularly if there is increased activity on a bone scan, the patient is placed in a cast or Boston brace to assist the healing of the pars defect.

There are occasional patients with a spondylolisthesis of less than 50% in which the symptoms persist at an unacceptable level. Fusion *in situ* of L5 to the sacrum using a posterolateral fusion technique, pre-

ferably with the Wiltse approach, is the preferred method of treatment and has a high success rate for fusion.

In those with a pars defect without a slip, but continuing symptoms, repair of the defect can be achieved using a bone graft and the Scott technique of wiring between the transverse process and the spinous process on both sides or alternatively a screw across the defect augmented with a bone graft.

Patients with a slip greater than 50% are likely to develop symptoms and progressive displacement, particularly during adolescent growth. Fusion is generally advised for these patients. The presence of tight hamstrings and neurological changes in the lower limbs do not necessarily require a decompressive procedure, and these settle in the vast majority of cases once fusion has been obtained. Exploration of the nerve roots is only advised in those in whom neurological symptoms persist or the tightness of the hamstrings does not resolve after a solid fusion.

Reduction of a spondylolisthesis with fusion is only rarely indicated if there is gross displacement. It has the advantage of improving the cosmetic result and allowing fusion of L5–S1 only. The posterior elements are removed, the spinal dura and L5 nerve roots are kept in view and a posterior lumbar interbody fusion is performed. The L5–S1 disc space is distracted to allow the vertebral bodies to slip backwards. The use of a traction wire on the posterior elements of L4 lifting the spine upwards helps in reduction. Although this is an attractive concept the high rate of neurological complications suggests that it should be used only in unusual circumstances, and certainly only by those expert in techniques using pedicle fixation. Before reduction of a spondylolisthesis an MRI is performed because degenerative changes in the disc at L4–5 would indicate a fusion at that level.

Postoperatively, after posterolateral fusion or reduction and fusion, immobilization is recommended using a cast incorporating one leg. This cast immobilization should be continued for three months, after which the cast is removed and the patient is carefully rehabilitated.

REFERENCES AND FURTHER READING

Bradford DS. Treatment of severe spondylolisthesis. A combined approach for reduction and stabilisation. *Spine* 1979; **4**: 423–429.

Edgar MA. Back pain in childhood and adolescence. *Curr Orthop* 1987; **1**: 194–208.

Harrington PR. Surgical instrumentation for management of scoliosis. *J Bone Joint Surg* 1960; **42A**: 1448.

King HA, Moe JH, Bradford DS, Winter RB. The selection of fusion levels in thoracic idiopathic scoliosis. *J Bone Joint Surg* 1983; **65A**: 1302–1313.

Luque ER. The anatomical basis and development of segmental spinal instrumentation. *Spine* 1982; **7**: 256–259.

Mehta MH. The rib vertebral angle in the early diagnosis between resolving and progressive infantile scoliosis. *J Bone Joint Surg* 1972; **54B**: 230–243.

Terminology Committee Scoliosis Research Society. A glossary of scoliosis terms. *Spine* 1976; **1**: 57–58.

Weinstein SL, Zavala DC, Ponseti IV. Idiopathic scoliosis. Long-term follow-up and prognosis in untreated patients. *J Bone Joint Surg* 1981; **63A**: 702–712.

Wiltse LL, Newman PH, Macnab I. Classification of spondylolysis and spondylolisthesis. *Clin Orthop Rel Research* 1976; **117**: 23–29.

Chapter 22
Upper Limb Trauma

H Kerr Graham

Orthopaedic surgeons need a clear understanding of the nature and management of upper limb injuries. Fractures of the upper limb are common and many injuries are prone to complications and a poor clinical outcome.

Incidence

The most common reason for admission to hospital in childhood is for manipulation of an upper limb fracture. These fractures do not occur evenly throughout the year because in most countries there is a seasonal peak corresponding to school summer holidays, higher ambient temperature and increased hours of daylight. Certain activities have been associated with 'epidemics' of upper limb fractures including roller blading and skateboarding. Complete prevention of the large number of upper limb fractures in childhood is clearly not possible. However, education and preventive measures such as protective equipment are important factors in limiting this number.

Aetiology

The majority of upper limb fractures are sustained as the result of indirect violence, usually a fall on the outstretched hand during play at school or sport or at home. A minority result from direct violence and are associated with multiple injuries from causes such as motor vehicle accidents or falls from a height.

Open injuries and comminution are uncommon and the majority of fractures can be managed by simple closed treatment as an outpatient. However, the large numbers involved mean that maintenance of a uniformly high standard of management can be difficult and requires good organization. A 'minor' fracture to the orthopaedic surgeon can cause a major family upset.

Classification of Epiphyseal Injuries

The classification of epiphyseal injuries by Harris and Salter in 1963 is widely accepted and for most cases useful (*Figure 22.1*). It is based on a simple four group classification by Poland dating from the last century (Poland, 1898). The two lines of failure are horizontally through the physis and vertically across the physis. The Salter–Harris types 1–4 can be constructed from these two lines of failure. The type 5 injury is only occasionally a primary entity; more often it is a sequel of injury types 1–4.

Rang has added a Type 6 injury to this classification. This is a peripheral perichondrial ring injury that is often associated with open injury and growth arrest. Degloving injuries from hover lawnmowers

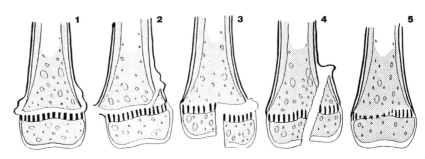

Figure 22.1 Salter–Harris classification of epiphyseal injuries. Type 1 is along the growth plate and can be displaced. Type 2 is through the metaphysis and along the growth plate. Type 3 is along the growth plate and through the epiphysis. Type 4 is through the metaphysis, through the growth plate and through the epiphysis.

produce some of the most devastating injuries of this type.

SHOULDER GIRDLE INJURIES

Clavicle

Fractures of the clavicle are the most common fracture in childhood.

Fractures of the middle one-third are rarely severely displaced and heal and remodel quickly and reliably. Formal reduction is not required and management is by supportive slings. Some use a 'figure of eight' immobilization bandage, but its use has not been shown to produce better results than a simple broad arm sling. The only indications for open treatment are open fractures and neurovascular compromise from a severely-displaced closed fracture. There is often a visible or palpable lump at the fracture site for about one year after injury, consisting of the fracture displacement or angulation with a vigorous callus response.

Fractures of the medial one-third or lateral one-third of the clavicle should be differentiated carefully from epiphyseal injuries and sternoclavicular or acromioclavicular dislocations. Plain radiographs of the medial end of the clavicle can be difficult to interpret, but computerized tomography (CT) is helpful. Age is often the best guide. Under the age of 12 years the majority of injuries are metaphyseal fractures or epiphyseal separations (Salter–Harris Type 1 or 2). Adult pattern acromioclavicular dislocations are associated with adolescent sporting activity and are managed as adult injuries.

Sternoclavicular dislocations are rare. Acute posterior dislocations can present as life-threatening emergencies because of pressure on the trachea or great vessels, and should be reduced by open methods. Chronic anterior dislocations are sometimes seen and there is no satisfactory approach to management.

Scapula

Fractures of the scapula are rare in children. The majority are caused by falls from a height or motor vehicle accidents. They are associated with child abuse, crush injuries, rib fractures and pulmonary contusion, and these injuries are more important than the scapular fracture, which does not usually require specific management unless there is involvement of the glenoid.

Glenohumeral Dislocation

Traumatic glenohumeral dislocation is rare in childhood and almost unknown under the age of 12 years. However, once an anterior dislocation has occurred in the growing child, persistent instability requiring reconstructive surgery is almost inevitable.

Atraumatic dislocation in childhood is more common and may be voluntary or involuntary. Many of these children have multidirectional instability and generalized joint laxity. Some have pathological ligamentous laxity (e.g. Marfan syndrome). Management should include a consideration of the emotional and psychiatric factors and is always non-operative in the first instance. A vigorous programme of shoulder rehabilitation will be successful for many adolescents. Under no circumstances should voluntary dislocators be offered surgery (see Chapter 15).

PROXIMAL HUMERAL FRACTURES

Injuries to the proximal humeral epiphysis and metaphysis are common following falls on the outstretched hand.

Management

Management is dictated by age, site of injury and degree of displacement. The majority of injuries in skeletally-immature children are managed by simple immobilization using a sling, collar and cuff, or Velpeau bandage. Healing is rapid (about three weeks) and remodelling tends to be rapid and complete. This is because the proximal humeral physis is so active, contributing 80% of humeral growth. There is also a wide range of motion at the glenohumeral joint, so a functional deficit due to malunion of the fracture is exceptionally rare. Most fractures at this site in children can therefore be treated in this manner and posttraumatic growth disturbance is rare.

A few injuries in older children benefit from closed reduction, but it should be appreciated that only a few injuries require reduction, not many are reducible, and even less are stable after reduction.

Open reduction and fixation is reserved for displacement of more than 50% or angulation of more than 30° in children with less than two years of growth remaining.

DIAPHYSEAL HUMERAL FRACTURES

Diaphyseal fractures are uncommon compared to fractures of the proximal and distal humerus. The age distribution is bimodal with the first peak from 0–3 years (birth injuries and child abuse) and the second in those over 12 years (sports injuries, motor vehicle accidents). Fractures in children aged 3–12 years are often pathological (i.e. due to unicameral bone cyst, osteogenesis imperfecta). The majority of these fractures are not severely displaced, and open injuries and radial nerve palsy are uncommon.

Management

Management is usually closed, using gravity to align the fracture in external splintage using a collar and cuff, Velpeau bandage (undisplaced or minimally displaced fractures), sugar-tong plaster slabs or a 'hanging cast.' The latter requires careful application and adjustment to correct malalignment. Persistent malalignment can be managed in a cast brace once the fracture has become sticky at about 7–10 days after the injury. Severely-displaced diaphyseal fractures are sometimes seen in multiply-injured children who have been in car accidents. Open fractures can be managed by external fixation and unstable closed fractures by internal fixation (intramedullary rod or plate).

A fracture at the junction of the distal diaphysis and metaphysis, the 'M–D' fracture, is not uncommon. Unlike supracondylar fractures, closed reduction and percutaneous Kirschner wire fixation is rarely practical and traction is sometimes required.

DISTAL HUMERAL FRACTURES

Injuries to the distal humerus are common and a wide variety of fractures and epiphyseal injuries are seen. Precise anatomical diagnosis is essential to ensure the most appropriate management.

Supracondylar Fractures of the Distal Humerus

Supracondylar fractures are common between the ages of 4–10 years, and are usually the result of a fall on the outstretched hand.

Classification

The injury is classified according to the direction of displacement and the degree of displacement.

In the common extension pattern the distal fragment is displaced backwards and the sharp proximal fragment can injure the neurovascular structures. In the much less common flexion injury, the distal fragment is displaced forwards and injuries to the median nerve and brachial artery are unusual, but ulnar nerve injuries are more common.

The Gartland grade assessed from the lateral radiograph offers a guide to both prognosis and management.

- Grade 1 fractures are essentially undisplaced and stable.
- Grade 2 fractures are partially displaced on the lateral radiograph, but there is some remaining contact. The soft tissue injury is correspondingly greater, but neurovascular problems are rare.
- Grade 3 injuries are completely displaced and there is no contact between the proximal and distal fragments on the lateral radiograph. The degree of soft tissue injury is correspondingly higher with the major risks being to the brachial artery and median nerve.

Complications

Early complications include:

- Arterial injury, which is indicated by an absent or reduced pulse and a temperature or colour difference. The late signs are motor and sensory deficits.
- Compartment syndrome producing pain at rest and in excess of that expected for an uncomplicated fracture. The pain is worsened by passive extension of fingers and there is a loss of active movements, with swelling, tenderness and raised pressure within the compartment.
- Nerve palsy, which is indicated by sensory loss or impairment, loss of sweating, motor palsy and a loss of active movements, but passive movements are unimpaired.

Late complications include:

- Volkmann ischaemic contracture, which is rare, with an incidence of less than 1%. Nevertheless, the effects are crippling and must be avoided. Ischaemia can result from an arterial injury, a compartment syndrome, or a combination of both. In an established Volkmann contracture, the ischaemic muscle becomes scarred and fibrotic and therefore short, making hand function virtually useless. If the wrist is extended the fingers are tightly flexed. If the wrist is passively flexed to its limit the fingers can be partially straightened demonstrating the short flexor tendons.

- Malunion, usually with cubitus varus or a gunstock deformity. This is often associated with a rotational malalignment and results in an unsightly deformity, often with the ability to perform party-trick manoeuvres.

Management

Immediate management
Grade 1 fractures are easily managed by simple immobilization in a collar and cuff for three weeks. The addition of a backslab may give comfort to the child and parent.

Grade 2 fractures are managed by closed reduction and either immobilization in flexion or percutaneous Kirschner wire fixation. Fractures with a simple extension deformity that are stable after reduction without severe swelling may not require fixation (*Figure 22.2*). Many of the remainder are better managed by percutaneous Kirschner wire fixation to avoid the risk of displacement and malunion. Serious neurovascular injuries are unusual with grade 2 injuries; however, cubitus varus is paradoxically more common after grade 2 injuries than grade 3 injuries because grade 3 injuries are usually managed more aggressively by closed reduction and Kirschner wire fixation or traction.

Grade 3 extension supracondylar fractures can be difficult to manage because of associated soft tissue injury, severe swelling, neurovascular injury, or forearm fractures. Complications can be minimized by giving higher priority to the management of the soft tissue injury than to the management and anatomic reduction of the fracture. An absent radial pulse demands immediate reduction, and anaesthesia should be planned so that there is no delay.

The traditional management of closed reduction and immobilization in flexion is hazardous because the margin between the flexion that will secure the reduction and the flexion that will compromise the circulation is so small. Almost all cases of Volkmann's ischaemia are caused by immobilization of a swollen elbow in flexion and not by an arterial injury *per se*. Closed reduction and percutaneous wire fixation is the best management for the majority of these injuries (*Figure 22.3*). Providing the fracture is reducible, the position can be held by two Kirschner wires and a position of high flexion is no longer required. The risk of neurovascular injury is reduced. The K wire fixation affords good control of the carrying angle and the risk of cubitus varus deformity should be less than 5%.

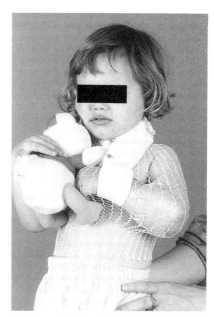

Figure 22.2 Management of the supracondylar fracture by closed reduction and immobilization in flexion. There is a collar and cuff sling, adhesive tape around the elbow to maintain flexion, and a 'string vest' to prevent undue movement. (Reproduced with permission from Graham HK, Glasgow JFT. *Injuries in Children*. British Medical Journal, London.)

Some surgeons still prefer to avoid the use of percutaneous wires because of the risk of nerve injury and infection. Closed reduction and immobilization in flexion may be appropriate when the reduction is stable and a position of more than 90° flexion can be obtained without circulatory compromise.

A few Grade 3 fractures cannot be reduced by closed means, often because of a delay in presentation. Some children present late because of unsuccessful attempts at reduction elsewhere or a loss of position after closed reduction and immobilization in flexion. These fractures can be difficult to manage and each should be considered carefully. Open reduction should only be undertaken by experienced surgeons and the principal indications are open fractures, arterial injuries and compartment syndromes. A pulse that disappears immediately after reduction may indicate entrapment of the artery within the fracture and is an indication for exploration and open reduction.

Olecranon screw traction is still a useful method for managing difficult fractures despite the disadvantage of a prolonged stay in hospital. It is rarely necessary to maintain traction until bony union. Usually traction can be discontinued in favour of a collar and cuff after 7–10 days.

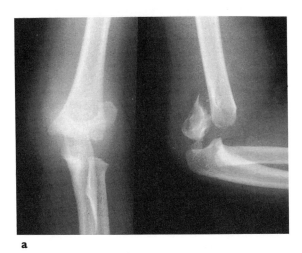
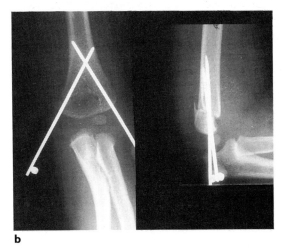

a   b

Figure 22.3 a Gartland Grade 3, completely displaced extension supracondylar fracture. **b** The injury shown in Figure 22.3a has been treated with closed reduction and crossed percutaneous K wires. (Reproduced with permission from Graham HK, Glasgow JFT. *Injuries in Children.* British Medical Journal, London.)

The flexion supracondylar fracture accounts for less than 5% of supracondylar fractures. Displacement is usually less severe than with extension injuries, and neurovascular injuries are less frequent, except ulnar nerve palsy. Reduction is more difficult and requires a position of extension during manipulation. If an anatomical reduction is achieved, percutaneous Kirschner wire fixation can be used. Irreducible fractures can be managed by open reduction or traction in about 30° of flexion.

Assessing the child

After a supracondylar fracture most children are frightened and in pain. Pain levels are important, but difficult to assess if the child is apprehensive. Passive extension of the fingers is a helpful monitor of compartment pressure. Symptoms and signs become difficult to interpret when nerve palsies and compartment syndrome coexist. For example, a median nerve palsy may mask the pain of ischaemia and all the findings may be attributed to the nerve palsy.

Assessment of any neurovascular compromise is extremely difficult in the acute stages in the child under four years of age. Loss of sweating and therefore sensory loss may be the only clue to a nerve lesion. Over the age of four years most children can be persuaded to make a fist or at least to attempt to curl the fingers. A palsy of the median nerve or the anterior interosseous nerve results in the 'pointing sign' where the lateral three fingers flex down, but the index finger and thumb are left straight. Loss of thumb extension indicates a posterior interosseous nerve palsy and may be less painful to test than wrist extension because the muscle does not cross the fracture site. Loss of finger separation indicates ulnar nerve palsy. Over the age of eight years sensory testing is more reliable.

Arterial injury

The most common presentation of a vascular complication is a cold, white, pulseless hand after a Grade 3 extension injury. The pulse will return in the majority of cases after a prompt closed reduction of the fracture. If the pulse does not return, but the distal circulation is satisfactory, the treatment can be expectant. The fracture is fixed with percutaneous wires so the arm can be immobilized in extension and is then carefully observed for signs of compartment syndrome. If the pulse does not return and there are any signs of circulatory compromise the brachial artery should be explored. Most explorations will reveal that the brachial artery is trapped in the fracture site and the circulation is restored after correction of the anatomy. Sometimes the artery remains in spasm for a few minutes after its release and some topical local anaesthetic can help overcome this. If the spasm cannot be reversed and the circulation restored, there is often an intimal tear in the artery. The circulation should be restored by a vein bypass graft and the help of a vascular surgeon is useful. Fortunately a complete tear of the brachial artery is extremely rare.

Weakness or absence of the pulse at later stages after reduction and pinning is more difficult to manage. If there are any other signs of vascular insufficiency such as pain from compartment syndrome or circulatory compromise to the skin of the hand, an exploration should be carried out. There is a small role for arteriography. Because the indications for exploration are clinical, arteriography often causes delays and the anatomical site of the arterial lesion is always known (i.e. opposite the fracture in the antecubital fossa).

Compartment syndrome

It is probably more important to detect raised compartment pressure than arterial insufficiency. Presence or absence of the radial pulse is an unreliable sign. Pain, especially with passive finger extension, is the most reliable. Pressure in the flexor compartment can be measured by the Whiteside technique using readily-available equipment or with a portable monitor. In the past, decisions have been made on the compartment pressure with 30 mmHg or more taken as an indiation for immediate exploration. Following work on tibial fractures (McQueen and Court-Brown, 1996) it would seem more appropriate to calculate diastolic pressure less the compartment pressure and if the difference is less than 30 mmHg exploration should be undertaken.

Management is by urgent decompression of the affected compartments. The antecubital fossa is explored by an anterior Henry approach. The proximal vertical limb allows inspection of the brachial artery and median nerve as well as direct access to the fracture, which is reduced and fixed with Kirschner wires. The distal limb permits direct inspection of the muscles of the flexor compartment and direct decompression.

Nerve lesions

The majority of nerve injuries are traction injuries in continuity and management is expectant. Recovery is bimodal. Some palsies recover in a few days (neuropraxias) others in 3–6 months (axonotmesis). If there has been no improvement of a nerve palsy within six months of the injury then exploration should be considered. Release of the nerve from fracture callus or decompression from adhesive scar tissue may be helpful. A complete tear of the nerve (neurotmesis) is very rare and when it occurs microscopic repair is required; but delay in diagnosis is common.

Volkmann ischaemic contracture

The management of the established condition is extremely difficult. Tendon lengthening and bone shortening have been tried without great success. A slide or proximal release of the fibrotic muscle has been used to increase the length of the short tendons. Recently, there has been more success using microvascular free tissue transfer with a vascularized innervated gracilis transfer to replace the forearm flexors, but experience is limited to a few centres of expertise.

Malunion

Assessment of the carrying angle clinically during the acute stages of treatment is difficult because direct palpation of bony landmarks is unreliable, and when the elbow is flexed the carrying angle cannot be seen. Assessment has to be radiological, with an anteroposterior (AP) radiograph of the distal humerus using Baumann's (humerocapitellar) angle (*Figure 22.4*). This can be carried out after pinning or manipulation with the elbow flexed. The normal range is 64–81° and angles above 81° are likely to result in cubitus varus. It is reproducible even with minor alterations in the degree of angulation of the X-ray beam in relation to the distal humerus. A special grid is available and is a useful piece of equipment in children's fracture clinics.

Even with optimum management an alteration in the carrying angle is a common residuum of a childhood supracondylar fracture. These are usually malunions and not the result of a growth disturbance.

A mild increase in valgus is usually acceptable. However, significant cubitus valgus can be cosmetically unacceptable and result in tardy ulnar nerve palsy.

Cubitus varus is much more ugly and may require corrective osteotomy. It is preferable to wait for about two years after the injury until full motion has returned and the outcome is quite clear. The most popular technique is a lateral closing wedge osteotomy of the distal humerus, but the technique must be precise and fixation adequate. Some surgeons use a medial approach to avoid the more obvious lateral scar. Various methods of internal fixation have been described including a screw in each fragment with wire looped around both, plate fixation and cross K wires. Most series report high complication rates including a loss of correction and nerve injuries. Often the most disfiguring aspect of the deformity is the rotational malalignment and the bump of the prominent lateral condyle. These aspects are difficult to correct with a standard closing lateral wedge.

Associated injuries

About 5% of supracondylar fractures are complicated by an ipsilateral forearm fracture. This injury has been called the 'floating elbow' because the elbow is effectively dissociated from the rest of the upper limb skeleton. It is associated with an increased incidence of neurovascular injuries, Volkmann ischaemic contracture and open fractures. Both fractures should be managed by reduction and fixation. Usually this can be closed reduction and percutaneous Kirschner wire fixation, but sometimes open reduction and fixation is required (*Figure 22.5*).

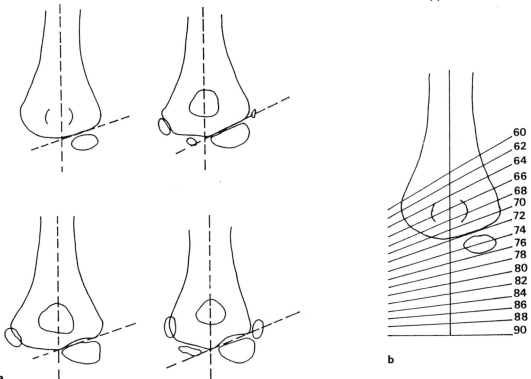

Figure 22.4 a Baumann angle at different maturities of the distal humerus.   **b** Measurement of Baumann angle with an overlay grid of the angles. (Reproduced with permission from the *Journal of Pediatric Orthopedics.*)

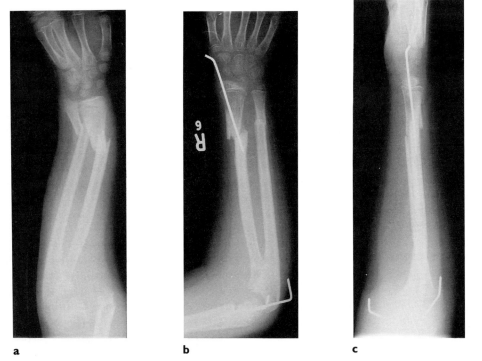

Figure 22.5 a The 'floating elbow' with a grade III extension supracondylar fracture and displaced fractures of the distal radius and ulna.   **b,c** Both fractures were reduced and fixed with percutaneous wires. (Reproduced with permission from Graham HK, Glasgow JFT. *Injuries in Children*. British Medical Journal, London.)

Epiphyseal Injuries of the Distal Humerus

These used to be considered rare, but with more accurate radiological studies including ultrasound, arthrography, and magnetic resonance imaging (MRI), more cases are recognized. They are usually Salter–Harris Type 1 or 2. They are much less common than supracondylar fractures of the distal humerus in all age groups except in infancy. They may result from birth injury, child abuse and previous supracondylar fractures. Because the fracture surfaces are broader and less sharp than those of a supracondylar fracture, neurovascular injuries are less common and reduction is often easier. Union is rapid and the only major complication is cubitus varus.

Fractures of the Medial Epicondyle

The epicondyles of the elbow are traction apophyses giving origin to the collateral ligaments and important muscle groups. Injuries are usually the result of traction or avulsion forces. Medial epicondylar separations are common and are seen most frequently in children aged 8–12 years, the male to female ratio being higher than for other elbow injuries at 4:1.

Complications

Up to 50% of these fractures are associated with elbow dislocation and 15–20% with incarceration of the medial epicondyle within the elbow joint (*Figure 22.6*).

Ulnar nerve palsy accompanies a significant number of medial epicondylar separations, especially those injuries with incarceration of the fragment within the elbow joint.

Misdiagnosis of a displaced injury of the medial condylar physis as an epicondylar injury is not uncommon, particularly in the younger patient before ossification of the medial condyle has occurred. These require open reduction and internal fixation.

Management

The majority of these injuries are managed by a short period of immobilization followed by an active range of movement exercises. Conservative management of displaced injuries frequently results in a non-union or fibrous union; however, this is usually asympto-matic and the range of movement may be better than that of those injuries managed by open reduction and fixation.

Indications for open reduction and internal fixation include incarceration within the elbow joint, complete ulnar nerve palsy and fractures with more than 5 mm displacement in the dominant arm of a throwing athlete. A small screw is preferred in this subcutaneous site to percutaneous or buried Kirschner wires.

Fractures of the Lateral Epicondyle

The lateral epicondylar apophysis ossifies late, just before skeletal maturity, and injuries are rare. Some may go unrecognized.

Injuries to the Lateral and Medial Condylar Physes

Injuries to the lateral condylar physis are common, but those involving the medial condylar physis are uncommon and affect an older age group. Otherwise these are 'mirror image' injuries, with similar biological behaviour and similar management principles.

Classification

Separations of the condylar physes are Salter–Harris type 4 injuries, running from the metaphysis, through the growth plate and across articular cartilage into the elbow joint. There are two main patterns of lateral condylar fractures according to whether the fracture line runs through the lateral condylar physeal ossification centre (Milch type 1) or across the top of the ossification centre, along the growth plate and then through the articular surface (Milch type 2).

Radiology

Displaced injuries in older children are easily recognized, but there can be difficulties in the younger child and in the presence of other injuries and if there is elbow dislocation (*Figure 22.7*). Distinguishing lateral condylar physeal injuries with elbow dislocation from Salter–Harris Type 2 separation of the distal humeral physis can be particularly difficult. Good quality AP and lateral radiographs of the elbow are essential, but oblique views, comparison views and contrast arthrography are sometimes necessary.

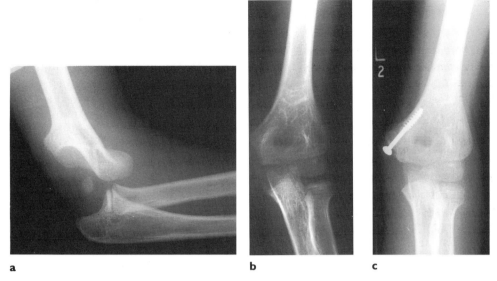

a   b   c

Figure 22.6 **a** Lateral radiograph showing posterior dislocation of the elbow with separation of the medial epicondyle. **b** On the anteroposterior view after closed reduction the medial epicondyle has been incarcerated in the joint. **c** After open reduction and internal fixation of the medial epicondyle. (Reproduced with permission from Graham HK, Glasgow JFT. *Injuries in Children*. British Medical Journal, London.)

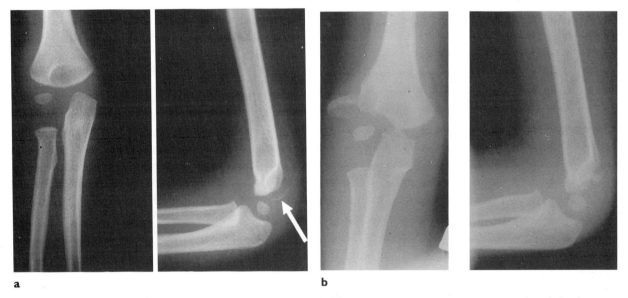

a   b

Figure 22.7 **a** Lateral condylar fracture in a four-year-old. The anteroposterior view is normal and the fracture shows up as a 'flake' of bone on the lateral view. This was managed in a collar and cuff sling. **b** Two months later showing an established non-union with gross displacement. Recognition of the fracture and then adequate reduction and fixation is essential. (Reproduced with permission from Graham HK, Glasgow JFT. *Injuries in Children*. British Medical Journal, London.)

Prognosis

There is a considerable contrast between the biological behaviour of these fractures and that of supracondylar fractures of the humerus. Supracondylar fractures have a good blood supply and union is rapid and assured. The articular surface is not involved and joint motion usually returns to normal eventually. In contrast lateral condylar physeal injuries seem to have a tenuous blood supply, union is always slower, and non-union is a recognized complication. The articular surface is involved and permanent stiffness is a greater risk.

Management

Undisplaced and stable injuries require three weeks of immobilization and careful radiographs taken out of the cast to assess union. Longer periods of immobilization are sometimes necessary, but increase the risk of permanent loss of elbow motion, especially the final 30° of extension.

Displaced fractures require prompt open reduction and internal fixation, usually with two Kirschner wires. Screw fixation may be necessary in the older child (*Figure 22.8*), but is usually unnecessary and impractical for most of these injuries because the metaphyseal fragment is so small.

There is an in-between group of slightly displaced injuries for which the management is controversial. Most authorities consider that a fracture with more than 2 mm displacement should be treated with open reduction and internal fixation.

The metaphyseal fracture line is oblique and a standard AP view does not demonstrate the true maximum displacement, which is shown best on a lateral oblique view. Stability is just as important as the amount of displacement. Some guide to stability is gained from a careful clinical examination (bruising, swelling, irritability, joint range of motion), but

the best assessment is a varus stress radiograph under anaesthesia. Slightly displaced and unstable fractures can be managed easily by percutaneous Kirschner wire fixation and the results are uniformly good. The penalty for undertreatment of these fractures can be delayed union, non-union and progressive displacement. These problems can be more difficult to manage than a simple fresh injury and an aggressive policy for the minimally-displaced injury is justified.

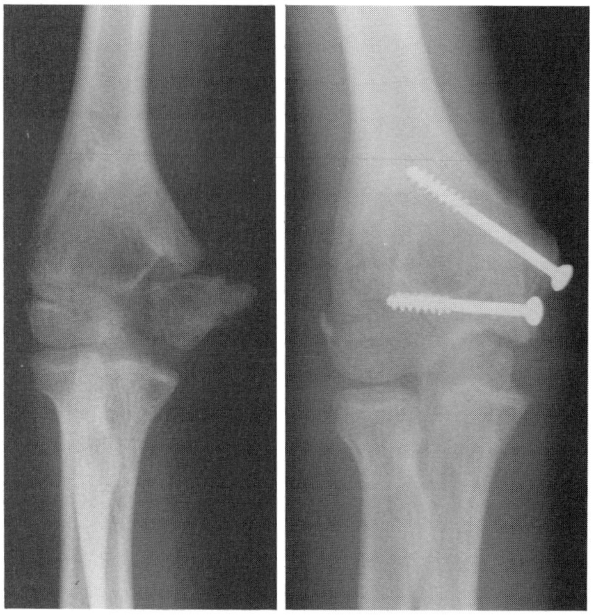

T and Y Condylar Fractures of the Distal Humerus

These are uncommon compared to supracondylar or isolated condylar fractures, and they occur more frequently in adolescents than children. Comminution and displacement are less severe than in adult-pattern injuries.

Closed reduction and percutaneous fixation is appropriate for some of these injuries, but most require open reduction and screw fixation.

OLECRANON FRACTURES

Fractures of the olecranon in children are uncommon; the majority are minimally displaced greenstick fractures and treatment comprises only about three weeks of cast immobilization. About 50% of olecranon fractures are accompanied by other fractures in the elbow region and many of these will require more aggressive treatment than the olecranon fracture itself. These include dislocation of the radial head (Monteggia fracture) and fractures of the radial neck, medial epicondyle, and lateral condyle.

Displaced fractures should be examined carefully under fluoroscopic screening. Once the pull of the triceps is negated by placing the elbow in extension, some will reduce and can be managed in an extension cast for 2–3 weeks before gently flexing the elbow for a further two weeks of immobilization.

Widely separated olecranon fractures require open reduction and internal fixation. A tension band construction is useful, but in many cases the 'band' can be a heavy absorbable suture (No. 2 Vicryl) rather than a wire loop. This simplifies hardware removal to a stab incision to remove two Kirschner wires.

a   b

Figure 22.8 a Fracture of the medial condyle of the humerus with considerable displacement and rotation. **b** Following open reduction and screw fixation. The screws have been placed to avoid the growth plate and the olecranon fossa. (Reproduced with permission from Graham HK, Glasgow JFT. *Injuries in Children*. British Medical Journal, London.)

CORONOID FRACTURES

Coronoid fractures are rare in children, occurring as isolated brachialis avulsions or as part of a traumatic elbow dislocation. Open reduction and fixation are only exceptionally required.

FRACTURES OF THE RADIAL NECK

In contrast to the adult, fractures of the radial head are rare in children. Most result from a fall on the outstretched hand and the direction of angulation is related to the position of the hand in relation to the ground reaction force and to the position of forearm rotation at the time of impact. Most injuries are fractures of the radial neck, including metaphyseal fractures and Salter–Harris Type 1 and 2 epiphyseal injuries.

The degree of angulation and displacement can be graded into four groups to guide management (*Figure 22.9*). The displacement is the maximum displacement seen during fluoroscopic screening at various positions of forearm rotation as a single oblique film may underestimate the true degree of displacement.

Over 50% of radial neck fractures are associated with other fractures of the elbow. These injuries may require more active management than the radial neck fracture and ultimately have a greater bearing on the outcome.

Management is by simple immobilization (Group 1), closed manipulation or percutaneous leverage (Groups 2 and 3) or open replacement, avoiding internal fixation if at all possible (Group 4). Percutaneous leverage is a means of achieving reduction by manipulating the displaced head–neck fragment using a Kirschner wire under fluoroscopic control. It is successful for the majority of Grade 2 and 3 fractures if closed reduction fails and open reduction can be avoided. In general, fractures that are only partially displaced are managed by closed means and have a good prognosis. The more severely displaced fractures, those associated with other injuries, and those managed by open reduction and internal fixation have a variable outcome. Stiffness, particularly loss of forearm rotation, is the main residual problem.

FOREARM FRACTURES IN CHILDREN

Fractures of the forearm bones are the next most common bony injury in childhood after fractures of the clavicle. Fortunately the majority are easily managed and proceed uneventfully to full recovery. They are important injuries because of the large number presenting and the few particular injuries that give rise to significant complications.

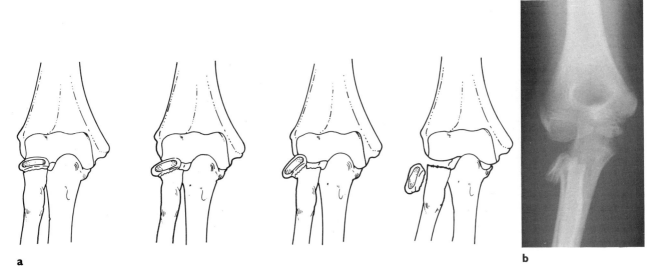

a

b

Figure 22.9 **a** Classification of radial neck fractures according to the amount of displacement (Steele and Graham, 1992). Group 1 are virtually undisplaced and are treated by simple immobilization. Groups 2 and 3 are displaced and angulated and are treated by reduction and immobilization. Group 4 is completely displaced and requires open replacement and fixation as stability dictates. **b** A Group 3 fracture with 70° of angulation and 60% displacement. If closed reduction fails this can be treated by percutaneous leverage with a K wire. Following reduction this fracture is usually stable. (Reproduced with permission from the *Journal of Bone and Joint Surgery*.)

Distal Third Fractures

The distal third of the forearm bones is the most common site of injury, usually as the result of a fall on the outstretched hand. The injury pattern is often asymmetrical in that each bone fails in a different manner (e.g. a displaced fracture of the distal radius is accompanied by a greenstick fracture of the ulna or a fracture of the ulnar styloid). This may make reduction more difficult and less stable. There are four basic fracture patterns:

* Buckle or torus injuries. These are minimally displaced and stable. Cast immobilization for three weeks is usually adequate treatment.
* Greenstick fractures. These require reduction if the angulation is more than about 20°, although clinical deformity is much more important than radiological deformity.
* Epiphyseal injuries. These are usually Salter–Harris Type 1 and 2 and displacement is variable (*Figure 22.10*). Healing and remodelling are rapid at this site and significant degrees of primary displacement or redisplacement in the cast can be readily accepted in younger children. Forceful late remanipulations may result in physeal damage and growth plate arrest, which is a more serious outcome than a minor degree of displacement. The incidence of growth arrest following distal radial or ulnar physeal injury is low, but the injury is so common that a significant number of children present some years after the injury with a

progressive deformity. There has usually been a radial growth arrest with continued growth in the ulna, giving rise to a post-traumatic Madelung deformity. Reconstructive options include excision of physeal bars, epiphysiodesis, osteotomy and shortening or lengthening procedures.

* Displaced fractures. These are managed by closed reduction and cast immobilization. Incomplete reduction and redisplacement are common. Careful follow-up and cast care are necessary. Any residual deformity usually remodels rapidly and fully so that permanent deformity is uncommon. A few injuries are irreducible as a result of soft tissue interposition and open reduction and Kirschner wire fixation may be required (*Figure 22.11*). Some fractures are so unstable and prone to redisplacement that percutaneous K wire fixation should be considered as a primary option. These include the completely displaced isolated fracture of the distal radius and fractures of the distal radius in association with supracondylar fractures (floating elbow).

Diaphyseal Forearm Fractures – Middle and Upper Thirds

These are less frequent than distal third fractures, but can be much more difficult to manage. Proximal fractures are more often complete, more difficult to reduce, and more prone to losing their position in the cast. Union and remodelling are much slower, and

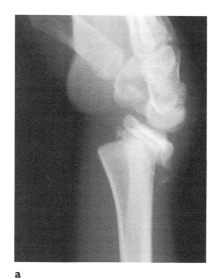
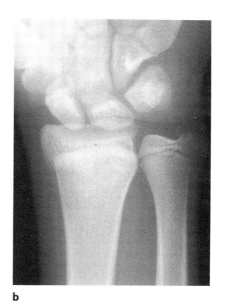

a   b

Figure 22.10   a Salter–Harris Type 2 injury to the distal radial epiphysis with dorsal displacement and angulation.   **b** Note the slightly displaced fracture of the ulnar styloid.

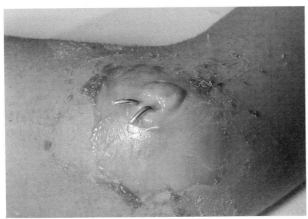

Fig 22.11 Percutaneous K wire fixation is widely used in the management of upper limb fractures in children. Pin site infection is a constant risk. Guidelines to avoid infection are: (1) avoid tension by careful positioning and release of the skin; (2) bend the wires clear of the skin and allow for postoperative swelling; (3) immobilize the affected part to prevent skin–pin movement; (4) leave for a maximum of three weeks without an inspection. (Reproduced with permission from Graham HK, Glasgow JFT. *Injuries in Children.* British Medical Journal, London.)

refracture following cast removal can be a problem. Remodelling in the diaphysis is more a process of smoothing the fracture outline than epiphyseal reorientation or major changes in alignment (*Figure 22.12*).

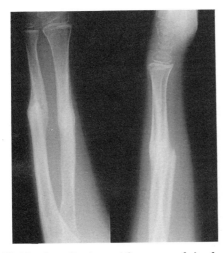

Figure 22.12 In a diaphyseal fracture of the forearm, bayonet apposition is acceptable if alignment and rotation are maintained. These appearances in a seven-year-old are compatible with normal function and appearance.

There is a considerable variation in fracture personality and each case should be studied in detail, taking into account the patient's age and sex before deciding on the management. Some complete fractures with severe angulation deformity are uniplanar deformities with largely intact periosteal tubes and good stability after reduction. In other cases the displacement, comminution and age of the patient dictate open reduction and internal fixation as the primary treatment option.

Many fractures are successfully managed by closed reduction and cast immobilization. General anaesthesia and image intensification are helpful for very unstable fractures; simple greenstick deformities can be managed by closed reduction under regional anaesthesia in the emergency department. By convention upper third fractures are immobilized in supination, middle third fractures in neutral, and distal third fractures in pronation. This is no more than a very rough guide and the stability of the individual fracture should be assessed in various positions. Immobilization in extreme positions of rotation should only be used until the fracture is sticky and not until union. Therefore a change of cast after three weeks is usually required.

The degree of displacement or angulation that can be accepted varies with the site of the fracture and the age of the patient. Angulation of the middle third of the ulna is very obvious because the bone is subcutaneous. In contrast the upper third of the radius is well covered with muscle and residual angulation is less obvious. Angulation and displacement are easily seen on radiographs, but rotation can only be judged clinically. Malrotation deformity undergoes very little remodelling and can produce an ugly deformity as well as a permanent loss of forearm rotation. If in doubt take the cast off and have a look!

If open reduction is required, fixation is also necessary, but need not be as robust as in adult fracture fixation. In children, casting is almost always used to supplement plating of forearm bones, and if the anatomical position is obtained, early movement is not essential to full recovery. The scars from plating are considerable and should be minimized by using short plates and careful surgery. Intramedullary fixation is sometimes used, and on occasions fixation of only one bone may be adequate.

Diaphyseal fractures are clinically and radiologically united after 6–8 weeks in the majority of children. However, consolidation can be slow and refracture is not uncommon. If a child is judged as unreliable a below-elbow plaster cast may be required for an extra 2–4 weeks.

MONTEGGIA FRACTURE DISLOCATION

Monteggia lesion is a combined fracture of the ulna and a dislocation of the radial head. It is important to recognize the combination of these injuries because the radial head dislocation is one of the more common missed injuries of childhood. The ulnar fracture is usually in the mid or proximal third and sometimes through the olecranon. The direction of angulation is always related to the direction of radial head dislocation, but this can be obscured by first aid repositioning and splinting measures.

Radiology

There are two golden rules. Firstly, a line drawn on a radiograph through the radial shaft and head should bisect the capitellum in any view: AP, lateral or oblique. Secondly, never accept evidence of an 'isolated' fracture of the radius or ulna without checking the status of the elbow or wrist joints, both clinically and radiologically (*Figure 22.13*).

Monteggia's lesion is classified according to the direction of the radial head dislocation (Bado).

- Type 1: anterior, immobilize in flexion and supination.
- Type 2: posterior, immobilize in extension for about four weeks.
- Type 3: lateral, immobilize in flexion and supination.

- Type 4: anterior, but a radial neck fracture occurs, not a dislocation of the radial head. This rare injury is more likely to require open reduction.

Management

In the acute stage
The majority of Monteggia lesions can be reduced by closed manipulation and are reasonably stable. Open reduction of the ulnar fracture is necessary for an irreducible or grossly unstable injury. Sometimes this automatically reduces the radial head, but if there is any doubt on perioperative radiographs the lateral side should be opened to look at the reduction of the radial head.

In the late stage
Late-presenting cases are more difficult to manage, though late manipulations up to three weeks after injury can be successful. Thereafter open reduction of the radial head is necessary, but the most important point is to correct the ulnar deformity by osteotomy. In the case presenting late the ulnar fracture may have remodelled straight, but to ensure the radial head stays in position the ulnar osteotomy should be left with an exaggerated angle to keep the radial head in position. Some centres reconstruct the annular ligament at the same time with part of the triceps tendon. With increasing delay in diagnosis the outcome becomes progressively less favourable and early diagnosis is the key to successful management.

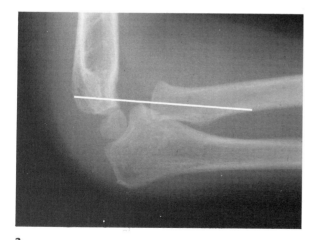
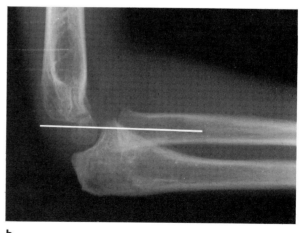

a   b

Figure 22.13 a Monteggia fracture dislocation, Bado type I, in an immature elbow. There is a greenstick fracture of the ulna and anterior dislocation of the radial head. A line drawn along the axis of the upper radius does not pass through the capitellum. **b** After a closed reduction. A line drawn along the upper radius now passes through the capitellum indicating that the radial head has been reduced.

GALEAZZI FRACTURE DISLOCATION

Galeazzi lesion consists of a fracture of the radial shaft, usually in the middle or distal third, and a dislocation or subluxation of the distal radioulnar joint. It is a much less common injury than Monteggia injury and usually occurs in adolescents rather than children. Closed treatment is possible, but less likely to succeed than for Monteggia lesions. The radial fracture must be reduced and held in anatomical alignment by open or closed means. The position of the distal radioulnar joint will then be satisfactory.

HAND AND WRIST INJURIES

Serious hand injuries in children are unusual, but the hands, like the face, are always on view and deformity is not easily accepted.

Distal Phalanx

Terminal crushing injuries are common in toddlers and children. Technically these are open fractures, but good care of the soft tissues is the main focus of management. Burst lacerations require cleaning and dressing. Suturing usually provokes more tissue devitalization and is rarely required. Minor to moderate degrees of tissue loss from the pulp are well tolerated and best managed conservatively by a period of dressing rather than local flap reconstruction.

Fingertip flexion injuries can produce a spectrum of mallet finger-equivalent injuries, with Salter–Harris Type 1, 2 or 3 growth plate separations at the base of the proximal phalanx. Careful reduction and fixation is required for many of these injuries, but the results may still be poor as a result of growth arrest and recurrent deformity.

Other Phalanges

Fractures of the phalangeal shafts can usually be managed by strapping to the neighbour or 'buddy taping,' but malrotation must be excluded on clinical grounds because it may not be noted radiologically.

The 'extra-octave' injury is an abduction injury to the epiphysis at the base of the proximal phalanx of the little finger. Reduction is usually easily achieved by flexing the digit to 90° (tightening the collateral ligaments) and then adducting the finger towards its neighbours. This manoeuvre is usually more effective than the 'pen between the fingers' manoeuvre. Position is maintained by neighbour strapping.

Metacarpal Injuries

Isolated metacarpal shaft fractures are usually splinted by their intact neighbours and interosseous muscles. Multiple fractures result from crushing injuries. Elevation to reduce swelling, splintage in the position of function, and soft tissue care are the priorities.

Fractures at the base of the thumb metacarpal heal and remodel quickly, and minor degrees of residual angulation do not impair the result. The exception is the rare paediatric Bennett fracture, a Salter–Harris Type 3 injury, which requires open reduction and internal fixation.

Dislocations in the Hand

Dislocations most commonly involve the metacarpophalangeal and interphalangeal joints of the thumb, index and little fingers, the 'outboard digits.' Simple dislocations are not associated with bony avulsion fractures, there is no soft tissue entrapment, reduction is easily accomplished and the results are uniformly good following simple immobilization. Complex dislocations are associated with avulsion of collateral ligaments or the volar plate. Sometimes there is 'buttonholing' of the displaced joint through a capsular tear and reduction is blocked by interposed volar plate or extensor tendons. This is particularly seen in the child's first metacarpophalangeal joint. Open reduction is required. The main dangers are failure to recognize the injury and accepting a less than perfect closed reduction of a digital dislocation.

Carpal Injuries

In the child the carpal bones consist of a relatively small ossific nucleus surrounded by a thick layer of cartilage. This cushions the carpal bones to such a degree that fractures are rare. Ossification of the scaphoid starts at six years of age and fractures are uncommon before ten years of age. Nevertheless fractures are seen in older children and adolescents and may occasionally result in the complications that are well recognized in adults such as non-union and avascular necrosis of the proximal pole.

REFERENCES AND FURTHER READING

Gartland JJ. Management of supracondylar fractures of the humerus in children. *Surg Gynecol Obstet* 1959; **109**: 145–154.

Graves SC, Canale TS. Fractures of the olecranon in children: long-term follow-up. *J Pediatr Orthop* 1993; **13**: 239–241.

Letts M, Rowhani N. Galeazzi-equivalent injuries of the wrist in children. *J Pediatr Orthop* 1993; **13**: 561–566.

Lincoln TL, Mubarak SJ. 'Isolated' traumatic radial-head dislocation. *J Pediatr Orthop* 1994; **14**: 454–457.

McQueen MM, Court-Brown CM. Compartment monitoring in tibial fractures. *J Bone Joint Surg* 1996; **78B**: 99–104.

Mintzer CM, Waters PM, Brown DJ, Kasser JR. Percutaneous pinning in the treatment of displaced lateral condyle fractures. *J Pediatr Orthop* 1994; **14**: 462–465.

Ogden JA. Injury to the growth mechanisms. In: *Skeletal Injury in the Child*, second edition, pp. 97–174. WB Saunders, Philadelphia, 1990.

Petersen HA. Physeal fractures: Part 3 classification. *J Pediatr Orthop* 1994; **14**: 439–448.

Pirone AM, Graham HK, Krabjich JI. Management of displaced extension type supracondylar fractures of the humerus in children. *J Bone Joint Surg* 1988; **70A**: 641–650.

Poland J. *Traumatic Separations of the Epiphyses*. Smith Elder and Company, London, 1898.

Rang M. *Children's Fractures*, 2nd edn. J.B. Lippincott, Philadelphia, 1983.

Rockwood CA, Wilkins KE, King RE. *Fractures in Children*, 3rd edn. J.B. Lippincott, Philadelphia, 1991.

Salter RB, Harris WR. Injuries involving the epiphyseal plate. *J Bone Joint Surg* 1963; **45A**: 587–622.

Steele JA, Graham HK. Angulated radial neck fractures in children: a trial of percutaneous reduction. *J Bone Joint Surg* 1992; **74B**: 760–764.

Templeton PA, Graham HK. The floating elbow in children. Simultaneous supracondylar fractures of the humerus and of the forearm in the same upper limb. *J Bone Joint Surg* 1995; **77B**: 791–796.

Williamson DM, Coates CJ, Miller RK, Cole WG. Normal characteristics of the Baumann's (humerocapitellar) angle: an aid in assessment of supracondylar fractures. *J Pediatr Orthop* 1992; **12**: 636–639.

Younger ASE, Tredwell SJ, Mackenzie WG, Orr JD, King PM, Tennant W. Accurate prediction of outcome after pediatric forearm fracture. *J Pediatr Orthop* 1994; **14**: 200–206.

Chapter 23
Lower Limb Trauma

Mark D O'Sullivan

Fractures and associated injuries in children differ significantly from those in adults. There are major anatomical and physiological differences, which must be taken into account when treating these injuries.

Children's long bones have growth plates and epiphyses. Fractures are particularly common around the growth plate and can be difficult to detect due to the variable radiolucency. A good knowledge of the possible injuries is therefore important as well as the use of special investigations to diagnose these problems. Growth plate injuries can lead to limb length discrepancy and progressive angulation of the limb.

The child's periosteum is much thicker and stronger than that of adults and is more biologically active, producing more abundant callus in a shorter time. The younger the child, the more rapid the healing time.

The remodelling potential in a child's fracture is extensive. Following growth in the affected bone, deformity can be corrected by resorption of the convexity and filling in of the concavity, and this appears to be a response to normal stress. Overgrowth of the bone is common. A femoral fracture will result in 1 cm of overgrowth.

Another important factor to consider when treating children's fractures is how fracture patterns vary with age. Upper limb fractures are much more common than lower limb fractures in the child. Fragile bone diseases such as osteogenesis imperfecta are usually diagnosed at birth or during the first few years. Child abuse is most common during the first two years.

PELVIC FRACTURES

Most pelvic fractures in children are caused by motor vehicle accidents, and associated injuries are common. The mortality rate is 8%. The associated injuries are listed in Table 23.1.

Table 23.1 Injuries associated with pelvic fractures (from Rang, 1983)

Local injuries	Haematuria (30%)
	Urological injury (10%)
	Abdominal injury (11%)
	Perineal or gluteal lacerations (7%)
Distant injuries	Head (61%)
	Chest (9%)
	Fractures of the upper extremity (17%)
	Fractures of the lower extremity (17%)

Classification

In the emergency situation, fractures of the pelvis can be classified into three categories (Quinby, 1966):

- Uncomplicated fractures.
- Fractures with visceral involvement requiring transfusion.
- Fractures associated with immediate massive haemorrhage, which are the most severe and associated with a high mortality rate. The children present in shock, require massive transfusion, and often die.

The classification of Key and Conwell enables these fractures and their management to be standardized and a comparison of results (*Table 23.2*).

Fractures Without a Break in the Pelvic Ring

Avulsion fractures occur in children or young adults participating in sporting activities. Avulsion of the anterior superior iliac spine (ASIS) due to traction on the sartorius usually occurs in athletics. Avulsions of the anterior inferior iliac spine (AIIS) classically

Table 23.2 Classification of fractures of the pelvis (Key and Conwell, 1951)

1. No break in the continuity of the pelvic ring
A. Avulsion fractures
  1. Anterior superior iliac spine
  2. Anterior inferior iliac spine
  3. Ischial tuberosity

B. Fractures of the pubis or ischium
C. Fractures of the wing of the ilium
D. Fractures of the sacrum or coccyx

2. Single break in the pelvic ring
A. Fractures of two ipsilateral rami
B. Fracture near or subluxation of the symphysis pubis
C. Fracture near or subluxation of the sacroiliac joint

3. Double break in the pelvic ring
A. Double vertical fractures or dislocation of the pubis (straddle fracture)
B. Double vertical fractures or dislocation (Malgaine fracture)
C. Severe multiple fractures

4. Fractures of the acetabulum
A. Small fragment associated with dislocation of the hip
B. Linear fracture associated with non-displaced pelvic fracture
C. Linear fracture associated with hip joint instability
D. Fracture secondary to central dislocation of the acetabulum

occur with kicking sports (soccer and rugby). Avulsion of the ischial tuberosity, due to traction on the hamstrings, is usually seen in athletes, particularly gymnasts.

Radiographs show displacement of the fragment to a varying degree (*Figure 23.1*). The treatment is usually bed rest for a couple of days, followed by crutches with guarded weight-bearing until comfortable. This usually takes 3–4 weeks, and then there can be a slow resumption of sporting activity.

Fractures of the pubis, ischium, wing of the ilium, sacrum and coccyx usually require bed rest until comfortable, followed by crutches until healed. Fractures of the sacrum are occasionally associated with damage to the sacral nerves, resulting in a loss of bowel and bladder function.

Single Breaks in the Pelvic Ring

Fractures of two ipsilateral pubic rami constitute a true break in the pelvic ring, and can only be caused by considerable force. Associated injuries are therefore common. In the child, these fractures tend to heal rapidly, but bed rest is required for 2–4 weeks, followed by crutches until pain free.

Fractures near or subluxation of the symphysis pubis and sacroiliac joint are rare in children, and are only caused by considerable force.

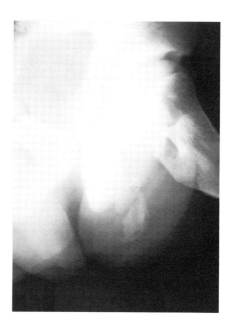

Figure 23.1 Avulsion of the ischial tuberosity. This 12-year-old gymnast sustained an avulsion of the hamstring origin. It healed with conservative treatment.

Double Breaks in the Pelvic Ring

The importance of diagnosing double breaks lies in the recognition of the severe trauma required to cause the injury (e.g. motor vehicle accidents or serious falls) and the risk of associated injuries. By definition they are unstable. They can be divided into:

- Double vertical pubic ring fractures (straddle or floating fractures).
- Malgaine's fracture.
- Multiple crushing injuries for which classification is impossible.

Double breaks may require traction and internal or external fixation, depending on the type of fracture.

Acetabular Fractures

These are uncommon in children. There are four types:

- Small fragments, which most often occur with traumatic dislocations of the hip.
- Stable linear fractures.
- Linear fractures with hip instability.
- Fractures secondary to central dislocation of the acetabulum.

These account for approximately 10% of pelvic fractures. Treatment is reduction of the hip and acetabular fragments where possible. The fractures are treated closed if stable, but larger fragments must be anatomically reduced and fixed to ensure congruity and stability.

TRAUMATIC DISLOCATION OF THE HIP

This is rare. There is a bimodal age distribution, with children aged 2–8 years dislocating with trivial injuries. In the teenager they occur as a result of significant trauma such as a motor cycle accident. Occasionally there are associated fractures in the older age group, and a post-reduction computerized tomographic (CT) scan is important to rule out any intra-articular loose fragment. They are easily reduced under general anaesthetic, and as long as this is carried out in the first eight hours after injury, avascular necrosis is unusual.

FRACTURES OF THE HIP

These fractures are uncommon in children, and make up less than 1% of hip fractures. Unlike the comparable fractures in the adult population, they usually result from high velocity trauma. The fractures have a poor prognosis and complications are frequent. For displaced fractures immediate reduction and fixation with evacuation of the intra-articular haematoma is advised to try to prevent avascular necrosis.

Classification (*Figure 23.2*)

Fractures of the hip are classified as:

- Type 1: transepiphyseal fractures (with or without dislocation).
- Type 2: transcervical fractures (displaced and non-displaced).
- Type 3: cervicotrochanteric (displaced and non-displaced).
- Type 4: intertrochanteric (displaced and non-displaced).

Type 1 are the least common of the proximal femoral fractures. About 50% are associated with dislocation of the femoral head. Severe trauma is required to cause the injury and the injury may be a

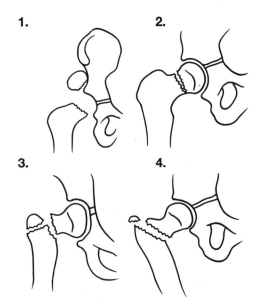

Figure 23.2 Classification of femoral neck fractures. **1.** Transepiphyseal with or without dislocation from the acetabulum. **2.** Transcervical. **3.** Cervicotrochanteric. **4.** Trochanteric.

result of child abuse. Diagnosis of these fractures may be difficult before there is ossification of the femoral head, but should be suspected if there has been significant trauma or if there are clinical signs of shortening and external rotation. Transepiphyseal fractures with dislocation are associated with a high incidence of poor results due to avascular necrosis, growth arrest and non-union. They usually require open reduction and secure internal fixation, but in the younger age group a single attempt at closed reduction may be tried. In those without dislocation, closed reduction with or without internal fixation is performed.

Type 2 (transcervical) fractures are the most common proximal femoral fracture, accounting for about 50% of hip fractures in children. The complication rate of these fractures is high due to a 40% rate of avascular necrosis, which appears to be related to the amount of initial displacement. Management is by anatomical reduction (open or closed) and internal fixation. It is generally believed that these fractures should be treated as soon as possible in an attempt to avoid avascular necrosis, and if the fracture is to be treated closed, the hip should be decompressed by aspiration or capsular release (*Figure 23.3*).

Type 3 (cervicotrochanteric) fractures account for 30% of children's hip fractures. Avascular necrosis occurs in 20–30% of cases. Closed reduction and internal fixation with a small hip screw is the treatment of choice for displaced fractures. For undisplaced fractures, the treatment is controversial; internal fixation is advised because of the risk of displacement.

Type 4 (intertrochanteric) fractures account for 10–20% of hip fractures. Traditional treatment has been skin or skeletal traction followed by a spica cast with the hip in abduction. Internal fixation is now more popular, particularly if the fracture cannot be reduced or held reduced in the spica.

Subtrochanteric fractures also occur in childhood and can be treated by internal fixation or closed reduction and hip spica.

Complications

The complications include the following:

- Avascular necrosis, which may affect the epiphysis and resemble Perthes disease, or in the transcervical fractures may affect the whole of the proximal fragment.
- Non-union, particularly in those treated without internal fixation.
- Premature growth plate arrest, which is common and can cause leg length discrepancy and if partial, coxa vara.
- Secondary osteoarthritis, particularly in those affected by avascular necrosis.

AVULSION FRACTURES OF THE UPPER FEMUR

Avulsion fractures of the greater and lesser trochanters can occur as a result of sudden muscular contracture. Lesser trochanteric avulsion occurs in the teenager before the epiphysis fuses at the age of

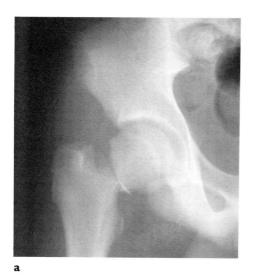

a

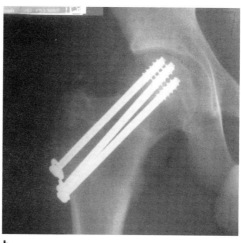

b

Figure 23.3 **a** Displaced transcervical fracture of the left neck of femur in a 15-year-old boy. **b** Closed reduction and internal fixation with cancellous screws resulted in uncomplicated union of the fracture shown in Figure 23.3a.

about 18 years. Despite significant displacement it is treated symptomatically with a return to normal activity after 4–6 weeks. Internal fixation is unnecessary. Avulsion of the greater trochanter in this age group is less common. If significantly displaced some advocate internal fixation rather than immobilization in abduction in a hip spica.

FRACTURES OF THE SHAFT OF THE FEMUR

Femoral shaft fractures are common in the paediatric age group. They may occur following major or minor trauma and must be considered serious injuries because of the possibility of shock following blood loss. Femoral shaft fractures in children differ from adult injuries in many important ways. They heal quickly, longitudinal deformity usually remodels, and there is usually overgrowth of the femur by 1 cm. The fractures can be classified according to the following criteria:

- Open or closed.
- Level.
- Pattern.
- Degree of displacement.
- Angulation.
- Simple or complex.
- Unusual features (birth fractures, child abuse, pathological fractures, or associated fractures).

Management

Birth fractures
These heal quickly, usually within ten days. Strapping of the affected limb onto the abdomen can give adequate immobilization as healing takes place and a hip spica is unnecessary.

Infants
These are often managed by Gallow traction (*Figure 23.4*). Fractures tend to heal very quickly in this group (within three weeks). Some describe the use of this traction at the patient's home to shorten the hospital stay. These patients must be monitored closely for fracture alignment and the development of any ischaemia of the limbs such as a compartment syndrome. Gallow traction should not be used in children over 10 kg or two years of age as the risk of vascular complications is unacceptable. We rarely use prolonged Gallow traction in this age group, but usually aim for early discharge in a hip spica.

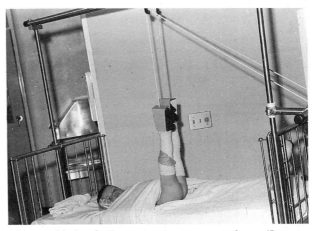

Figure 23.4 Gallow traction in an infant. (Reproduced with permission from Williams PF, Cole WG. *Orthopaedic Management in Childhood.* Chapman & Hall, London.)

Children less than eight years of age
This group in general is reasonably easy to treat with a hip spica. The child is admitted, a femoral nerve block is used to relieve pain and the limb is placed in simple traction. The spica is applied under general anaesthetic on the next available list, usually the day after admission (*Figure 23.5*). Once the parents are happy to look after the child at home, the patient is discharged, usually after 48 hours. One cm of shortening is aimed for as the femur tends to overgrow by that amount during the first year. The position is checked radiologically during spica application and again at one week. The spica is removed at six weeks and checked clinically and radiologically for union.

Indications for surgery: there are occasional indications for fixing femoral fractures in children under eight years of age. Management of an irritable child after a head injury can be very difficult in traction. Internal fixation may also be indicated if there is an associated vascular injury, the fracture is pathological, there is a large soft tissue component or with multiple injuries. These can be managed with the use of an external fixator or flexible intramedullary rods avoiding the growth plates. Antegrade femoral nailing is contraindicated in this age group because of the high rate of growth arrest in the greater trochanter.

Children over eight years of age
This group is the most difficult to manage because of the complications of malunion. Hip spica treatment can result in excessive shortening, and remodelling is poor in this age group. Traditional treatment was to persevere with traction until union took place. Other

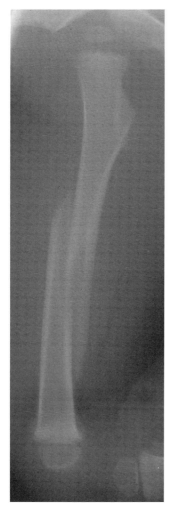

Figure 23.5 This two-year-old child with a spiral fracture of the shaft of the femur was treated by early spica application.

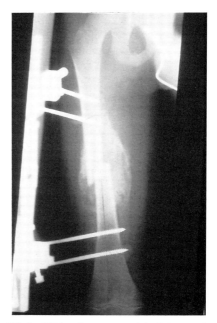

Figure 23.6 This nine-year-old girl sustained a fractured femur in association with a head injury. Note the abundant callus around the fracture at six weeks. An external fixator was used to control the fracture.

options include skeletal traction for 2–3 weeks until the fracture is 'sticky' followed by spica treatment and external fixator (*Figure 23.6*) or intramedullary nailing using flexible intramedullary nails. Flexible nails avoid the risks of growth plate damage as they are inserted from medial and lateral supracondylar regions. These fractures take 6–12 weeks to unite. The advantages of surgical treatment are early joint mobilization to prevent knee stiffness and early discharge using crutches. Early discharge from hospital is being increasingly encouraged as costs escalate.

Adolescents

In general adolescents are treated in the same way as adults with closed intramedullary nailing. This is particularly true for patients who are two years or less from skeletal maturity (*Figure 23.7*). Possible problems with intramedullary nailing include damage to the greater trochanteric growth plate and possibly the distal growth plate leading to growth arrest and angular deformity. There may be rotational malunion and there have also been reports of avascular necrosis of the femoral head.

FRACTURES AND DISLOCATIONS OF THE KNEE

Fractures about the knee are important because of associated injury to the growth plates. The lower femoral growth plate contributes 70% to the length of the femur and approximately 37% to the length of the lower limb. The proximal tibial physis contributes 55% to the length of the tibia and 25% to the length of the limb. Injuries to these can have serious sequelae if there is a growth plate arrest.

Fracture–Separation of the Distal Femoral Physis

This is an uncommon injury and is usually caused by a motor vehicle accident or a sporting activity. There are two types:

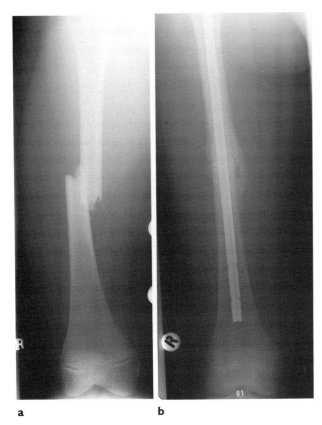

a   b

Figure 23.7 **a** A transverse fracture of the midshaft of the femur in a 14-year-old boy. **b** The fracture shown in Figure 23.7a was treated by intramedullary rodding and had united at eight weeks.

- Anterior displacement caused by hyperextension of the knee. Neurovascular damage may occur as the femoral shaft is displaced into the popliteal fossa.
- Medial or lateral displacement due to the knee being forced into abduction or adduction. Neurovascular structures are usually spared.

There is a high incidence of growth plate arrest following these injuries (*Figure 23.8*).. The Salter–Harris classification does not necessarily provide a prognosis for these fractures. The age of the patient, the severity of the trauma, the magnitude of the displacement, and the adequacy of the reduction are more important. Most of these fractures are Salter–Harris Type 2, with the fracture line extending across the growth plate and then extending obliquely across the metaphysis Salter–Harris Type 3 and 4 injuries in particular require anatomical reduction and internal fixation to prevent growth plate arrest and joint incongruity. These injuries are usually unstable, and require open reduction and internal fixation, either with K wire fixation or interfragmentary lag screw fixation avoiding the physis. Manipulation and cast immobilization should only be used for the minimally displaced and completely stable fractures. Osteochondral fractures of the articular surface should be reduced open and internally fixed. Careful follow-up is required for at least

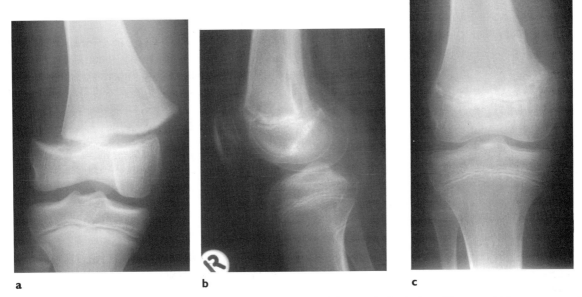

a   b   c

Figure 23.8 **a** This Salter–Harris Type I fracture of the distal femoral physis in a 12-year-old boy occurred in a motor vehicle accident. It was reduced and held in a plaster cast for six weeks. **b,c** At eight weeks, it is apparent that there has been a central growth arrest of the distal femur.

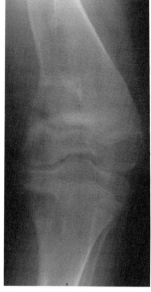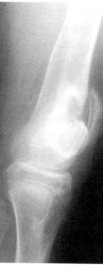

Figure 23.9 At age 14, ten years after an open injury to the distal femur, there has been a growth arrest with varus deformity of the distal femur. The growth plate of the proximal tibia is also abnormal, resulting in recurvatum of the proximal tibia. This deformity was treated by an osteotomy of the distal femur.

two years to watch for any growth plate damage (*Figure 23.9*).

Fracture–Separation of the Proximal Tibial Physis

This is a much rarer injury than that of the distal femur. The mechanism of injury is usually a hyperextension force that displaces the tibial metaphysis posteriorly. Most are Salter–Harris Type 2 fractures and can be treated by closed reduction and immobilization in a long leg cast. Salter–Harris Type 3 and 4 fractures should be anatomically reduced and internally fixed. If the fracture cannot be reduced closed, open reduction and internal fixation should be performed. An above-knee cast is worn for 6–8 weeks.

Avulsion of the Tibial Tubercle

This is uncommon and is due to flexion of the knee against a contracted quadriceps muscle. It occurs most commonly during sport in the 13–16 year age group. Watson–Jones described three types.

- In type 1, a small fragment of the tibial tubercle is avulsed and displaced upward.

- In type 2, the whole anterior portion of the tibial tubercle is displaced upward.
- In type 3, the fracture extends upward into the joint surface (*Figure 23.10*).

Treatment depends on the amount of displacement. Undisplaced fractures can be treated in a plaster of Paris cylinder for six weeks, while displaced fractures should undergo open reduction and internal fixation using cancellous screws or a tension band wire fixation.

Fractures of the Intercondylar Eminence of the Tibia

In children, injuries that would rupture the anterior cruciate ligament in an adult cause avulsion of the intercondylar eminence. The most common cause is a bicycle accident that causes forced hyperextension of the knee. They are most common in boys aged 8–14 years. Three types of fractures are recognized based on the amount of displacement and the fracture pattern seen on the initial radiographs.

- Type 1 is non-displaced.
- Type 2 has a posterior hinge with an elevated anterior portion.
- Type 3 is fully displaced and rotated. These are the most common, accounting for 45% of these injuries.

The goal of treatment is to obtain a stable knee with a full range of motion. For a non-displaced or minimally displaced fracture (types 1 and 2), the treatment is by plaster of Paris cylinder. Displaced fractures (type 2) are managed initially by aspiration of the joint and extension of the knee. If the fragment cannot be reduced and for type 3 fractures, arthroscopic or open reduction of the fragment is carried out (*Figure 23.11*). The fragment is fixed with suture, wire or screw. Failure of reduction is usually due to interposed meniscus or rotation of the fragment.

Complications include ligamentous laxity, which is very common after these injuries, but in this age range is seldom sufficient to limit activities or require treatment.

PATELLAR FRACTURES

Patellar fractures are uncommon in children. As in adults, they occur as a result of a direct blow or sudden contraction of the extensor mechanism of the knee, or both. Patellar fractures are classified accord-

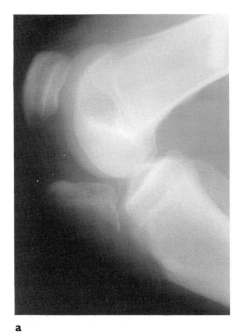
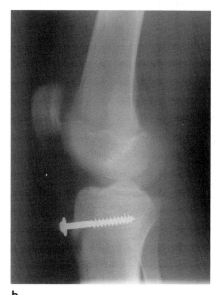

a   b

Figure 23.10 a Fracture of the tibial tubercle in a 15-year-old boy sustained during a football match. It is a type 3 fracture. **b** The fracture was fixed by open reduction and internal fixation. A plaster cast was used for six weeks and the fracture united uneventfully.

ing to their location, pattern and degree of displacement of the fracture.

The sleeve fracture of the patella only occurs in adolescents. There is an avulsion of a small bony fragment from the distal pole of the patella together with an extensive sleeve of articular cartilage and retinaculum pulled off the body of the patella.

Treatment of patellar fractures is generally non-operative for undisplaced fractures with cast immobilization for at least four weeks. Displaced fractures

are treated by open reduction and internal fixation. Sleeve fractures require open reduction and internal fixation of the fragment and repair of the retinaculum.

FRACTURES OF THE TIBIA AND FIBULA

Classification

Classification of fractures of the tibia and fibula is shown in Table 23.3.

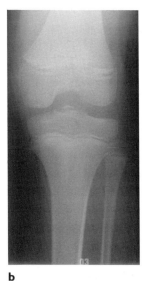

a   b

Figure 23.11   A type 2 fracture of the intercondylar eminence of the tibia in an 11-year-old boy.

Table 23.3   Classification of fractures of the tibia and fibula

A. Fractures of the proximal tibial and fibular physes

B. Fractures of the proximal tibial metaphysis

C. Fractures of the tibial and fibular shafts
    1. Isolated fractures of the tibial shaft
    2. Fractures of both tibial and fibular shafts
    3. Isolated fractures of the fibular shaft

D. Fractures of the distal tibial metaphysis

E. Fractures of the distal tibial and fibular physes

Fractures of the Tibial and Fibular Shafts

These are the most common injuries of the lower limb in children and are often caused by indirect injuries such as twisting and less commonly by direct force. Isolated fractures of the tibia make up 70% of these injuries and most are at the junction of the middle and lower one-third. The intact fibula prevents shortening, but angulation, particularly into varus, may develop. Fractures of the tibia and fibula are less stable. Shortening can be a major problem and there is a tendency for the fracture to drift into valgus.

Management

Fractures of the tibia and fibula in children are usually uncomplicated and can be treated by manipulation and long-leg plaster. Healing occurs in 4–6 weeks in most cases. Open reduction and internal fixation are occasionally required, particularly with open fractures or when the child has an associated head injury.

Complications

There may be a compartment syndrome, which is difficult to diagnose in the child. In children with persistent severe pain after closed reduction of a tibial fracture, the compartment pressures should be measured, and if raised, a fasciotomy of the compartment should be performed. Rarely in the severe injury there may be a vascular injury requiring repair.

In the long term the fracture may have delayed union, or in exceptional circumstances, a non-union. There may be a malunion with shortening, angular deformity or rotational deformity.

Particular Fractures of the Tibial Shaft

Toddler's fracture in the distal part of the tibia often presents because the toddler is unable to walk. There may be no history of trauma. Examination may suggest a fracture, and if radiography does not reveal a fracture line, a bone scan may be warranted. Treatment is an above-knee plaster for 3–4 weeks (*Figure 23.12a*).

Stress fractures nearly always affect the upper one-third of the tibia in children. They are most common in the 10–15 year age group. Plain radiographs may

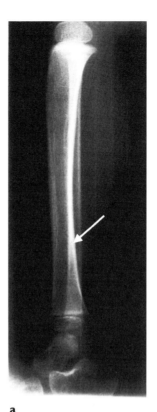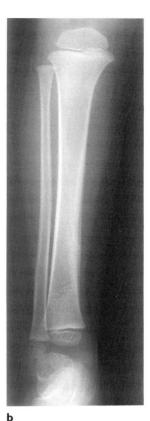

a   b

Figure 23.12 a Toddler's fractures are common fractures, but can be difficult to see on the original radiographs (arrow). If they are not visible on plain films, a bone scan is very helpful in making the diagnosis. **b** Two weeks later, there is a periosteal reaction and the fracture line is more obvious.

not show any abnormality initially, but the bone scan is reliable.

Fractures of the proximal tibial metaphysis
These fractures are caused by trauma to the lateral aspect of the extended knee. The most common sequel is the development of a valgus deformity of the tibia and parents should be warned that angular deformity can occur despite appropriate treatment (*Figure 23.13*). The cause of this is unknown, but possible theories include:

- Tibial overgrowth.
- Inadequate reduction due to soft tissue interposition.
- Early weight-bearing.
- Asymmetrical growth stimulation (increased medial growth in comparison to lateral growth).

There is disagreement about the appropriate treatment for valgus deformity. At our institution, it is generally thought that the deformity corrects itself.

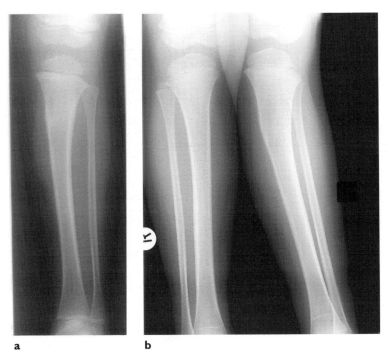
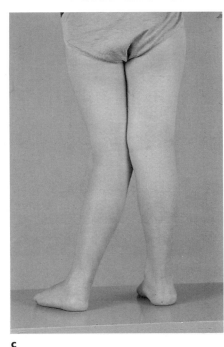

a   b   c

Figure 23.13 **a** This undisplaced fracture of the upper tibial metaphysis was treated in an above-knee plaster and united uneventfully. **b** Six months later there is a marked valgus deformity of the upper tibia. **c** Clinically, there is a severe valgus deformity of the left knee. This resolved spontaneously over the next four years.

Other surgeons feel that a varus osteotomy is required. If the deformity is still present towards the end of skeletal maturity, an osteotomy or epiphyseal stapling can be performed.

Fractures of the Distal Tibial and Fibular Physes

These are common injuries and are often complicated by growth arrest of the physis. Various classifications have been used, but the Salter–Harris classification remains the one most commonly used. The distal fibula injury may be a Type 1 with virtually no displacement and can be easily overlooked.

At the distal tibia the Salter–Harris Type 1 and 2 injuries have a good prognosis, but Type 3 and 4 are associated with a high incidence of partial growth plate arrest and progressive deformity. The Tillaux fracture with detachment of the anterolateral fragment of the distal tibial epiphysis is occasionally seen in adolescents. This is a Salter–Harris Type 3 fracture and occurs because the lateral part of the epiphysis is the last to fuse. The triplanar fracture is a variant of epiphyseal injuries peculiar to ankles. It was not described in Salter and Harris' original description, but has become known as the Salter–

Harris Type 7 injury. The triplanar fracture occurs in three different planes. It starts in the frontal plane in the metaphysis, comes forwards in the transverse plane along the growth plate, and then passes in the sagittal plane through the epiphysis into the joint space (*Figure 23.14*).

Assessment is by plain radiographs, but CT scans can improve the imaging to display the amount of articular surface displacement. Stress views may show up an epiphyseal separation at the distal fibular growth plate.

Management

Treatment varies according to the type of injury, age of the patient, and the mechanism of injury. In general, if the fracture is a Salter–Harris Type 1 or 2 it can be managed by a closed reduction, and then a plaster of Paris for 4–6 weeks. If the reduction is unsuccessful an open reduction should be undertaken with internal fixation so that the growth plate is not damaged.

For the Salter–Harris Type 3, 4 and 7 injuries with displacement, treatment is by open reduction and internal fixation to reduce the chance of a bony bar across the growth plate, and also to restore joint congruity. Lag screws can be used intraepiphyseally, but no screws should be placed across an open

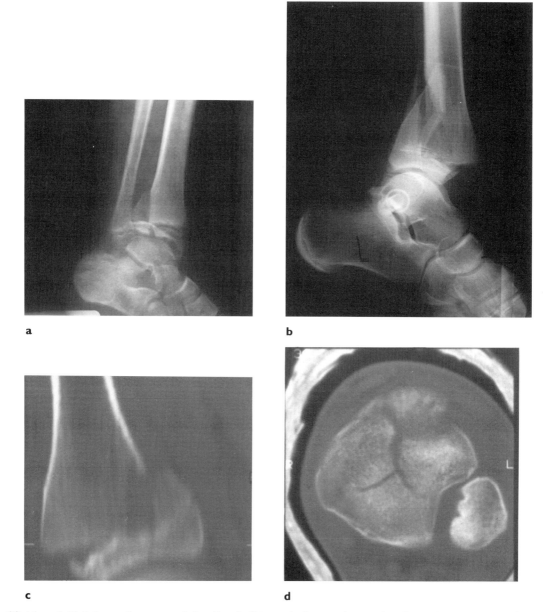

Figure 23.14 a,b Triplanar fracture of the distal tibia and plain radiographs show the three dimensions of the fracture. **c,d** Computerized tomography scans are useful in demonstrating the displacement of the fracture, particularly the intra-articular portion of the injury.

growth plate. Some use K wires across the growth plate and remove them at 4–6 weeks.

FRACTURES AND DISLOCATIONS OF THE FOOT

Fractures of the foot in children generally cause little trouble in treatment. Fractures involving the tarsal and metatarsal bones are much less common than in the adult population. Fractures at the base of the fifth metatarsal are relatively common and can be confused with the os vesalianum, a normal sesamoid. A short leg plaster for 3–6 weeks is generally sufficient treatment.

PATHOLOGICAL FRACTURES

Pathological fractures may result from local or generalized pathology as discussed below.

Local Bone Lesions

Simple bone cyst lesions typically occur in the upper humerus and upper femur. The fractures may cause deformity and occasionally growth disturbance, but heal readily. Most of these lesions require treatment when healing has occurred, and occasionally smaller lesions are healed by the fracture.

Non-ossifying fibroma is a common lesion and may be present in up to 40% of children. Pathological fractures heal readily and tend to partially heal the lesion. Bone grafting is used occasionally if the lesion is very large or if there is any doubt about the diagnosis.

Generalized Bone Disorders

Osteoporosis may be secondary to neuromuscular disorders such as spina bifida, cerebral palsy and muscular dystrophy. Plaster treatment is usual, but care must be taken to prevent pressure areas in those patients with altered sensation. In patients with altered sensation (e.g. spina bifida) the fracture may present as a hot swollen limb. These fractures tend to heal with hyperplastic callus.

Osteogenesis imperfecta fractures are extremely common and treatment is usually by splintage. Recurrent fractures are often treated by intramedullary rodding, particularly in type 3 osteogenesis imperfecta (see Chapter 5).

Osteopetrosis is an uncommon disease that may present with a pathological fracture. While the bones appear dense radiologically, they are actually weaker than normal and fracture readily.

Non-Accidental Injury

Non-accidental injury is becoming an increasingly recognized problem that is often not diagnosed until too late, and the child may die.

Clinical Features

History
The diagnosis is difficult, but is based on the history of previous injury, the circumstances of the present injury, and evidence of sequential injuries. The history may be inappropriate or may change with questioning. It is rare for children under two years of age to sustain broken bones accidentally and parents should be questioned carefully. Children rarely break bones by falling out of bed or when left alone, but a common way for children under one year of age to sustain a femoral fracture by accident is when the parent holding the child falls downstairs and lands on the child's leg. Late presentation may be a feature of non-accidental injury, and injury when under someone else's care is suspicious.

Examination
Bruising may be present in a different area to that expected from a fall. Facial bruising from a fall is uncommon in a child because they can usually manage to put their arms out to break a fall. Old bruising should be sought, and bruising indicating a strong grip identified. Often these children are malnourished and unusually quiet even when the examination is painful, indicating a chronic problem; however, this is not always the case.

Radiology

When the diagnosis is suspected a skeletal survey with plain films of the limbs should be undertaken. A bone scan may show areas of increased uptake and plain radiographs can then be taken. Bone scanning is more sensitive at picking up recent fractures.

Typical radiological injuries are metaphyseal injuries, which may be a greenstick buckle (torus fracture), transverse or at the metaphyseal corner. There may be epiphyseal separation or just sclerosis or irregularity of the metaphysis. Periosteal elevation may indicate a recent fracture or rough handling, but may be present to a mild degree in infants particularly between 1–3 months of age. Diaphyseal fractures are the most common non-accidental fractures and are usually transverse, but can be spiral with a twisting force. Rib fractures are common and skull fractures occur in about 10%. Subdural haematomata and widespread cerebral damage can result from violent shaking.

Management

The child should be admitted for investigation and protection and the relevant departments notified. Photographs should be obtained of all visible signs of injury. It is most appropriate to involve paediatric colleagues to assist in the management of the family. With appropriate back-up, which may be arranged through the family courts, most of these children are returned home to their parents in the long term. Management of the skeletal injury is along standard lines.

Differential Diagnosis

Non-accidental injury may be confused with osteogenesis imperfecta and occasionally haemophilia and leukaemia, where easy bruising may occur. These considerations should not deter the clinician from making a diagnosis of non-accidental injury because the risk of death in the unrecognized case is approximately 5%.

REFERENCES AND FURTHER READING

Canale ST, King RE. Pelvic and hip fractures. In: Rockwood CA, Wukins KE, King RE (eds) *Fractures in Children*. pp. 991–1120. JB Lippincott, Philadelphia, 1991.

Garvin KL, McCarthy RE, Barnes CL, Dodge BM. Pediatric pelvic ring fractures. *J Pediatr Orthop* 1990; **10**: 577–582.

Heeg M, Klasen HJ, Visser JD. Acetabular fractures in children and adolescence. *J Bone Joint Surg* 1989; **71B**: 418–421.

Key JA, Conwell HE. *Management of Fractures, Dislocations and Sprains*. CV Mosby, St Louis, 1951.

Ogden JA. *Skeletal Injury in the Child*. WB Saunders, Philadelphia, 1990.

Quinby WC. Fractures of the pelvis and associated injuries in children. *J Paediatr Surg* 1966; **1**: 353–364.

Rang M. *Children's Fractures*. JB Lippincott, Philadelphia, 1983.

Sugi M, Cole WG. Early plaster treatment for fractures of the femoral shaft in childhood. *J Bone Joint Surg* 1987; **69B**: 743–745.

Chapter 24
Limb Length Inequality

Ian P Torode

Limb length inequality is a common sequel of many congenital and acquired musculoskeletal diseases. Once it has been recognized, it is important to identify the cause, predict the future and prescribe a plan with the most appropriate management of the inequality. There is no other area of paediatric orthopaedics that has progressed so significantly over the last ten years. The development of limb lengthening and realignment procedures with the precision now afforded by the more complex external fixation devices allows major deformities to be corrected. However, it is important to remain aware of the rationale of treatment and the place for simple, more traditional equalization techniques in the management of these children.

Aetiology

Congenital

Congenital conditions causing limb length inequality include the following:

- **Femoral deficiencies** have been covered in Chapter 4. The growth inhibition in these limbs is relatively constant so the inequality remains proportional to the length of the limb.
- **Tibial and fibular deficiencies** have been discussed in Chapter 4. The growth inhibition is again relatively constant. Treatment for congenital pseudarthrosis of the tibia may contribute to the shortening.
- **Neurofibromatosis** is often associated with overgrowth of the affected limb.
- **Vascular malformations** such as diffuse haemangiomas and arteriovenous fistulae often cause overgrowth of the affected limb, but this is seldom more than about 5 cm at maturity.

Trauma

Traumatic causes of limb length inequality include the following:

- **Diaphyseal fractures** due to overlap of fragments and malunion. Many fractures of the femur in children under ten years of age heal with overlap, but there is rarely a discrepancy in the long term because homeostatic mechanisms correct the shortening. Most of the overgrowth occurs in the first three years after the fracture.
- **Epiphyseal injuries** with growth plate injuries can result in partial or complete growth plate arrest. This is seen in Salter–Harris Type 3 and 4 injuries and in any epiphyseal injury sustained through considerable force. The distal femoral growth plate is particularly prone to growth plate arrest after trauma. Partial growth plate arrest can not only cause limb length discrepancy, but can also cause progressive angular deformity if the arrest is peripheral because growth in the unaffected part of the growth plate continues.
- **Avascular necrosis** following treatment of developmental dysplasia of the hip (DDH) or a femoral neck fracture can cause a leg length discrepancy. Often growth continues normally and then a growth plate arrest takes place at a later stage. If the arrest is eccentric it may deform the upper femur, as described by Kalamchi and McEwen (1980) (see Chapter 16).

Infection

Infection may lead to growth plate arrest. This is most frequently seen in the upper femur and humerus where the osteomyelitis can be combined with a septic arthritis because the capsule extends beyond the growth plate. The leg length discrepancy following a septic hip may also be due to septic dislocation, as seen in Tom Smith disease. Growth plate abnormalities often follow the fulminant infections seen in multiple sites in neonates and meningococcal septicaemia. However, they are not common after the subacute osteomyelitis of childhood, which is often seen to transgress the growth plate.

Osteomyelitis of the diaphysis has in the past resulted in overgrowth of the bone, presumably due to hyperaemia. With the early control of sepsis this is now unusual.

Neurological conditions

Leg length discrepancy occurs in neurological abnormalities. Discrepancies in poliomyelitis range up to as much as 8 cm. The discrepancies in spina bifida often occur where there is asymmetrical neurological involvement, but this is rarely clinically significant. The shortening seen in spastic hemiplegia may not disadvantage the child if it accommodates a fixed equinus deformity.

Tumour and tumour-like conditions

Tumours and tumour-like conditions causing limb length inequality include:

- **Malignant tumours** because hyperaemia can cause limb overgrowth and involvement of the growth plate may cause growth arrest, but these effects are irrelevant to the clinical management. The effects of treatment with excision of joints and the use of radiotherapy may cause problems in survivors.

- **Multiple exostoses**, which frequently cause growth abnormalities. Angular deformities of the lower limbs and abnormalities of the alignment of radius and ulna are the usual manifestations of the growth abnormalities rather than limb discrepancies, although sometimes the forearms are very short.
- **Other skeletal dysplasias**, for example fibrous dysplasia, which causes shortening and also angular deformities. Enchondromatosis (Ollier disease) often causes shortening and significant deformities (*Figure 24.1*) (see Chapter 5).

Hemihypertrophy and hemiatrophy syndromes

Hemihypertrophy can occur as an idiopathic finding. This usually remains proportional to the length of the limb so the discrepancy at maturity is predictable.

- The Klippel–Trénaunay–Weber syndrome is characterized by asymmetrical limb hypertrophy and haemangiomas, and the overgrowth of the limb can be quite gross (see Chapter 7).
- Russell–Silver syndrome with short stature, café au lait spots and small in-curved little fingers is

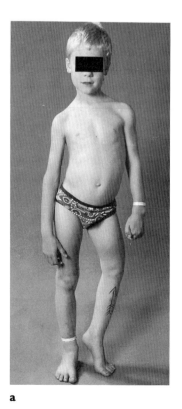
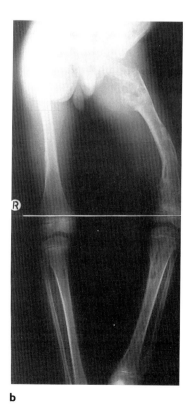

a   b

Figure 24.1 **a** Enchondromatosis (Ollier disease) in an eight-year-old boy with shortening and bowing of the femur. His left arm is also affected. **b** The long leg radiograph showing diffuse enchondromatosis of the femur and tibia. The femur was 5.7 cm short and the tibia 4.3 cm short. (Reproduced with permission from Menelaus M. *The Management of Limb Inequality*. Churchill Livingstone, Edinburgh, 1982.)

frequently associated with up to 6 cm of lower limb shortening.

- The Proteus syndrome is a particularly virulent form of limb hypertrophy. It may involve the trunk or spine, with one limb, usually a leg, enlarging at an alarming rate. Amputation may be the only answer.

Non-septic inflammatory conditions

Juvenile chronic arthritis (JCA) and haemophilia often develop overgrowth at affected joints, presumably as a result of hyperaemia at a chronically inflamed joint. If the onset is late, the growth plates of the affected joints may fuse prematurely. The knee and ankle are most frequently involved.

Radiotherapy and thermal injuries

Radiotherapy used in the treatment of malignant tumours such as Ewing sarcoma or osteosarcoma can result in premature fusion of the growth plate. Frostbite, burns and electrical injury have also been reported as producing premature fusion.

Clinical Features

History

A careful history is important and should include the timing of the discrepancy and relevant information to decide on aetiology. Other information that may prove useful includes the heights of parents and siblings, physical signs of maturation in the patient and the time of onset of menses.

Clinical examination

The examiner assesses the stature of the patient in general. Vascular abnormalities, café au lait spots, Klippel–Trénaunay–Weber and Russell–Silver syndromes may be apparent. The gait of the patient is important and the short leg gait should be differentiated from a Trendelenburg gait. While standing any scoliosis or pelvic obliquity should be noted. The examiner should note temperature variations of a limb suggestive of hyperaemia in JCA and haemophilia.

Once a leg length discrepancy is suspected, apparent discrepancy is differentiated from a real discrepancy (see Chapter 1). Any joint deformity is noted. If there is a real length discrepancy, a Galleazzi test demonstrates whether this is above or below the knee. If the difference is in the femur, palpation of the greater trochanter and anterior superior iliac spine demonstrates whether this is above or below the trochanter.

Often children are presented by their parents in the first year of life because of concerns about leg length inequality. The assessment at this stage can be difficult because of the relatively short fat limbs and the poor cooperation of the child. In this age group it is important to rule out hip dysplasia by examining for instability and imaging the hips. Regular follow-up helps to confirm any discrepancy as the limb grows.

The use of blocks to estimate the height necessary to make the iliac crests level is probably the most relevant measure. This amount is the 'functional difference' between the lower limbs and takes into account the limb length including the foot, any contribution from the pelvis and any contribution from joint deformity.

A non-stretch tape measure can be used to measure the distance between two bony landmarks. The anterior superior iliac spine to the medial malleolus is commonly used. However, care must be exercised in positioning the patient to equalize any joint deformity. The landmarks may prove elusive in the obese or after an innominate osteotomy. The use of the medial malleolus does not take into account the heel height, which may be significant in congenital deficiencies.

The measurement of the upper limbs does not usually require the accuracy of that of the lower limbs. A satisfactory estimation can be obtained with the patient undressed to the waist, erect and with the limbs hanging by the side. The relationship of the fingertips to the knee will indicate a discrepancy, and by flexing the elbows the relative lengths of the humeri can be estimated. The non-stretch tape measure will reliably measure forearm length.

Radiology

Skeletal maturity is assessed using a radiograph of the child's left hand. The appearance is then compared to those in the atlas devised by Greulich and Pyle, which gives the skeletal age to the nearest six months for boys and girls. This can be quite different from the chronological age and gives an indication of how much growth would be expected to take place.

Teleradiography

A plain radiographic plate is placed behind the limb and the tube is placed at a considerable distance from the patient. Divergence of the beam causes distortion of the image and enlargement. The enlargement has been calculated at 6.6%; however, this will vary with different techniques.

X-ray scanography

This is a variation of teleradiography in which the X-ray tube is moved. By moving the tube over a long plate, the distortion and magnification is significantly reduced.

Orthoroentgenography

A radio-opaque ruler is placed adjacent to the long film. Exposures of the hip, knee and ankle are made and the measurements can be taken directly from the exposed film.

Computerized tomography

Using the scout film a cursor is placed over the bony landmarks and the lengths can be read directly by the computer. The accuracy of this method depends on the positioning of the patient and the placement of the cursor and has been estimated to be within 0.2 mm. The foot, pelvis, upper limbs or other body segments can also be measured in this way (*Figure 24.2*).

Prognosis

The behaviour of a leg length discrepancy depends on its aetiology. The discrepancy in the common congenital deficiencies and hemihypertrophy stays in proportion to the length of the limb, so it increases with age. After a diaphyseal femoral fracture that heals with overlap, there is a discrepancy, which stays the same or improves due to increased growth. The child with avascular necrosis of the femoral head may have a discrepancy that then remains static and then increases close to maturity as a result of premature growth plate arrest of the upper femur.

The treating surgeon should attempt to estimate the expected discrepancy at maturity and predict the effect of surgical intervention. If the diagnosis is made at an early stage the child should be seen annually on at least three occasions. The discrepancy is plotted and if the behaviour of the discrepancy is expected to be proportional to the length of the limb, a straight line to maturity gives the expected adult discrepancy. The estimation of skeletal maturity is obtained from the Greulich and Pyle atlas with skeletal maturity at a skeletal age of 14 years in girls and 16 years in boys.

The choice of treatment for limb length inequality varies according to circumstances. In general terms discrepancies at maturity of less than 2 cm can be ignored. Where the discrepancy is 2–6 cm it is appropriate to shorten or slow down the growth of the long limb epiphyseodesis. Where the estimated discrepancy at maturity is expected to be more than 6 cm lengthening techniques should be considered, although these may be used in conjunction with an epiphyseodesis of the long leg.

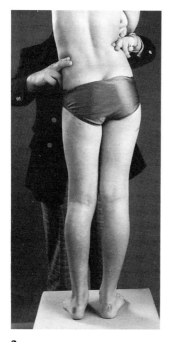 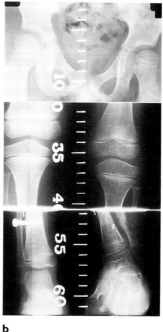 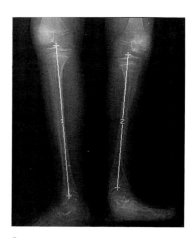

a   b   c

Figure 24.2   a Asssessment of leg length discrepancy. A short left leg: the examiner's fingers demonstrate the difference in height of the iliac crests. Also note the postural scoliosis.   **b** An orthoroentgenogram of a short left leg, demonstrating that the shortening is in the tibia. Measurements can be taken against the metal ruler. **c** Tibial length measurement using computerized tomography. (**a** & **c** reproduced with permission from Menelaus M. *The Management of Limb Inequality.* Churchill Livingstone, Edinburgh, 1982.)

Prediction of the effect of epiphyseodesis is therefore important. Calculations can be made as to whether epiphyseodesis can be successful in correcting the deformity and when and where it should be performed.

We have used the Menelaus and Westh (1981) technique, which is the simplest of the published methods. The growth in this period is assumed to be a straight line to maturity and skeletal maturity has been taken to be 14 years in girls and 16 years in boys. The distal femoral growth plate has been assumed to contribute 3/8 inch (0.9 cm) to growth each year and the upper tibial growth plate 1/4 inch (0.6 cm) each year. By epiphyseodesis up to 5/8 inch (1.5 cm) can be obtained per year to skeletal maturity in achieving leg length symmetry.

Green and Anderson have produced growth remaining charts of the distal femur and upper tibia, which take into account the slow down of growth around maturity (Anderson *et al.*, 1964). The surgeon also incorporates the percentage of growth inhibition of the shorter limb, which is then graded as mild, moderate, marked or severe. There is an upper line for tall children and a lower line for short children.

The Moseley graph technique is more complicated, but may be more accurate in predicting the final discrepancy and the effect of various epiphyseodeses (Moseley, 1987). It has now been produced as a computer program. A number of accurate measurements are made to create the lines of best fit. The more recordings made, the more accurate the prediction.

Management

Orthotics and prosthetics

A patient with a leg length difference of even several centimetres may not want nor need any aids to function normally. The concept that the child's spine will be 'put out' if the legs are not precisely equal in stance should be firmly rejected because there is no evidence for this. To a child the addition of something to their shoes where he or she does not appreciate any benefit will simply be an encumbrance and an unnecessary expense to the parents. Table 24.1 gives some idea of the limitations of conservative management of leg length discrepancy.

Shoe modifications: a raise can be added either within the shoe or on the heel or sole. A raise within the shoe is limited to 1–1.5 cm otherwise the heel continually leaves the shoe. The amount that can be added to the heel and sole is only limited by the instability created by increasing heights and the acceptance of the appearance.

Table 24.1 Conservative management of limb length discrepancy

Discrepancy (cm)	Management
Up to 1.5	Raise heel only (inside or outside)
1.5–5	Raise heel and sole
5–12	Patten and boot
12–20	Patten and ankle–foot orthosis, or extension prosthesis
Over 20	Extension prosthesis

Patten: to reduce the weight of large heel and sole raises an alloy patten can be fitted to the sole. Stability and their appearance have limited their use; however, they may have a role if durability is important.

An extension prosthesis is a useful means of providing a large addition to length, as is needed for congenital deficiency of the femur. The prosthesis holds the foot in equinus and it is necessary to make sure that the patient works on maintaining the range of dorsiflexion at the ankle. This prosthesis is also known as an O'Connor boot. A solid-ankle–cushion-heel (SACH) foot is attached to simulate ankle motion.

Amputation and prostheses

The Syme amputation is described in detail in Chapter 4. After a Syme amputation in young children a SACH foot is used. This may be replaced by a more sophisticated unit in older children with demands for greater responsiveness. Proximal suspension can be provided by a patellar tendon-bearing fit (PTB) with a supracondylar strap, or by a patellar tendon supracondylar fit (PTS), or by a silicon suspension system (3S).

After a knee disarticulation for tibial hemimelia, it is helpful if there is a difference in femoral lengths to accommodate a prosthetic knee. Suspension is similar to above-knee prostheses and is easier if the femoral condyles are not too bulbous.

The above-knee prosthesis is commonly used after malignancy and for children with a proximal femoral focal deficiency (PFFD) following Syme amputation and knee fusion. Good stability of the socket is important. A knee joint and prosthetic foot are incorporated to suit the patient's needs.

Limb shortening

The long limb can be shortened to equalize the leg lengths. This can either be carried out in the growing child by restricting growth by epiphyseodesis or by cutting out a segment of the bone to produce an acute shortening. Discrepancies up to 8 cm can be satisfactorily managed by a limb reduction procedure. In general bone-shortening procedures are reserved for skeletally-mature patients and an epiphyseodesis is used if there are open growth plates. The ideal candidate for acute shortening has overgrowth of one segment of a limb.

Epiphyseodesis Eradication of one or more growth plates is one of the most useful methods of managing a leg length discrepancy and may be used for a child with an expected discrepancy at maturity of 2–8 cm. Growth plate arrest may be used as an adjunct to lengthening either to address a residual discrepancy after a lengthening or to reduce the amount of lengthening required. The traditional method is as described by Phemister, but we now use percutaneous methods almost exclusively.

Phemister technique of growth plate arrest In a bloodless field, two 3 cm incisions are made over the appropriate growth plate. The periosteum is elevated, the growth plate exposed, and a block of bone incorporating the plate is excised. The underlying growth plate is removed with a curette and the block impacted into the defect after changing its orientation by 180°. The wounds are closed and a dressing applied incorporating a plaster splint to prevent inadvertent injury in the postoperative period.

Percutaneous technique of growth plate arrest The growth plate is identified on an image intensifier and a drill is introduced through a 1 cm incision. A large drill such as the 4.5 mm AO drill should be used. The growth plate is damaged extensively by drilling across the plate and by sweeping the drill through an arc anteriorly to posteriorly. The position and direction of the drill are controlled by the image intensifier and a similar approach is made to the other side of the growth plate. For the proximal fibular growth plate an open approach is made to avoid injury to the common peroneal nerve.

The complications are failure of closure of the plate and asymmetrical closure. Regular radiological review is necessary in the postoperative period. If an asymmetrical closure is suspected on the radiograph, prompt reoperation on the appropriate side of the growth plate can avoid the need for corrective osteotomy.

Growth arrest by staples While recognizing that there have been numerous reports of using staples for correcting limb length discrepancies it has been our practice to reserve the use of staples for correcting angular deformities.

Femoral shortening A discrepancy of 2.5–7.5 cm can be dealt with by resecting an appropriate segment of bone; however, resections of more than 4 cm will result in an extensor lag for some time afterwards.

Proximal metaphyseal shortening is performed on a standard radiolucent operating table. A lateral approach is made to the subtrochanteric area of the long femur, and the nail or screw of the surgeon's choice is introduced into the femoral neck. The lateral aspect of the femur is marked to control rotation. A segment of the femur is resected with the upper osteotomy at the level of the lesser trochanter. The plate is then fixed to the femoral shaft (*Figure 24.3*). The patient is mobilized on crutches within a week and full weight-bearing is achieved by six weeks.

Diaphyseal shortening was originally performed with an open approach and retrograde nailing. The technique has now been improved so that intramedullary instruments designed specifically for this are used to resect 2.5–5 cm of the diaphysis with a closed technique. A double osteotomy is made, the segment of bone split and pushed aside, and the ends of the femur fixed by an intramedullary rod.

Distal metaphyseal shortening in the femur can be satisfactorily achieved using the technique described by Wagner. A step cut osteotomy is performed and fixation obtained using an AO blade plate. Care must be taken to avoid inadvertent angular deformities due to poor plate placement.

Tibial shortening The ideal patient for tibial shortening has overgrowth of the below-knee segment and is skeletally mature. However numerous patients with a deficiency in length below the knee have had the 'normal' tibia shortened to approximate leg length equality by removing segments up to 4 cm in length.

A number of techniques are suitable and include the stepcut technique (*Figure 24.4*) as described by Broughton *et al.* (1989b), resection and compression plate fixation, resection and intramedullary rod fixation (Wagner), and metaphyseal resection and plate fixation. The latter approach may be useful if there is an angular deformity of the proximal tibia that requires correction, though skin closure may be difficult with this technique. The muscles look 'baggy' afterwards and take a considerable time to adjust. Tibial shortening is best limited to a maximum of 4 cm.

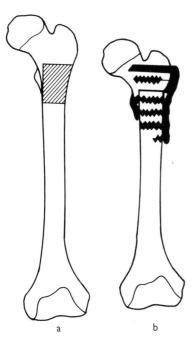

Figure 24.3 Proximal metaphyseal femoral shortening with an angle blade plate.

Intrapelvic shortening When a patient has acetabular dysplasia and an ipsilateral long leg of modest degree the Kalamchi modification of the Salter pelvic osteotomy may be useful. A slightly wider exposure

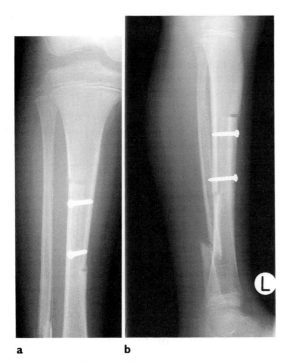

Figure 24.4 Tibial shortening using a stepcut and screw fixation. (**a** reproduced from Menelaus M. *The Management of Limb Inequality.* Churchill Livingstone, Edinburgh, 1982.)

is necessary to see the posterior part of the iliac wing. A wedge of bone with the base placed posteriorly is excised and about 1 cm of shortening can be obtained. The distal fragment is then rotated, brought forward slightly and impacted into the proximal fragment.

Limb lengthening

Limb lengthening can be accomplished by correction of deformity, by stimulation of growth, and by physically lengthening a bony segment of a limb. These are all complex procedures and a thorough knowledge of the mechanical principles and the many possible complications are imperative before they are undertaken.

The prospect of stimulating growth in a short limb has given rise to many innovative, but sadly ineffective ideas. The creation of arteriovenous fistulae and sympathectomy have been tried unsuccessfully. In some centres there has been interest in circumferential metaphyseal periosteal resection to stimulate growth. The results are unpredictable and this has not gained wide acceptance.

Acute distraction with interpositional grafts A simple method of gaining a modest amount of length of approximately 1–1.5 cm is by acute distraction. A distracter is applied and then an osteotomy is made across the bone. The distracter lengthens the bone, a bone block is interposed and the bone plated using the standard AO technique. Further bone graft is applied around the osteotomy site to reduce the risk of non-union. This is commonly used in the forearm to equalize the radius and ulna lengths but there are some advocates for its use in the femur.

Intrapelvic lengthening Where a patient presents with a modest discrepancy or where a hypopolastic hemipelvis is part of a limb length problem, a modest gain can be obtained through a pelvic reconstruction. This modification of the Salter innominate osteotomy was described by Millis and Hall. It involves the standard approach for a Salter osteotomy, but the bone graft is trapezoidal in shape, thereby distracting the transiliac osteotomy.

Lengthening by gradual distraction Many attempts have been made over this century to lengthen limbs by distraction. The Wagner technique gained wide acceptance in the 1970s. The bone was divided and acutely distracted by up to 5–6 mm. This was followed by daily distraction of 1.5 mm. At 4–6 weeks, when the desired length had been achieved, the bone was fixed by a large plate with a bone graft

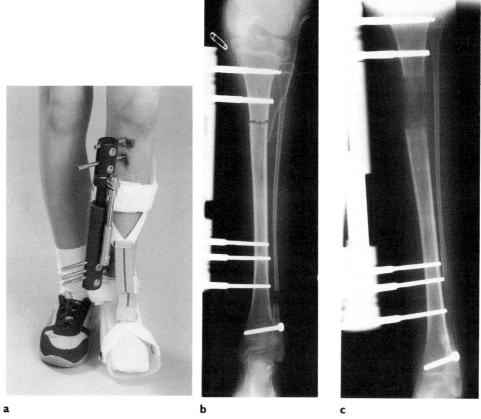

a   b   c

Figure 24.5 **a** The Orthofix uniplanar frame for tibial lengthening.   **b** The osteotomy has been performed, the frame attached, and lengthening is started after about ten days.   **c** Following lengthening and with new bone formation. (**a** & **c** reproduced from Menelaus M. *The Management of Limb Inequality.* Churchill Livingstone, Edinburgh, 1982.)

across the callus bridge. Although satisfactory results were obtained by skilled surgeons the rate of complications was high and the technique has largely been supplanted by slower distraction techniques.

The development of limb lengthening techniques owes much to the pioneering work of de Bastiani of Italy and Ilizarov of Siberia. These men improved our knowledge of the method of bone division, the rate of distraction, and the mechanics of the frames to hold the limb and allow the distraction. Ilizarov's work in this area was remarkable because he developed his techniques through the 1950s and 1960s and they only came to widespread attention in the 1980s.

Osteotomy: it is important to preserve the periosteal and endosteal blood supply so that callus forms quickly. Small osteotomes are preferably used; power saws are no longer used. Subcutaneous Gigli saw division of the bone is also described, which gives a low velocity division that repairs quickly. A metaphyseal division gives a bigger cross section for healing, but a diaphyseal division allows larger fragments for control with the frame.

Rate of distraction: Wagner advocated an immediate distraction of 5–6 mm and later distraction of 1.5 mm per day. Kawamura suggested that distraction should be delayed until the laying down of procollagen is established. De Bastiani and others have advocated a delay of 14 days in adults and 10 days in children to allow callus formation. The most commonly employed techniques now use a distraction rate of 1 mm per day in divided increments after an initial delay of 10–14 days. Radiographs are performed every week or two and if the callus looks poor, distraction can be restricted or even compressed until a reasonable amount of callus is obtained. The radiographs also ensure that no deformity is developing as the limb is lengthened.

The frame: Wagner popularized the unilateral frame, which has been modified by de Bastiani as the Orthofix system (*Figure 24.5*). Circular frames such as the Monticelli Spinelli and the Ilizarov systems are now more commonly used (*Figure 24.6*). The circular frames are applied with pretensioned wires passing through the bone. These are particularly adaptable for the correction of angular or

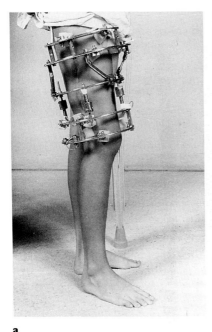
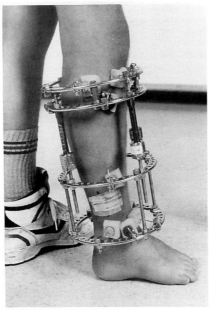
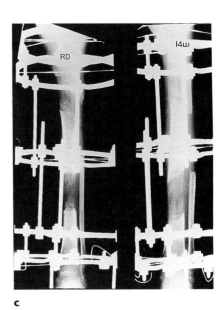

a   b   c

Figure 24.6 **a** Ilizarov frame on the femur. **b** Ilizarov frame on the tibia. A fibular osteotomy has been performed and lengthening is planned in the upper metaphysis. **c** Tibia following bifocal lengthening using the Ilizarov frame. (Reproduced with permission from Menelaus M. *The Management of Limb Inequality*. Churchill Livingstone, Edinburgh, 1982.)

rotational deformity, bone transport, and lengthening at two sites in the one bone. The small wires give rise to fewer complications than the larger pins used for unilateral frames, and weight-bearing is possible in the circular frames. However, the circular frames are more complex to apply and have to be adapted for the femur with half-circle frames and pins around the groin area (*Figure 24.7*).

The duration: the time taken from surgery until removal of the frame should be expressed in terms of time per unit length obtained. Although times around four weeks per centimetre have been suggested, in our experience the time the patient should be prepared for is approximately six weeks per centimetre gained.

Complications: these include:

• Pin tract infections. These vary in severity from those requiring oral antibiotics as an outpatient to those requiring inpatient intravenous antibiotics to the need for pin removal. Only neglected pin infections should require sequestrectomy of the pin tract.

• Deformity of adjacent joints. All patients must be observed closely, particularly during the lengthening phase, for the development of soft tissue tightness causing deformity of adjacent joints. Equinus at the ankle is common in tibial lengthenings. These deformities can usually be treated by

aggressive physiotherapy, although sometimes it is necessary to temporarily slow or stop the distraction.

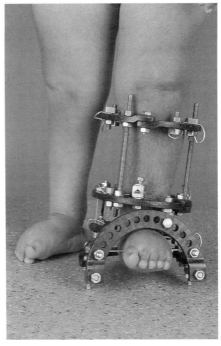

Figure 24.7 A small Ilizarov frame has been used to stabilize the correction obtained after revision surgery to a club foot in a two-year-old child.

- Joint subluxation. This is of major concern and must be treated urgently. Soft tissue release may be required; however, consideration should be given to adequate splinting and to the addition of further fixation points and extension of the frame across the involved joint. In proximal femoral focal deficiency there is usually a deficiency of the cruciate ligaments. During a femoral lengthening the tibia may subluxate posteriorly on the femur, and if the acetabulum is deficient the femoral head may subluxate laterally and superiorly.

- Deformity of the involved bone. Any frame can provide asymmetrical forces in distraction, particularly unilateral frames as the distraction force away from the long axis of the bone will also provide a bending moment to that bone. This must be looked for and appropriate alterations made. A femoral lengthening with a unilateral frame on the lateral side can produce a varus deformity of the femur. This is also a possible complication after frame removal if the new bone is not mature. Immediate manipulation under anaesthesia and cast application may salvage the situation in the tibia.

- Nerve palsies. Nerves may be injured by direct injury when the pins are inserted, by distraction of a nerve onto a pin, or by stretching during distraction. Caution must be exercised when correcting longstanding deformities. There is a significant risk of injuring the peroneal nerve during extension of the knee if the joint has been chronically flexed.

- Vascular injuries. Vascular injury is a serious, although infrequent occurrence. Systemic hypertension may occur during lengthening and result from a vascular or neurogenic cause.

- Lack of bone formation. The rate of distraction should roughly parallel the production of regenerated bone. If the appearance of callus on serial radiographs is poor, the rate of distraction should be reduced or stopped. It may be necessary to reverse the distraction and compress the gap to stimulate callus formation before starting the distraction again. Some centres have used ultrasound to look for cysts in the new bone and to gauge strength, and others have used double X-ray assessment (DEXA) scanning. We rely on plain radiographs to assess when to remove the frames.

Other techniques include:

- Chondrodiatasis. This term is applied to the method of applying the distraction force across the epiphyseal plate. It has limited application, but may be used where a growth plate is already partially injured or when the child is close to the end of growth and subsequent closure of the plate is not a problem. The new bone tends to be well formed.

- Implantable intramedullary distracters. These have had success. In the Bliskunov method the patient's movement between the femur and pelvis provides the distraction force. There are also techniques in which the implanted intramedullary device distracts after rotating the distal fragment of the limb backwards and forwards through a quarter of a turn.

- Distraction over an intramedullary nail. This technique will probably find greater acceptance over the next decade. A locking intramedullary nail is implanted at the time of application of the distraction frame and osteotomy. After the desired lengthening has been obtained the nail is locked. This method allows early removal of the distraction device and is particularly useful in larger bones, which can accommodate the fixation pins and an intramedullary nail.

PREMATURE GROWTH PLATE ARREST

Total Growth Plate Arrest

Total growth plate arrest produces shortening of the limb segment, but no angular or rotational deformity.

Management

The management of this situation depends on the expected discrepancy in limb length and one or more of the techniques of limb shortening or lengthening are used.

Partial Growth Plate Arrest

Aetiology

A partial growth plate arrest is most commonly caused by trauma, particularly Salter–Harris Type 4 fractures and high-energy Type 2 fractures. Injuries that involve crushing of the plate should also be observed closely. Infection can cause a partial arrest, but often the infective process is diffuse and the plate damage widespread, leading to a total arrest. Exceptions are infections that result in a septicaemic state (e.g. meningococcal septicaemia). An asymmetrical growth plate arrest can also result

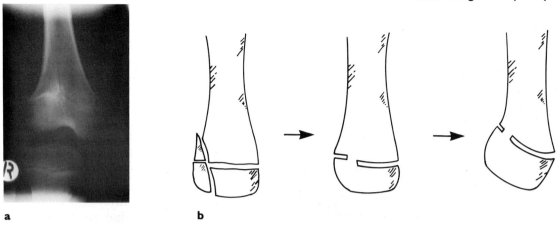

a   b

Figure 24.8 a Partial growth plate arrest in the distal femoral physis. This produced a valgus flexion deformity of the femur. **b** Mechanism of progressive angular deformity and shortening after a displaced Salter–Harris Type 4 epiphyseal injury.

from a thrombotic or embolic mechanism or ischaemia due to an arteritis. Non-traumatic causes include Ollier disease, Blount disease and unicameral bone cysts.

Classification

The site of the partial growth plate arrest can be classified as central, peripheral and linear.

- Central partial growth plate arrest leads to a tenting of the growth plate with distortion of the epiphysis and articular surface. It slows longitudinal growth, and if eccentric produces angular deformity (*Figure 24.8*).
- A small peripheral bar can give rise to a rapidly progressive angulatory deformity.
- Linear partial growth plate arrest most commonly follows a Salter–Harris Type 4 injury and its effects depend on its site.

Clinical Features

There is angular deformity, which is assessed using a standard goniometer, and leg length discrepancy, which is assessed in the usual way.

Radiology

Plain radiographs demonstrate the growth plate distortion and the amount of angular deformity, while standard anteroposterior (AP) and mediolateral tomograms are used to map the plate. The percentage of plate involved and the precise site is identified (*Figure 24.9*). CT scanning has now superseded plain tomography. The cuts should be taken in

the sagittal and coronal planes and three-dimensional reconstruction may be helpful.

Management

Treatment for a partial growth plate arrest has to aim at correcting the angular deformity, correcting the limb length discrepancy, and ensuring that this correction is maintained until maturity. Removal of the bony bar by epiphyseolysis may produce all these effects and may be combined with an osteotomy for angular correction. Where epiphyseolysis is unlikely to be successful the rest of the plate may be arrested to stop any progression. Angular deformity is corrected by osteotomy. Limb length discrepancy can be addressed by shortening the long leg or lengthening the short leg as described above. The angular deformity and limb length discrepancy can be corrected at the same time by chondrodiatasis.

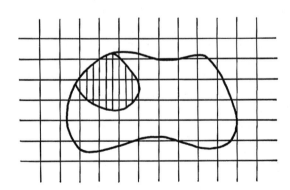

Figure 24.9 Mapping out the exact position of the bony bar is essential for planning the method of correction and approach to excise the bar.

Epiphyseolysis is unlikely to be successful if more than 50% of the plate is involved. Epiphyseolysis should only be used if more than two years of growth are likely at the plate and the operation can be carried out through healthy skin. These guidelines may be broken in particular circumstances. Epiphy-

seolysis is particularly useful in the distal femoral and the proximal and distal tibial growth plates, and central bars give better results. Epiphyseolysis should be strongly considered if the child is very young and the other options are repeated osteotomy or limb lengthening procedures because a failed

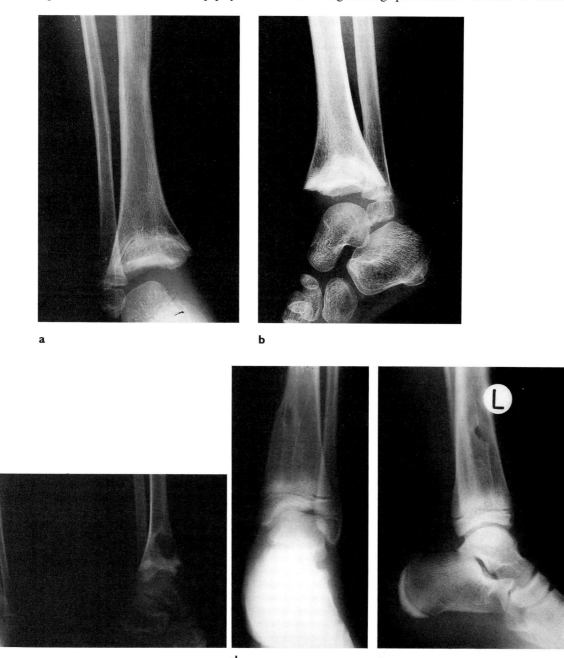

a   b

c   d   e

Figure 24.10   a,b Girl of four years of age with a central tenting lesion of the distal tibial physis following a Salter–Harris Type 4 lesion at the age of two years. She has half an inch of shortening and a varus deformity (anteroposterior and lateral views).   **c** The bar has been excised through a large metaphyseal window.   **d,e** Seven years later, growth plate activity has been restored and there is no leg length discrepancy. The proximal migration of the metaphyseal window confirms the growth at the distal tibial physis (anteroposterior and lateral views). (Reproduced with permission from Menelaus M. *The Management of Limb Inequality*. Churchill Livingstone, Edinburgh, 1982.)

epiphyseolysis does not compromise subsequent treatment.

Epiphyseolysis

Excision of the bony bar or epiphyseolysis to reestablish normal growth plate function was first described by Langenskoild in 1967 (Langenskoild, 1981). The bar is excised and the gap is filled by an interpositional material to prevent recurrence. Various interpositional materials have been described including fat, silastic and methylmethacrylate. All seem to be similarly successful, but the silastic and methylmethacrylate have less chance of displacement by postoperative haematoma.

Technique: peripheral bars are approached directly and central bars through a metaphyseal window placed to avoid damage to the perichondrial ring. Good exposure, a bloodless field and a good light are important. Some use a fibreoptic light source and some a headlight, and others carry out the procedure under the operating microscope. An arthroscope can provide light and visualization. We use a high speed burr and remove bone until the healthy white plate can be seen around where the bar was. A dental mirror can be helpful to check complete removal. The interpositional material is then applied. Postoperatively the patient should non-weightbear for six weeks to protect the bone weakened by the excision.

Results: most authors report a success rate of about 80% but the results reflect the selection of patients (*Figue 24.10*). We would generally combine this procedure with an osteotomy to correct an angular deformity of more than 20°.

Completion of the epiphyseodesis

If the injury has occurred in an older child with less than two years of growth left and more than 50% of the plate involved then completion of the epiphyseodesis is usually more appropriate. Contralateral epiphyseodesis may also be undertaken in these circumstances to maintain equal limb lengths.

Osteotomy and leg lengthening

An angular deformity and a leg length discrepancy should be addressed by osteotomy and limb equalization techniques. The use of the former growth plate as the distraction zone may be useful in the technique of chondrodiatasis.

Vascularized growth plate transfer

The transfer of the proximal fibula with its growth plate and epiphysis has been reported from our institution to replace a proximal humerus and a distal radius (Taylor *et al.*, 1988). This procedure may have wider application in the future.

REFERENCES AND FURTHER READING

Aldegheri R, Trivella G, Lavini F. Epiphyseal distraction. *Clin Orthop Rel Research* 1989; **241**: 117–127.

Anderson M, Green WT, Messner MB. Growth and predictions of growth in the lower extremities. *J Bone Joint Surg* 1964; **46A**: 1197–1202.

Broughton NS, Dickens DRV, Cole WG, Menelaus MB. Epiphyseolysis for partial growth plate arrest. Results after four years or at maturity. *J Bone Joint Surg* 1989a; **71B**: 13–16.

Broughton NS, Olney BW, Menelaus MB. Tibial shortening for leg length discrepancy. *J Bone Joint Surg* 1989b; **71B**: 242–245.

Carey RPL, de Campo JF, Menelaus MB. Measurement of leg length by computerised tomographic scanning: brief report. *J Bone Joint Surg* 1987; **69B**: 846–847.

De Bastiani G, Aldegheri R, Renzi–Brivio L, Trivella G. Limb lengthening by callus distraction (callotasis). *J Pediatr Orthop* 1987; **7**: 129–134.

Ilizarov GA. The tension stress effect on the genesis and growth of tissues: Part I. The influence of stability of fixation and soft tissue preservation. *Clin Orthop Rel Research* 1989; **238**: 249–281.

Kalamchi A. Modified Salter osteotomy. *J Bone Joint Surg* 1982; **64A**: 183–187.

Kalamchi A, McEwen GD. Avascular necrosis following treatment of congenital dislocation of the hip. *J Bone Joint Surg* 1980; **62A**: 876–888.

Langenskoild A. Surgical treatment of partial closure of the growth plate. *J Pediatr Orthop* 1981; **1**: 3–11.

Millis MB, Hall JE. Transiliac lengthening of the lower extremity. *J Bone Joint Surg* 1979; **61A**: 1182–1194.

Moseley CF. Leg length discrepancy. *Othop Clin N Am* 1987; **18**: 529–535.

Paley D. Problems, obstacles, and complications of limb lengthening by the Ilizarov technique. *Clin Orthop Rel Research* 1990; **250**: 81–104.

Taylor GI, Wilson KR, Ries MD, Corlett RJ, Cole WG. The anterior tibial vessels and their role in epiphyseal and diaphyseal transfer of the fibula: experimental study and clinical application. *Brit J Plastic Surg* 1988 **41**: 451–469.

Westh RN, Menelaus MB. A simple calculation for the timing of epiphyseal arrest. A further report. *J Bone Joint Surg* 1981; **63B**; 117–119.

Winquist R, Hansen S. Closed intramedullary shortening of the femur. *Clin Orthop Rel Research* 1978; **136**: 54–61.

Index

Note: page numbers in **bold** indicate tables and numbers in *italics* indicate illustrations